CONTENTS

D1092597

To my family, friends, Ruby, and to all of the health educators past, present, and future; all of you have allowed me to stand on the shoulders of "giants."

PREFACE

I VALUE MY health. Sometimes, however, I take my health status for granted. I have had the good fortune of growing up relatively healthy and in a supportive, healthful environment. As a younger adolescent, I competed in cross-country running, track and field, and eventually marathons and road races. In my younger twenties, I happened upon weights and began aggressively pursuing strength training in addition to cardiovascular health. As I became more involved with health and fitness, I realized that many other people were not. Friends and family members did not share the same zeal for health and fitness that I did. Was I out of the ordinary? As the years progressed, I noticed that many of my male friends did not seem to be aging well in comparison to their female counterparts. Expanding waistlines, poor eating habits, little to no exercise, and a continual barrage of questions often were topics of discussion during our gatherings.

In my professional practice I felt compelled to help family, friends, and other people achieve the best health possible. People want to be healthier, but they also want to balance their lives with other aspects of health and

Figure P.1   Dimensions of Health and Wellness

Source: Adapted from Hettler (1976)

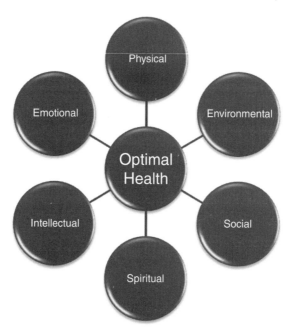

wellness outside of gym memberships and treadmills. I changed my practice to reflect the six dimensions of health and wellness: physical, environmental, social, spiritual, intellectual, and emotional (Figure P.1).

Any book is a static resource or a tool. Like a wrench or any other tool, it is up to the reader to use this book by putting its concepts and suggestions into action every day. I have included the most recent research and evidence-based science to help readers along in the quest for optimal health and better health-related outcomes. Health is an ever-changing reflection of the balances and imbalances of our everyday existence. It is my sincere wish that readers use this book in good health or find good health while using it.

PURPOSE

Why a book on male health? Male health encompasses 50% of the world's medical issues; it is an important topic to study and address in the classroom and beyond. First, let me clarify why this book refers to *male health* rather than *men's health*. One of the primary purposes of this book is to help readers become familiar with the multitude of sociobiological aspects and influences that affect male health and quality of life across the life span. The term *men* connotes a specific age range. Yet health begins at the time of conception (and sometimes before) and is a process experienced until individuals die. The term *male health* best captures and encompasses all the life stages of the male sex rather than one particular life stage.

This book addresses issues in male health using data-driven, epidemiological information presented in an easy-to-understand format. Each stage of male health, from birth and infancy until the elder years and death, is discussed in detail. Topics range from physical health and wellness to emotional and psychological health. Others include intellectual health, environmental health, occupational health, and spiritual health. *Concepts in Male Health* provides a comprehensive, practical approach to teaching and learning about issues affecting male health across the life span.

BOOK DEVELOPMENT

Development of this book began like that of many others. A passing discussion with a colleague, a cup of coffee with a friend, much personal reflection on lived experiences, and many other normal life processes initiated and provided the impetus for this book. After being challenged by my former department chairperson to develop a course dedicated to issues in men's health, I went about writing a course syllabus, finding appropriate resources and activities, and selecting course readings. The latter proved more difficult than expected. There were no adequate textbooks for the course. I set out on a mission, casing several listservs, to see if anyone could point me in the best direction. Responses to many of the discussions and questions I posed were met with a similar level of frustration. My conclusions were that men's health was a topic embedded in gender studies or human sexuality courses and only received a passing mention. Moreover, most instructors appeared to be using a medley of articles and internet resources to facilitate their courses. I was trying to put together a course reading packet. A cohesive textbook and resource was needed for students in my classes.

ORGANIZATION OF THE BOOK

Covering important health topics as they pertain to males is the primary intent of this book. However, *how* the content is presented to the reader is a strong focal point. Each chapter presents a particular life stage and the health challenges many males face during this stage. The information in each chapter is practical, usable, and applicable in daily life.

Key Features

Throughout the text, you will notice the following features that will help you assimilate the chapter concepts in a more meaningful and practical way:

- *Chapter Learning Objectives.* Each chapter includes learning objectives consistent with Bloom's Taxonomy for each main point of the chapter. Learning objectives are presented in an easy-to-follow format and sequence.

- *Myths/Facts.* Many areas of health are surrounded by a shroud of intrigue, mystery, and simply misinformation. The Myth/Fact feature in each chapter presents common myths, misinformation, and half-truths about a topic and follows with the related facts. These features allow readers to question what they may have assumed or learned in the past and "unlearn" their assumptions based on fact-driven, evidence-based resources.

- *Vignettes.* A brief vignette in each chapter presents a real-world example of a pertinent health issue that many males face. Examples include physical issues such as heart disease and cancer; other areas address occupational and social health determinants such as job stress and relationships.

- *Key Terms.* A list of relevant terms for each chapter is provided to assist the reader in developing a comprehensive and working understanding of the chapter information. Terms are defined in the glossary at the end of the book.

- *Discussion Questions.* Review questions are provided at the end of each chapter. These questions address health-specific content included in the chapter, spanning both the scope and breath of the information.

Additionally, the book's website (www.josseybass.com/go/leone) includes instructor support materials that can be adapted to course content and instructor teaching style.

The resources included with this book will help advance not only the knowledge of male health, but also the study of it. Through the teaching resource repository and chapter PowerPoints on the book's website, students and instructors will find it simple to integrate the main concepts pertaining to male health. Presenting the facts in an easy-to-follow format enables students to assess their knowledge of the topic so as to develop a healthier perspective of male health.

DISCLAIMER

This book is meant to serve as a textbook for students in classes that support male health. Not all diseases are presented; many are presented in the chapters on periods of the life span when the diseases are most likely to occur. Some diseases may occur during different phases of life than where detailed in this book. This book does not claim to provide information that replaces qualified medical and professional consultation.

ACKNOWLEDGMENTS

The writing of a book is never possible without the support of others. I thank the following people, groups, and organizations for their input, kindness, and continued support of my work.

I am grateful to my grandparents, parents, all of my family, good friends, and my dog Ruby for understanding why I put so much time and effort into this piece of work. Though it is never easy to sacrifice life's other engagements, your love and support of me and my work helped me to stay focused and on task. Thank you to all of my colleagues at Bridgewater State University, Indiana State University, Southern Illinois University Carbondale, The George Washington University, and Northeastern University as well as those in academia who responded to my queries and surveys on this important topic; without your input and advice the direction of this work would have been impossible to accurately assess. Additionally, I am appreciative and indebted to the many health professionals at advocacy organizations for male health, such as the Men's Health Network, the Men's Health Caucus, the Men's Health Initiative, Women Against Prostate Cancer, and the Foundation for Male Studies, Inc., for their work and insight. Thank you to Patrick Lentz of Patrick Lentz Photography in Boston, Massachusetts, for his stellar graphics and photography.

I thank the following reviewers for their many thoughtful and helpful comments: Demetrius J. Porche, Henrie M. Treadwell, and Salvatore Giorgianni. Mal Goldsmith and Becky Smith also provided valuable feedback in the early stages of the manuscript.

I recognize the support of the American Association for Health Education (AAHE) for standing behind this book and its concepts. To my editors Andy and Seth, thank you for your guidance and patience in this process. I express an immense thank-you to the students in my male health classes, specifically, my inaugural class in male health at The George Washington University in Washington, D.C., and my special topics class at Bridgewater State University. Without their unique comments and insight I would have missed quite a bit of information in the process. Last, to anyone else whom I may have interacted with during this writing journey, I sincerely thank you; without these everyday experiences I would never have been able to generate the insight this book demanded.

THE AUTHOR

JAMES E. LEONE, PhD, ATC, CSCS, *D, CHES, is an assistant professor of health in the Department of Movement Arts, Health Promotion, and Leisure Studies (MAHPLS) at Bridgewater State University in Bridgewater, Massachusetts. He earned a bachelor of science degree in physical education and athletic training from Bridgewater State University (formerly College), a master of science degree in athletic training and research methods from Indiana State University, and a doctor of philosophy in health education from Southern Illinois University Carbondale. He has an extensive background in the health sciences, teaching courses ranging from health education and health behavior to orthopedic assessment and exercise science. Leone has authored numerous scholarly publications and three book chapters, and he has presented to national and international audiences on a variety of topics in health education and public health. He is an active member of several professional organizations, including the American Association of Health Education, the American Public Health Association, the National Athletic Trainers' Association, and the National Strength and

Conditioning Association. Leone serves as an editorial associate for *The Health Educator* and *Body Image: An International Journal of Research* and is a regular reviewer for several scholarly journals and academic publications. In addition to his academic work, Leone enjoys physical activity, culinary experiences, and travel. He presently resides in Waltham, Massachusetts.

Concepts in Male Health

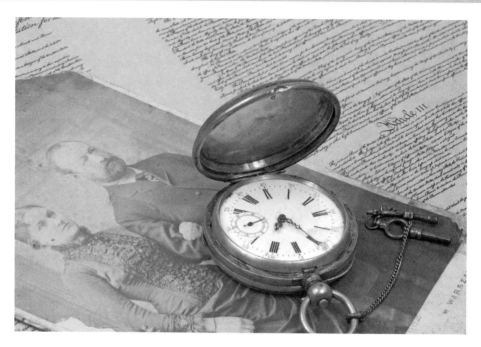

Historical Perspectives of Male Health

LEARNING OBJECTIVES

- Identify the main components of male health in the United States and internationally
- Understand male health in historical, cultural, and global contexts
- Interpret epidemiological and statistical evidence as it relates to male health
- Explain how culture can enhance or reduce health in males in the case of health-related disparities
- Analyze risk factors for being born male

M EN AND BOYS account for 50% of the world population, which translates into approximately 3.35 billion people! (International Data Base [IDB], U.S. Census Bureau, 2008). Yet, live infant male **birth rates** continue to trail those of females: in the United States, for every 1,000 live births among mothers ages 15–44 years old, 7.5 males die, compared to 6.2 females (National Center for Health Statistics [NCHS], 2005).

How and why do these numbers relate to health? First, let's take a look at the demographics of these baby boys. As of 2005, 4,138,349 babies were born to the following ethnic groups in the United States: 55.9% white/ Caucasian, 23% Hispanic/Latino, 14.1% black, 5.3% Asian, and 1.0% Native Americans and Alaskan Natives. With **mortality** data showing that the majority of infant premature deaths occur in non-white populations, it is easy to conclude that there are health-related disparities among these populations (Centers for Disease Control and Prevention [CDC], 2002). Families with low socioeconomic status (SES) are more likely to have issues accessing appropriate health care. In non-white populations there are more single-parent homes *without* adult males than there are single-parent homes *with* adult males (Clarke, Cooksey, & Verropoulou, 1998).

From a world perspective, males outnumber females until ages 45–49, when the numbers start taking a sharp downturn. By age 80+ women outlive their male counterparts by nearly 50% (IDB, 2008). What occurs between the ages of 0 and 44 and then from 45 to 80+? Age-adjusted rates remain relatively stable from birth until midlife for a variety of factors, such as **intentional and unintentional injuries,** disease and illness, and **homicide**. During the years 0–44, lack of **preventative health care** in some populations, such as marginalized or minority men, and reluctance to seek health care can drastically limit the health status of men (U.S. Agency for Healthcare Research, 2008). A recent survey of more than 1,000 men found that American men tend to delay medical care and also overestimate their health. Further, 92% of those surveyed said they wait a few days to seek medical care or advice when they are sick, in pain, or injured. Last, 55% reported not having a yearly physical examination and 42% said they had at least one chronic illness, yet nearly 80% described their health as being "good" or better (American Academy of Family Physicians, 2008). What do these data suggest? Are males delusional about their overall health status? Do males not want to acknowledge weakness or illness for fear of being viewed as unmasculine?

Many of these male notions and misconceptions about health begin in the early, formative years. Disease patterns that occur in youth and early adulthood that affect men as they age include cardiovascular disease, neoplasms (cancers), and unintentional accidents. According to 2004 data from the CDC, 321,973 men died of cardiovascular disease, including heart attack and stroke, 286,830 from cancers, and 72,050 from unintentional accidents (Heron, 2007).

Many of the aforementioned conditions and illnesses are preventable with aggressive **primary prevention**. A valid and reliable resource, such as this textbook, will help fill the need for a primary prevention tool. Throughout this book's thirteen chapters, readers will study not just the diseases, illnesses, and problems that afflict males throughout the **life span**, but more important, where they come from and how they can be addressed and prevented. Should a baby boy be circumcised? Does a toddler show signs and symptoms of autism or Asperger's syndrome? Does a boy show early signs of attention deficit disorder with hyperactivity? Why are more school-age boys than girls diagnosed with learning disabilities? Why do males have lower graduation rates from college than females? How does job **stress** add or detract from young adult health? What challenges do middle-aged men face beyond the "midlife crisis"? Why does the prostate continue to grow, yet some men continue to lose their hair? All of these questions and more are addressed from a **sociobiological** perspective for each life stage throughout this book.

This chapter provides an overview of what is meant by "male health," looking at historical contexts that have forged the way we view males and their health in contemporary society, Western and non-Western ideals of being male, and what it means to be born a male in society.

WHAT IS MALE HEALTH?

"Real men wear gowns." This was an advertisement in a popular health/ sports medicine magazine. The scene depicts a man standing next to a woman at a social function at which the other people are dressed up enjoying a bit of socializing. What makes the advertisement unique is that the man is wearing only a hospital gown! What is the relevance of this advertisement to this book? Let's break this advertisement down to its roots or elements.

First, the simple statement and accompanying image of a man wearing a gown has several connotations. What are they? Why do all of these possibilities surface? Many people would argue that the images and stereotypes conjured from this simple advertisement are a result of sociocultural bias. Others may argue that this image and terminology challenge what many cultures consider to be the **masculine** norm. In actuality, the advertisement is a public service announcement (PSA) aimed at promoting regular physical health checkups with primary care providers as men approach middle age.

What is a man? Defined, *man* is a term that describes a physically mature male; however, **male** refers to the biological traits of a person. Several aspects of being male and a man come into play, such as masculinity. The masculine norm can be elusive and has existed in a state of flux for centuries. Masculine standards have included being the provider, strong, silent, and practical, as well as the opposite of the female norm. While there certainly are many opposites between men and women, each has its own attributes that demand its attention.

The concept of **male health** is best described as the elements and components that converge and foster either a positive health outcome or a negative health outcome. Several elements factor into a male's overall health, including physical, emotional, occupational, spiritual, and financial. Health may be thought of as a confluence of these variables, similar to that of a Rubik's Cube™ puzzle (Eberst, 1984). A primary challenge of the puzzle is to align the scrambled sections according to various colors. Not unlike life's challenges, aligning one's elements of health, is a primary aim of advancing one's health. Balancing each section of one's health (the puzzle) is achieved through learning and experiencing life. Adapting to change often promotes a healthier life perspective.

The Healthy and Healthier Man

Traditionally, health was viewed as merely the absence of disease, and conversely, disease was looked at as the absence of health. By today's standards, these definitions could not be further from what constitutes health (Jadad & O'Grady, 2008). The term **health** and its close and inseparable counterpart, **wellness,** are comprised of many facets or prongs (Hawks, Smith, Thomas, Christley, Meinzer, & Pyne, 2008). Optimal health and wellness can be thought of as a balancing act among several key areas and concepts of wellness (see Figure 1.1).

- *Physical health* focuses on promoting a strong and vital body through good practices of nutrition, rest, exercise, avoiding harmful habits, and seeking medical care when needed.

- *Mental and emotional health* focuses on understanding one's emotions and feelings and making stable, healthy, and positive lifestyle choices. An emotionally healthy person is able to accept his or her limitations and draws from life experiences and inherent personal attributes.

Figure 1.1 Various Dimensions of Health and Wellness

Source: Adapted from Hettler (1976)

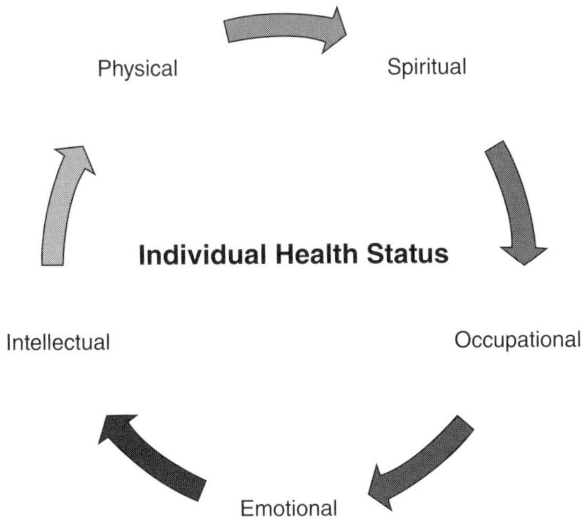

Physical

Spiritual

Individual Health Status

Intellectual

Occupational

Emotional

- *Occupational health* refers to workers' abilities to provide for themselves and their families in health-promoting employment settings. Healthy work settings include both emotional as well as environmental attributes that help employees achieve optimal health, such as work resiliency programs, employee assistance programs, and exercise programs.

- *Environmental health* focuses on the relationship between a person's physical environmental and its impact on his or her personal health. For example, protecting oneself from environmental hazards such as pollutants or poor air quality helps to promote better overall health.

- *Spiritual health* refers to a sense of connectedness with a greater power and gives life meaning and purpose. Spiritual health is enhanced by one's morals, values, and ethics.

- *Social health* involves the ability to communicate and relate well to others in society. Positive social health allows for a better sense of community and social growth of the individual.

- *Intellectual health* focuses on thinking, thought processing, learning, and interacting with one's world and environment in a creative manner.

The dynamic interplay among these concepts of health is what leaves a person with positive or negative health. It is rare that all aspects of health will be in alignment like a Rubik's Cube (Eberst, 1984); however, health is optimized when a majority of the components of health and wellness align with each side of the puzzle.

So what comprises the "healthy man"? Ultimately, if we stick to the dimensions of health and wellness discussed, the healthy man is one who values and maintains a physically healthy body, attends to challenges to his mental and emotional health, approaches his job in a healthy and positive manner, demonstrates environmentally responsible behaviors, views himself as a part of something greater than himself for spirituality, enjoys fulfilling social relationships and interactions, and engages in intellectual pursuits. Many of us would strive to attend to these facets of health. However, how many men attain this level of optimal health? Evidence-based research appears to tell a different story. Whether in life expectancy, years of quality life, disease, **health disparities,** violence and aggression, or drug use, males are failing to live up to the ideal of the healthy man. Perhaps individually and in a public health sense, we should be focusing on developing a "healthier" man versus an ideal.

MALE HEALTH IN HISTORY

The Account of Adam

Many of us would not think to look to the Old Testament in the Bible or similar religious texts for examples of male health. Genesis states that Adam (the first male) was created in the image of God (Gen. 2:10, 6:9; New International Version [NIV]). With this comes the assertion of power and reverence in that Adam represents an image of the most revered concept in religion (in this case Christianity), God himself. Power and ultimately all matters resulting from this, including health, can arguably be placed on the shoulders of Adam and all of his descendants. We also see examples of traditional male roles through Adam and Eve when Adam "leads" and Eve "follows." With leadership comes additional stress, both good and bad. Created in the image of God, as the first human being on Earth, and serving in the role of "leader," Adam must have been placed in a remarkable position of expectation and stress. Further, Eve bore Adam two sons, Cain and Abel. One might argue that Cain bore the original sin of aggression and ultimately **fratricide**. In today's society males are more likely to be homicide victims (nearly four times higher), commit violent crimes and general acts of aggression, and be perpetrators of domestic and intimate partner violence than their female counterparts (Heru, Stuart, Rainey, Eyre, & Recupero, 2006). The biblical account of course is only one account of the origin of man; many other written and oral traditions adhere to similar accounts of gender roles.

The role of the male in Western society remained virtually unchanged until recent times. Other cultures have embraced the male in different ways, with some theories and examples showing complete role reversals. To advance a healthy agenda for the modern male, we need to revisit our historical past and go beyond the scope of the Western, Judeo-Christian perspective.

Males in the Seventeenth Through the Twenty-First Centuries

For a majority of recorded history, patriarchal views were the predominant cultural tradition. To some extent, **patriarchy** still exists, albeit in other forms than what was once commonplace (Sanderson, 2001). For example, from the 1600s through much of the 1900s, a man was expected to be the provider ("breadwinner") of the family, the defender of home and nation, the architect of "life" with his seed, and ultimately the pilot of his own destiny. Examples may be seen as the strong father figure, the disciplinarian, and the soldier or warrior.

A paradigm shift occurred in the twentieth century. With gender equity came a silent release of the social keystones men have held for eons (Sanderson, 2001). The women's movements of the 1920s through the 1970s and present day have contributed to men redefining their roles in society, ranging from home and family to the definition of the healthy man.

With a redefining of gender roles and a shuffling of traditional Western cultural values, many psychiatrists argue that men may be more vulnerable than ever before (Boulding, 2000). Are men suffering an unspoken pain, and if so, in what ways? Lack of direction in the workplace has translated to all areas in which men have held positions of esteem and power. For example, with the women's rights and feminist movements, many men have relinquished positions of authority that they once occupied, often leaving them with a lesser sense of self-worth. Men are still held to traditional expectations of "macho" role models yet may lack appropriate outlets to be strong. (However, much of the feminist movement was viewed through a white/Caucasian "lens" and does not capture the experience of all female groups, that is, minorities.)

Employment and occupation have traditionally defined men (Boulding, 2000; Pope, Phillips, & Olivardia, 2000). One of the first questions typically asked of a man is, "So, what do you do [for work]?" Becoming unemployed has been described as the beginning of a socioemotional downward spiral in a man's life, often leaving him with an identity crisis. Additionally, if a man hurts, he must not cry or show excessive emotion or he is thought to be weak, emasculated, or feminine (Boulding, 2000). How a man does and should respond to these paradigm shifts are on completely opposite ends of the spectrum. On one end exists low self-worth, self-esteem, and frustration, among other negative emotions, whereas on the other end of the spectrum there is challenge, renewed opportunity for personal growth, and optimism. (See Figure 1.2.)

Unfortunately many men get caught up in the former rather than the latter end of the spectrum. Low self-esteem, self-worth, and frustration often translate to acting out and societal aggression, particularly in younger males. The latter can be seen with high rates of domestic violence, spousal or intimate partner abuse, drug use and abuse, and homicide (NCHS, 2008). According to a 2008 National Center for Health Statistics survey in the United States, by ages 15–24, males have a 2.76 relative risk of dying from suicide and homicide, as compared to females or males in other age categories. Moreover, black males have a 1 in 30 chance of being homicide victims, compared to 1 in 179 for white males (NCHS, 2008). This prompts an additional issue of minority and ethnic disparities.

These issues have been dubbed as a "silent health crisis in America" by noted physicians and **public health** advocates (Gremillion, personal communication, 2004). Health issues are over-represented in males throughout the life span; this fact is clear. Explanations are complicated, but the fact that men are encultured with masculine values such as **stoicism,** suppression of emotion, independence, and self-reliance adds to the complex intricacies of the issue (Parsons, 2009). Perhaps in order to develop a healthier male perspective, we need a new definition of masculinity.

CULTURAL PERSPECTIVES

The United States encompasses perhaps the most diverse population in the world (Boulding, 2000). Embedded in Western society are innumerable perspectives of how we view males. Recently in the United States there has

Figure 1.2   Gender Role Conflict Model

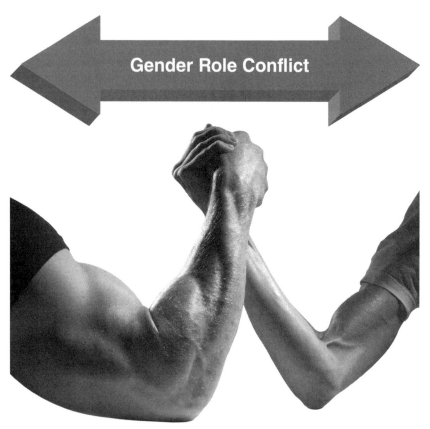

Traditional Masculine Values	Potential Consequences	Social Stigma (Challenges to Masculinity)
✓ Stoicism ✓ Providing/Protective ✓ Strength	✓ Low self-esteem ✓ Gender identity crisis ✓ Overcompensation ✓ Low self-worth ✓ Aggression	✓ Emotionality ✓ Femininity ✓ Weakness

been a renewed call and interest in advancing male health as a social movement in health care (Porche, 2009).

What Are *Masculine* and *Masculinity?*

The term *masculine* refers to being **male** or having male-like qualities and attributes. Biologically, a male is genetically defined as having an X and a Y chromosome and the supporting **androgens** such as testosterone; however, much of how a boy and eventually a man identifies with his sense of masculinity is constructed through social interaction (Stibbe, 2004). Does masculinity vary across cultures? Yes. What is more important than a definition of masculinity is what this term means for a male in a practical, worldly sense.

Models of masculinity in the United States have remained fairly stable since the country's founding. According to a model proposed by Badinter (1995), males must adhere to four primary areas of maleness:

1. Men must act like men, meaning that behaviors must fall within the acceptable sociocultural norms of a given society. For example, in Western culture it is acceptable for a male to be physically aggressive, whereas acting passive or appearing frail is considered to be a negative male quality.

2. Males are to be competitive and should demonstrate superiority through success.

3. Males are detached and impassive, often lacking an emotional response.

4. Males are willing to take on risks and risky behavior.

From this perspective, the risks of masculinity are numerous, including ignoring human aspects of caring, compassion, seeking assistance (medical care) when needed, being too aggressive to the point of violence, and taking risks that may place one's health and safety in jeopardy (Badinter, 1995; Parsons, 2009). Some males even react by super-compensating by harnessing masculine traits such as muscular development (Olivardia, 2001). The latter example coincides with the "threatened masculinity" theory presented by Mishkind, Rodin, Silberstein, and Streigel-Moore (1986). The theory posits that a growing parity with women in Western culture has left men to take charge of their level of muscularity, which often is the only factor that sets them apart from women. Bigger muscles may support a male's need for physical dominance and assertion of traditional patriarchy that has waned with modern Western culture. The latter can be seen in Western trends of **hypermasculine** male models and advertisements that promote unreal and idealistic male bodies (Pope et al., 2000; Pope, Olivardia, Gruber, & Borowiecki, 1999).

Myth: The terms *gender* and *sex* are the same and can be used interchangeably.

Fact: The more accurate term is *sex* to describe one's biology (that is, male or female), whereas **gender** refers to social constructs and influences such as femininity and masculinity.

International Male Health

Male health is certainly not just a Western concern. The international community also has begun to embrace the value of studying and advocating for male health initiatives. One of the primary global initiatives is focused on how to best engage males in their own health and health care. Community and occupational engagement efforts seem to be more effective than methods such as individual interventions. Many men identify with their jobs, occupational endeavors, and community and therefore see themselves as part of something greater. Knowing that their community or work may count on them as providers and producers, men may take more action and measures to advance and safeguard their health (Malcher, 2009). Taking a team approach in getting men to act on their health is likely to be more beneficial than simply promoting individualism. Engaging men in their territories, such as work, has led to several successes in countries such as Australia (Malcher, 2009). In 2002, the International Men's Health Week (IMHW) was proclaimed by representatives from various countries at the Second World Congress on Men's Health. Several multinational health organizations advocated for greater general awareness of issues related to the health of males and ways in which to enhance it. Long-term goals of this initiative are to connect international programs and resources with the goal of eliminating health concerns and disparities that affect men worldwide (International Men's Health Week [IMHW], 2009).

Several countries, including the United States, Canada, Great Britain, Australia, countries within the European Union, as well as nations in Africa, Asia, and South America, have begun to participate and advocate for global health. In 2005, the Vienna Declaration outlined a plan to proactively enhance the state of global men's health (Men's Health Network [MHN], 2009). The declaration mentions five major points:

1. Recognizing men's health as a critical issue and that there are health issues that only affect men

2. Promoting awareness of men's approach to health

3. Changing the way health care is provided to be more sensitive towards men's needs

4. Creating school and community programs that target boys and young men

5. Connecting health and social policies to better pursue men's health goals

These goals and initiatives have sparked interest in a variety of IMHW activities, including urological screenings, free health care screenings at events and locations that attract men, symposia and open forums to discuss relevant issues in men's health, workplace screenings, and public service announcements and campaigns, as well as a host of other programs and activities (IMHW, 2009).

Another example comes from Australia, where in June 2008 the government announced its first men's health policy in conjunction with the Royal Australian College of General Practitioners policy on men's health and the Australian Medical Association's position statement on men's health from 2005 (Parsons, 2009). The policy includes identifying the key roles of men in the community as fathers, sons, brothers, partners, and friends and the importance of these roles. Additionally, the policy encourages men to share their family histories of health with their doctors, know what a healthy weight is, have their blood pressure checked on a consistent basis, avoid smoking and excessive alcohol consumption, and maintain a healthy body and mind (Smith, Braunack-Mayer, Wittert, & Warin, 2008). Perhaps the most optimistic statement from this article says, "Improving men's health is not 'mission impossible' but will involve a concerted multipronged effort from government, medical and health promotion organizations, the health system in general, and primary care in particular. As a society we need to understand the changing roles of men in our society, foster positive expressions of masculinity and provide health care in a way that meets men's needs and takes into account their communication styles and the way they express illness and distress" (Parsons, 2009, p. 85).

The International Society for Men's Health (ISMH) also makes far-reaching efforts to promote awareness and advancement of male health issues. In sum, advancing male health is not futile or impossible. Challenges to male health are evident as data indicate, with higher mortality rates, greater relative risk of injury and death, and greater propensity for violence and aggression-related issues, such as imprisonment (MHN, 2009). From a global perspective, recognizing and preventing **morbidity** and mortality factors has the potential to positively affect not only men but society in general. Mothers, sisters, wives, children, and employers all have an international stake in men's health as we continue into the new millennium.

EPIDEMIOLOGICAL AND STATISTICAL EVIDENCE

Life Expectancy and Expectations of Life

Essentially, **life expectancy** is how long one expects to live and how long one does live. Data suggest a life expectancy of 75.2 years for males living in the United States. These data are in contrast to the 80.4 years of life for females living in the United States (NCHS, 2006, 2008). What is more important and less quantifiable is the *quality* of life experienced. **Health-related quality of life (HRQoL)** refers to a person's perception of his or her mental and physical health status over time (Richardson, Wingo, Zack, Zahran, & King, 2008; Drum, Horner-Johnson, & Krahn, 2008). For example, a man may live to be ninety years old but may incur a chronic disability or suffer from a disease such as cancer at age sixty-five; therefore, one may argue that only sixty-five years of HRQoL have been experienced. Conversely, a man may die at age sixty-five but still may have experienced excellent HRQoL.

Composer and jazz musician Eubie Blake (later quoted by baseball great Mickey Mantle) may have captured life expectancy best in this comment, "If I knew I was going to live this long, I would have taken better care of myself." So, what does a man expect out of his life? A solid career? A family legacy? A fancy sports car? Or is there something more that defines a man's lifetime? Most people tend to agree with the latter. The avoidance of suffering and the pursuit of happiness and joy underlie most people's goals in life; males are no different (Mehrotra, 2005). Perhaps the greatest of life's expectations for a man is simply being secure in himself as a person.

Social Perspectives of Male Health

In a 2003 article appearing in the *New York Times*, males were questionably dubbed the "weaker sex." Although written to spark interest and perhaps debate, the article offers compelling evidence concerning the social implications of being born male. **Epidemiology** is the study of trends and patterns of health in populations. For example, there are 115 males conceived for every 100 females; however, from that point on, the health of males takes a downturn, beginning with male infant mortality rates, with the male fetus at greater risk for miscarriage and stillbirth and with 5 males dying to every 4 females. Further, **sudden infant death syndrome (SIDS)** is 1.5 times more common in males; boys are more likely to be autistic, have Tourette's syndrome, be mentally retarded, have dyslexia, and be color blind. Into the teenage years, boys die at twice the rate of girls, with boys five times more likely to die from homicide, eleven times more likely to drown, and twice as likely to die in a car accident.

All ten leading causes of death defined by the CDC affect more men than women; 80% of the leading causes of death disproportionately affect African American men; men experience more life-limiting illness and premature death, with minority groups at an extraordinary risk level; and male health affects the community at large and limits the health of our nation as a whole. Additionally, as a man ages, he is twice as likely to lose his hearing, and because of higher levels of the sex hormone testosterone, he is at greater risk for elevated levels of LDL cholesterol (the bad kind) and lower levels of HDL (the good kind), which predisposes him to cardiovascular diseases. Some theories suggest that men have fewer T-cells for fighting infection and overall have weaker immune systems than women. The latter may be seen in higher death rates in males from influenza and pneumonia than in females. Rates of death and morbidity from cancer, diabetes, stroke, heart disease, and unintentional injury are all higher in males. Later in life (age 55+), men are more likely to die in automobile accidents, die from heart disease, and commit suicide. The *New York Times* article concludes by making light of the fact that if men live to be 100 years old, they tend to be in better shape than their female counterparts (Jones, 2003). When one analyzes these data and facts, the social implications of being born male appear dire. Is there a silent health crisis? (Gremillion, personal communication, 2004).

The news is not all bad, with some aspects drastically improving over time. With knowledge and advancements through science and biomedical progress, male health is becoming more of a public (and governmental) priority in the United States and abroad. For instance, **advocacy** efforts through the Men's Health Network, in addition to congressional efforts, have led to some exciting improvements, particularly in getting the awareness message out to the public sector. In 1994, with the assistance of Senators Bob Dole and Bill Richardson, Men's Health Week was initiated. These efforts, which center on the week ending on Father's Day in June, promote screenings and health fairs nationwide and involve declarations by state governors and participation by public health departments and major national corporations. Further, in 2003, a bill proposal (the Men's Health Act) for establishing an Office of Men's Health (OMH) through the U.S. Department of Health and Human Services (USDHHS) was proposed. The bill focuses on men's health activities, such as prostate cancer research and funding, state initiatives, and welfare reform; however, due to funding issues, the bill continues to sit in waiting, with revisions to the proposal made in 2005 and again in 2007.

Screening and targeting of men offer much hope for improving HRQoL; however, greater efforts need to be taken throughout a male's life span to prevent illness and health-related disparities from occurring in the first place.

The Functional Male and Gender Typing

Perhaps a fundamental cultural change is in order in how society views boys and men and what it means to be male. The male sex, body, and gender has been ascribed several meanings throughout time; for example, being male has meant strong, aggressive, a provider, tough, stoic, insensitive, emotionally suppressed, independent, and self-reliant, among other qualities (Parsons, 2009). Most notably, the popular view of the male has been one of his functionality in society. If society continues to view "male" as exclusively "functional," the slippery slope of detachment from humanistic values will continue, as will male health issues. Machines and computers, which have a functional capacity, break down, and people simply replace them; males are critically important in society and need to be understood, respected, and well maintained. Devaluing a male to his constituent parts and viewing them as functional components only perpetuates the social ills that befall males (Jones, 2003). Seeking help occurs only when the functional parts of a man break down and will continue to usurp proactive, primary prevention efforts in public health.

VIGNETTE

My family and I were sitting around the backyard fire pit on a cool but pleasant early September evening. My sister was due with her second child in December. The course of the evening's conversation jumped from my sister's two-year-old daughter to the final few weeks of the major league baseball season while the scent of hotdogs and hamburgers filled the early evening air. The conversation then jumped to my sister and her preference for the sex of her second child. She said, "It really does not matter, as long as he or she is healthy and normal." At that moment, I saw my brother-in-law smirking from his station at the grill. I asked him what he was up to over there. "Oh nothing," he replied.

(Continued)

After a few beverages I went into the house to use the bathroom and on my way noticed the inundation of all shades of blues in the new baby's room. Additionally, I noticed a new light with a base made of worn-looking baseballs and an autographed bat hanging on the wall. I knew my brother-in-law had been feverishly working on getting the new baby's room ready in his spare time. The baby was a boy!

Why did I assume the new baby was a boy? Colors and sports paraphernalia determined in my mind that I was expecting a nephew versus another niece. As I sat back down with my family, I smiled at my brother-in-law as if we both connected on the news of his new son and my new nephew. I still could not help but to think why I came to assume it was a boy. Had society engrained in me the same gender biases I taught about in my classes? Apparently so! As I gathered my coat and flip-flops ready to head home, I asked my sister what she thought about having a son. She immediately smiled and asked, "How'd ya know?" Briefly, I brought up the colors in the baby's room and the baseball items and she affirmed that indeed she was having a boy. She smiled, I gave her a hug and exclaimed, "You know, Sis, yellow is a nice color too!"

Racial, Ethnic, and Cultural Disparities Affecting Male Health

Males are at risk for a variety of physical, psychological, environmental, and psychosocial issues (Jones, 2003; Gremillion, 2004); however, specific racial, ethnic, and cultural groups are at an extremely high risk for negative health consequences. The more successful and higher status achieved by males, the longer and better HRQoL experienced (Redelmeier & Singh, 2001).

Birth data are perhaps one of the first pieces of vital information and statistics that illuminate racial, ethnic, and cultural health disparities. For example, U.S. data from the National Center for Health Statistics in 2005 show thirty-five-year trends for years of life for white and black men and women. White women, followed by black women, and then white men all converge in a near-common trajectory, whereas the linear trend for black males is far below the other three groupings. White males outlive their black male cohort by nearly 6.2 years (white = 75.7 years; black = 69.5 years). Black populations, particularly males, continue to reflect these disparities. Black populations had a 1.3 times higher age-adjusted mortality rate, 2.4 times higher infant mortality rate, 3.3 times higher maternal mortality rate, and 5.1 years lower overall life expectancy, and have 1,016.5 deaths per 100,000 people, compared to 785.3 per 100,000 in white groupings (Kung, Hoyert, Xu, & Murphy, 2008).

Health disparities in males are simply not just between white and black populations, but also among other ethnic and minority groups. The most stark contrasts, however, exist between white and black populations. Asian and Native American/Alaskan Natives data show tendencies equal to better years of life expectancy and mortality factors. Hispanic groupings also were better in health indicators than black populations, with the exception of Puerto Ricans, who had 822.5 deaths per 100,000 in data from 2005 (Kung et al., 2008). White males are more likely to commit suicide, although according to a recent report from *Community Voices,* a nonprofit seeking to improve health services and access to health care, black male suicide rates have risen from 5.6 per 100,000 to 13.8 per 100,000 over a fifteen-year period. These data point to a "secret epidemic" according to the authors of the report, in that black males are being omitted and marginalized by the mental health system, which partially explains the rise in suicides. The cumulative effects of racism also may explain the deterioration of the black male psyche in the United States (Xanthos, 2008). Additionally, black and Hispanic males were more likely to be victims and perpetrators of homicides.

These latter instances are significant in that they show the relationship between a person and his or her environment. Suicide generally falls within the realm of a psychological condition often associated with major depression, wherein a person acts (makes a choice) on his or her thoughts, emotions, and irrational motivations. In contrast, being the victim of a homicide is not within the direct control of a person. One could argue that lack of locus of control for black males and other minority groups in their environment and social positioning is a strong predictor of their mortality.

The phenomenon of ethnic and cultural disparities may be more marked in the United States than elsewhere in the world. First, in other countries and cultures, men occupy distinctive (and sometimes privileged) roles in society, whereas parity with females in U.S. society has been noted and alluded to by some researchers (Pope et al., 2000). Second, the U.S. population encompasses unprecedented heterogeneity of groups, ethnicities, and cultures, which often muddles gender and sex roles of males and females. Third, males in the United States have a less well-defined role in terms of their "functionality." Because we in the United States enjoy the conveniences of a modern, technological world, males may be viewed as less functional than their counterparts in developing nations, thereby affecting their self-esteem, self-worth, and gender roles.

It is evident that there is a social and health burden on minority males. Health disparities can be defined as differences in the **incidence, prevalence,** mortality, and burden and related adverse health conditions that exist among specific population groups in the United States (Brach & Fraser, 2000). Specifically, minority males occupy the top indicators of various health issues, ranging from heart disease and stroke to lung and prostate cancer. For example, black males have more than double the rate and mortality for prostate cancer than white males and even other minority groups (National Cancer Institute, 2009). Another pertinent finding concerns HIV/AIDS infections. While the national trend for HIV/AIDS transmission rates have decreased since first being tracked in 1977 to the present, new HIV/AIDS infections are increasing in gay and bisexual men and African American and Hispanic men (Holtgrave, Hall, Rhodes, & Wolitski, 2009). Asian males also may have higher risk and poor health outcomes, such as lung cancer due to smoking, which may be a coping mechanism for the stress of acculturation and racism. Cultural factors such as avoiding shaming one's family through weakness or poor health because of individual issues also may preclude Asian males from seeking health care (Frisbie, Cho, & Hummer, 2001; Gee, Spencer, Chen, & Takeuchi, 2007). There are a multitude of factors influencing males' motivation, attitudes, and receipt of treatment to maintain their health. Access to health care is one of the predominant and major barriers to receiving quality health care, simply due to socioeconomic position and status. The latter may be remedied by an augmented national health care system that ensures equal access and rights to health care for all citizens.

A man's level of education and lifestyle beliefs and behaviors also strongly predict his likelihood of being proactive in his health. For instance, men with lower educational levels (high school or less) have greater issues with their health (morbidity), ranging from obesity and substance abuse to cardiovascular disease and cancer. Mortality rates also are higher in these groups.

Minority male populations also hold different attitudes than majority populations toward health care and health care providers. Reluctance in seeking medical assistance is higher in males, but minority men may be even less likely to seek help when needed (Shavers & Brown, 2002). Black males have had a long-standing distrust for the medical community stemming back to mistreatment during times of slavery through unethical research practices in black male populations, such as the Tuskegee syphilis study (Kampmeier, 1972). Distrust is commonly encultured into newer generations. Other attitudes, such as *machismo* in the male Hispanic/Latino community also may preclude adopting healthy prevention behaviors and seeking medical consultation when needed (Stibbe, 2004; Pope et al., 2000; Bordo, 1999; Luciano, 2001). For example, a Hispanic man often is viewed as the patriarchal head of the household and is expected to sustain and fulfill the role of being superior and strong. In some instances, this attribute is even expected by women. The *machismo* cultural attitude often constrains Hispanic men from admitting that there may be an issue or problem with them physically or psychologically, thus delaying or precluding medical assistance.

Poor health in minority males ultimately trickles down to the family unit and society at large. Absence of male figures in minority family households sets forth a dangerous trend in perpetuating the social disease of negative health and health disparities. Strengthening father–son and male bonds may help avert the multitude of ills that affect minority families, particularly in African American communities. Community interventions, such as the University of Michigan Prevention Research Center study in Flint, Michigan, are examining the role male bonding can have in alleviating black males' disproportionate predisposition to violent behavior, early sexual encounters, substance abuse, and poor academic achievement (Caldwell, Wright, Zimmerman, Walsemann, Williams, & Isichei, 2004).

A healthy man is more likely to receive regular checkups from his physician, take proactive measures to assure his long-term health, care for his family, be a productive member of his community, and add to his family's overall HRQoL. Addressing health care delivery to minority groups is a solid step in securing the future success and health of the nation as a whole. We must avoid blaming the victim and acknowledge that health is not always a "choice" but rather results from a complex interaction of sociocultural determinants. Racism, segregation, redlining (a discriminatory practice of denying or increasing the costs of services to people), and many other variables often take the control away from minority groups, resulting in marginalization. Violence and aggression typically result from cumulative stress, often precipitated by racism and low socioeconomic status. Undocumented immigrant males present an even greater public health problem, because not being able to track their health status perpetuates uncontrolled long-term costs of health care. For example, undocumented groups often forgo seeing a health care provider for preventative and palliative treatments and frequently access emergency departments when in the most dire need of services. This drives up costs of services exponentially, often at the expense of taxpayers (Sanchez, Sanchez-Youngman, Murphy, Goodin, Santos, & Valdez, 2011). Tracking population health within these groups is a primary need and a public health challenge. Therefore, the pursuit of health is not a one-size-fits-all process. The time has come when males need not fear being viewed as weak or frail because they seek assistance with their health matters, because their health *does* matter.

Cultural Competence and Future Directions

One of the strongest (and cheaper) tools to advance the health of males from all backgrounds and walks of life is simply an understanding of their situations and positions in life. **Cultural competence** is the ability to effectively interact with people of different cultures and groups. This is a combination of an awareness of one's own worldview, examination of one's own feelings concerning other cultures, knowledge of other cultural practices, and the development of cross-cultural skills (Luquis & Perez, 2006). Strategies to reduce health disparities in males start with the delivery of a high **standard of care** for everyone, regardless of ethnic or cultural background. For example, in the U.S. penal system all men have the right to health care. This is not saying that health care ignores or excludes culture or ethnicity when delivering quality health care; just the opposite holds true to achieve a gold standard of care for all.

Minorities first need to value what the medical community can do to enhance their health and reduce their risks of illnesses and disease. A basic knowledge of activities and behaviors that can reduce the burden of disease is a great start in this fundamental cultural paradigm shift. The latter may be better accomplished by recruiting and including more minority groups, particularly minority males, to serve as health care providers such as doctors, nurses, and therapists. Using cultural leveraging also may prove efficacious by incorporating unique cultural contexts and values in the delivery of health care and interventions in minority communities (Fisher, Burnet, Huang, Chin, & Cagney, 2007). Health care coverage regardless of socioeconomic status, instead of catering only to elite groups who can afford the best access to health care, also will help ensure a better standard of care. Community coalitions, networks, advocacy, representation, and commitment from key community informants and stakeholders will help tailor more efficient and effective health outcomes for minority populations.

Targeting what minority males value and expect out of life can provide key insight as to what intervention strategies may work best (Fisher et al., 2007). For example, the social norms of black males may include close ties with family and religious groups and affiliations. Knowing this, health care workers and public health initiatives may concentrate energies and efforts that target these men in these settings, such as community block parties, sporting events, or church. Poor men and minority groups often live with a lot of pain, are demeaned and devalued, and die sooner than nonminority groups (Treadwell & Ro, 2003). The notion that poor men and minority men are more likely to perpetuate the social ills we all think will not affect us is simply wrong.

Whether it is substance abuse, lack of health care, violence, or any other health negative behavior or consequence, poor health affects *all* people in *all* communities. It may not affect your direct health, but it is your dollar bill. From a humanistic standpoint, society must invest in marginalized minority groups in order to advance society as a whole. Health-related disparities in minority men continue to be a stain on America's fabric. Many minority men are so concerned for their daily survival, caring for their families, and sustaining their jobs that they do not make health a priority.

Another challenge to the health care structure is the lack of quality and consistent data concerning the health of minority men (Treadwell, 2003). Because many minority men do not routinely seek medical care or are undocumented, there are very few chances to collect valid and reliable data to assess overall health and trends. One of the goals of public health is to assist minority males to be active participants in shaping their own health care and quite possibly their own destinies. To do this requires shifting the responsibility from solely the individual to government policies and other upstream factors affecting health policy decisions. A health care system that concentrates efforts on prevention versus treatment will go far in eliminating health disparities in the poor and underserved.

SUMMARY

In order to promote a healthier male in today's society, an understanding of how to best reach this group is needed. Understanding male health requires a working knowledge of causal factors of disease burden, psychological and gender-specific views on what health means to males, male sex role identity, sex role strain, and how ethnic and cultural factors affect male health. This chapter has detailed the health burden of males and the basics of what it means to be male, what it has meant to be male throughout history, and how males are viewed from Western and non-Western cultural perspectives.

KEY TERMS

Advocacy   Birth rate   Epidemiology

Androgen   Cultural competence   Fratricide

Gender

Health

Health disparity

Health-related quality of life (HRQoL)

Homicide

Hypermasculine

Incidence

Intentional and unintentional injuries

Life span

Life expectancy

Male

Male health

Masculine

Men

Morbidity

Mortality

Patriarchy

Prevalence

Preventative health care

Primary prevention

Public health

Sociobiological

Standard of care

Stoicism

Stress

Sudden infant death syndrome (SIDS)

Wellness

DISCUSSION QUESTIONS

1. Look for instances of how male health is viewed or treated in historical and religious texts such as the Bible, the Torah, the Quran, or others. Describe what you notice to be true in these texts. Do any of these points of view still hold true in today's society?

2. How has masculinity changed or remained the same since the 1600s in the Western world? Provide multiple examples to illustrate and justify your point.

3. Explain how the women's movements, such as women's suffrage of the 1920s era and the women's liberation movements of the 1960s and 1970s, have affected male health in the present day. Justify your answers.

4. Which cultures do you think do the best job in promoting male health? What makes their approach superior and how do you see this advancing a global male health agenda? Are there any cultures that devalue males or trivialize their health concerns? Explain your points of view.

5. Do you think that males are indeed the "weaker sex" as described in the *New York Times* article? Explain your position.

6. Explain how males can overcome health issues. What would be the top three areas that you would focus on to improve health status?

7. Explain the primary health issues of males in the following populations: black, white, Hispanic/Latino, and Native American. Detail at least one cultural bias that precludes good health.

8. If you were educating a new doctor or health care worker on male health issues, what would be your major emphasis?

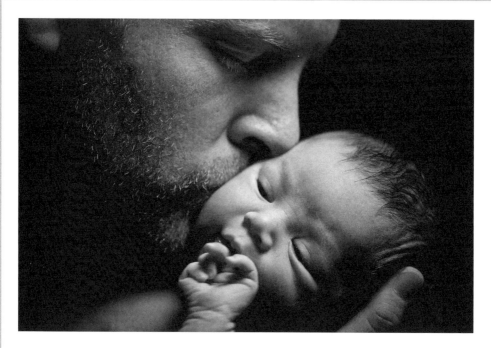

©iStockphoto.com/RonTech2000

2

Birth and Infancy

LEARNING OBJECTIVES

- Summarize challenges to male health starting at birth
- Identify biological and sociocultural underpinnings, factors, and risk in male health
- Summarize and analyze the various biological, social, cultural, and personal considerations concerning the practice of male circumcision, including public health and global perspectives

EXPECTANT MOTHERS, FATHERS, and family members often cannot wait to know the sex of an unborn child. More and more with today's phenomenal technology, particularly in prenatal imaging, parents can know the sex of their baby sooner and with more detail and accuracy than once thought possible. But what happens when the sex of a child is determined? How do these sociocultural factors affect the baby boy? What are the social and physical implications being born male? This chapter explores challenges to male health that begin at birth, the physical and sociocultural implications of being born male, and ways in which to enhance male infant health.

MALE INFANT MORTALITY AND HEALTH RISKS

The male sex and gender bring with them several challenges, even from the earliest stages of life. Some people assert that being born male begins a series of inherent risk factors (Tel Aviv University, 2009), whereas others highlight the effects of socioeconomic factors, such as race and class (Lean, 2008; Legato, 2006; Men's Health Network [MHN], 2009).

Statistically speaking, the male sex and gender carry with them significant risk factors for illness, injury, and even premature death. Biology plays a specific role; however, societal influences and determinants may play an even larger role in the development of males in society. For example, in Australia, one of the few countries that have actively advanced men's health policies in government, being born male still carries health risk factors such as cardiovascular disease, unintentional injuries, suicide, and obesity (Parsons, 2009). What can be done to address these issues? Are there genetic and biological factors we can address, or should greater efforts be placed on facilitating sociocultural change in how we view male health?

What Does the Biology Say?

A recent research study conducted in Britain found a connection between how much and what a mother eats prior to conception and the sex of her child. A mother's body can supersede the simple introduction of an X or Y chromosome from the male sperm into the egg, making the environment more favorable to one sex over the other. For instance, higher caloric energy intake prior to intercourse supported the conception of a male embryo; however, male birth rates are falling in industrialized countries such as the United Kingdom and the United States. This may be due to women restricting consumption of certain foods, calories, and nutrients because of dieting and body image concerns. The body in turn views the support of an embryo as nonfeasible and may revert to either not supporting conception or allowing access to the X chromosome, which requires less energy early on. Studies such as this clearly link the role of biology in the success of males and females even from the earliest moments of life (Parker-Pope, 2008).

Advancements in medical technology and health care overall have led to increased survival rates for mothers and their babies, but biology eventually takes over. We can keep baby boys and girls alive, but we cannot tell them how healthy they will be in their lives. Many of the biological issues men face occur later in life. Biologically, are boys the "weaker sex" as suggested in the previous chapter? We only list the facts and figures concerning this topic, but we also explore possible reasoning behind each statistic.

There are 105 male births for every 100 female births (MHN, 2009; National Center for Health Statistics [NCHS], 2008). Males are more likely to be **miscarried** and are at greater risk for being **stillborn** than females (Lean, 2008). The male infant death rate is around 22% versus 15% for females if born prematurely (MHN, 2009).

Research has identified a worldwide trend in many male species becoming more feminine from a biological perspective. The culprit: environmental chemicals and pollutants. For example, some mothers who were exposed to various chemicals and pollutants while pregnant gave birth to boys with smaller penises, ambiguous genitalia, and more feminine physical features (Lean, 2008). How a mother takes care of herself while pregnant greatly influences the viability of the fetus whether male or female (Shonkoff, Boyce, & McEwen, 2009); however, some researchers suggest exposure to chemicals and pollutants wreak havoc on male **chromosomes**, whereas female chromosomes may be more **resilient** (Lean, 2008; Tel Aviv University, 2009).

Risks with male fetuses are more common, as suggested from research based on 66,000 pregnancies and births. Prior to birth, male fetuses are more predisposed to rupture of the embryonic sac, which may cause premature delivery of the baby. Males who do make it to full-term status in utero are more prone to excessive growth, which can make delivery harder and more complicated for the mother. This latter fact can be seen with a greater number of cesarean births with boys than with girls (Tel Aviv University, 2009). However, research is quick to note that carrying a male fetus does not necessarily indicate a high-risk pregnancy. Vulnerabilities tend to persist in males throughout the life span, ranging from a shorter overall life span, greater susceptibility to infections, and less chance of withstanding disease than women (Legato, 2006; MHN, 2009; Tel Aviv University, 2009). Do these fetal and **neonatal** risk factors correspond to other risk factors later in life for a male? Are males set up to fail? The answers are yes and no and often are the topic of controversy in **gender studies**. Perhaps one of the more lucid quotes surrounding being born a boy or girl is the following: "It's almost like males and females are a different species. . . . They complete and complement each other, but a 'one-size fits all' medical approach does an injustice to both males and females. Men and women are different in so many respects, and these differences are more significant than the similarities between them" (Tel Aviv University, 2009).

Many aspects of why male fetuses and infants have a lower survival rate than females are still poorly understood. The rates of male births and a decline in viable male fetuses in industrialized countries suggest that they are attributable to more than just one factor. Some scientists point out that in **industrialized nations,** couples are delaying the start of a family until later in life. Research tends to support that as a male ages, so does his sperm, which lessens the likelihood of conceiving a male versus a female (Tel Aviv University, 2009). This area remains poorly understood.

Chances of survival are markedly increased for a male after birth; however, risks are still more prevalent than in female infants. Environmental risk factors, such as chemical exposures and pollutants, do not solely rest with a baby boy's mother. One study found statistically significant associations with childhood leukemia in both boys and girls when their fathers served in the military, with boys having higher rates (MHN, 2009). Infant boys are starting behind the proverbial eight-ball. We cannot simply change genetics to favor males, although biomedical advances are imminent. We can identify, understand, and potentially modify known risk factors (Shonkoff et al., 2009). Would men and women choose to have families earlier if they knew that risks of conceiving a male child who may have developmental or birth defects are much higher in older parents? Do men realize that as they age, the genetic information in their sperm also ages and goes through genetic mutations? Do expectant mothers realize that exposure to various environmental chemicals and pollutants may feminize their male fetuses? Do women understand that their interaction with the environment may cause deleterious consequences for a baby boy in the future? Most of these questions can be answered only on a personal level. What we in public health can do is advocate for better education for families concerning gender-based health issues.

SOCIOCULTURAL IMPLICATIONS OF BEING BORN MALE

The social aspects of being born male are perhaps more promising than the biological aspects. Although males still have more negative health consequences and shorter life expectancies than females, understanding and embracing social and cultural influences that affect these consequences can lead to better interventions, programming, and advocacy for male health. In public health, we tend to focus on primary prevention so as to advance individual, community, national, and global health. Yet primary prevention can only take us so far. We can try to genetically determine and alter mutations and risk factors for males; however, forging an understanding of how society shapes and influences what males do may be a better and more relevant form of primary prevention. For example, do we indoctrinate boys from the earliest of ages with a lifetime of rules, rituals, and expectations that if they choose to accept will cause them to be honored and respected, and if they decline, to be shunned, teased, and marginalized?

Typically, from a Western perspective, parents who learn the sex of the fetus begin an extensive preparation process that is inundated with sport equipment, blue blankets and sheets, toy trucks, and other stereotypical boys' toys. If parents swaddled their newborn baby boy in a pink blanket,

Figure 2.1   Common Western Masculine Values

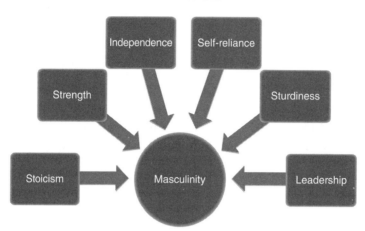

what would be the reaction of other people or family members? Strangers might simply assume it is a baby girl, whereas family members may voice their discontent about attempts to feminize the boy. These are social constructions and representations of what it means to be born male and all of the social implications that follow as a boy grows up. Many males have been **encultured** with traditionally masculine values, such as stoicism, suppression of emotions, independence, and self-reliance, and avoidance of anything that may be construed as feminine (Parsons, 2009). (See Figure 2.1.)

What do these traditional values mean for a male infant, young boy, adolescent, and man? Most research suggests that these sociocultural traits carry with them a lifetime of physical and psychoemotional consequences. For example, if a male is raised to be stoic and embrace the "suck it up and be a man" mentality, he is much less likely to seek health care services even when he may be in dire need of them (Parsons, 2009). Another example comes from the world of psychiatry. Males are not usually encouraged to discuss their feelings and emotions, which is evident from the nearly 70% of psychotherapy visits that are made by women. Thirty percent of the men who seek psychological consult only do so in the presence of a wife, girlfriend, or significant other (Baraff, 1991). These male values that are imbued in boys from the time they are born may exacerbate the already high risk factors males start with.

Everything about these values need not be viewed as bad or negative. Males embrace a sense of duty and honor in many occupations and services. For instance, the idea of psychological and physical toughness is a key attribute of military personnel and many civil service occupations (police, firefighters, and so on). Regardless, health risks because of social expectations have been well documented over the years and warrant further exploration and discussion, particularly when devising and implementing culturally sensitive and gender-specific **health promotion** programming.

Single-Parent and Nontraditional Families

What does the research say about males born into single-parent households? One of the stronger contributors to the health of a male infant, or any infant, is the structure of the family into which he or she is born. Family stability and a strong paternal figure who is involved in a baby's life lays the foundation for more positive life outcomes, such as going further in education, avoiding risky sexual practices, and resisting drugs and alcohol (Youth Risk Behavior Surveillance System [YRBS], 2008). Fatherless families in particular have been presented and discussed as a rampant social ill in the United States and abroad (fathers.com, n.d.). Various minority and cultural groups have disproportionate numbers of families without strong central male figures in the households (Treadwell & Ro, 2003). How does this lead male children astray? For the answers to this question we look at the data.

Negative health indicators for children of single-parent families include poverty and lower socioeconomic status (SES), drug and alcohol abuse, poor physical and emotional health, lower educational achievement, higher involvement in violence and crime, and greater incidence of sexual promiscuity, leading to increased rates of sexually transmitted infections and unwanted teen pregnancies (fathers.com, n.d.).

Fatherless households are five times more likely to be poor and live in poverty conditions and ten times more likely to be living in extremely poor conditions than households in which a father is present. More than 75% of children from single-parent and fatherless families will experience poverty by age eleven (U.S. Census Bureau, 2003). (See Figure 2.2.)

The obvious reasoning behind this is lack of income and resources compared with two-parent households. Many single-parent families are headed

Figure 2.2   Facts Concerning Fatherless Households

Fatherless households:
5 times more likely to be poor and live in poverty
10 times more likely to live in extremely poor conditions
75% of children in single-parent families experience poverty by age eleven
©iStockphoto.com/Sean_Warren

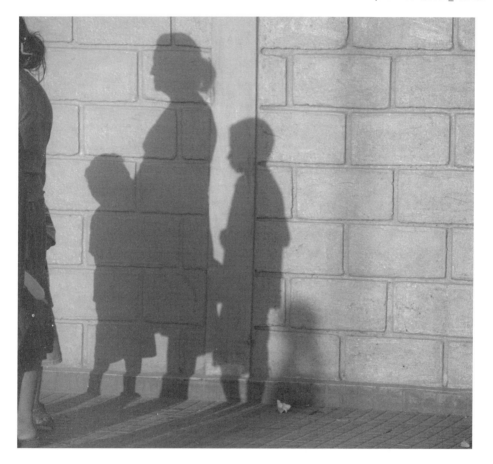

by women, with sparse to no contact with the babies' fathers. Lack of child support payments and other forms of support, such as time and emotional support, often drive families further into poverty. Some families lose their fathers or male figures due to untimely death, as can be seen in African American males' 7.1-year-shorter life expectancy than white males (Anderson & DeTurk, 2002).

Alcohol and drug use also disproportionately affects children, particularly males, from single-parent households. For example, children who come from fatherless homes and upbringings are 4.3 times more likely to smoke cigarettes and use other tobacco products than are children who come from homes in which a father is present (Denton & Kampfe, 1994; Stanton, Oci, & Silva, 1994). This fact is of no surprise, as many fatherless males often turn to peers and other sources for modeling, which can lead to the use of alcohol, tobacco, and other drugs. Alcohol and other drugs provide a **coping mechanism** (although unhealthy) with life stresses that may be linked to poverty and lack of male role models growing up.

Physical and emotional health also tends to lag behind in families in which fathers are absent. Women without partners are less likely to seek prenatal care due to lack of resources, particularly financial support. This in turn leads to greater health risks for the fetus and infant (Lean, 2008; MHN, 2009; Tel Aviv University, 2009). Children from single-parent households show higher rates of physical and mental illness, with rates higher in males than females. Boys also show higher rates of emotional disabilities and disturbances as well as learning disabilities such as dyslexia and attention deficit disorder. More suicides occur in males who come from households in which a father is absent or not consistently present (Hong & White-Means, 1993).

Educationally, boys from single-parent households are likely to drop out of school at nearly twice the rate of girls. Boys have higher rates of truancy, lower grades and grade point averages, and lower aspirations to further their educations. Boys also have been reported to be less engaged in educational programming and more often act out in inappropriate manners (Hong & White-Means, 1993).

Crime, aggression, and violence are more common in boys from single-parent families. The U.S. penal system is largely comprised of males, encompassing close to 95% of all incarcerated inmates (Treadwell & Ro, 2003). Boys are 1.7 times more likely to be criminal offenders and 2.1 times more likely to become chronic offenders in the legal system.

Last, boys from single-parent and absent-father households are more likely to be diagnosed with sexually transmitted infections (STIs) and contribute to unwanted pregnancies (Treadwell & Ro, 2003). The question of whether a male father figure matters from the time boys are born (or even before) and beyond is answered statistically in the affirmative. As social creatures we look to others for support and reinforcement from the earliest of ages. A baby boy born into a single-parent household, particularly one headed by a mother, is more likely to experience many social ills.

Racial disparities have a striking effect on single-parent families. Men of color often are marginalized in society, creating social and health inequities. A man who feels devalued and demeaned often reacts by dissociating from his reality, often at the expense of his family. Men of color are more likely to have lower education levels, be underemployed or unemployed, have more confrontations with law enforcement, be discriminated against, have poorer physical and emotional health, have less access to quality health care and health insurance, and often die sooner than white males (Treadwell & Ro, 2003). With all of these racial factors against him, it is difficult for a male to focus on setting good examples for his sons when he himself is up against tremendous odds.

Public health has to look beyond simply the individual perspective and take into account the social determinants of health. It is not adequate to say that a person should be accountable for his actions; a greater understanding of what prompts these social ills needs to be undertaken (Smedley & Smedley, 2005). Breaking the cycle of fatherless families will improve the health of future generations of boys.

Other areas that have less research backing are nontraditional families, such as gay and lesbian parents. Findings are mixed about whether or not a baby boy experiences more or less positive health outcomes in these situations. Loving and balanced families are probably the most crucial factors leading to well-adjusted boys; however, boys do look to other male role models. We as a society need to stress the need for fathers and other male figures to be present in boys' lives so as to foster healthier individuals in the community; otherwise, we are doomed to have boys raising themselves.

With many of the sociocultural issues exposed, researchers, scientists, and social scientists stand at a paradoxical precipice of male health. Males are encouraged to be brave, persevere in the face of illness, injury, and adversity, and seek occupations that have higher risk for danger and psychoemotional stress (Legato, 2006). Provocatively, Legato has asked, "Are we being sexist with men as we have with women over the past century? Do we ignore male health issues with only the fleet mention of prostate cancer and awareness?" (Legato, 2006). Do we simply see males and their health as a functional component of an ever-changing social system? Focusing an agenda on the unique challenges of males seems to be warranted in order to close the gap in cultural, racial, and economic disparities. Are males being underserved, ignored, marginalized, or simply being told to "man up"? Knowing what threatens males from the earliest of ages, both biologically and socially, will help advance the health of society as a whole.

CIRCUMCISION

Sometimes health decisions are made for people beginning at birth. Vaccinations and immunizations against infectious diseases often litter the calendar of any new parent. Most would agree that parental responsibility for providing the best medical advantages for their newborn is expected; however, where does a sex-specific procedure such as male circumcision factor in? Do parents have the right, or in some cases, the responsibility, to have their newborn sons circumcised? What are the medical, social, and ethical factors and considerations surrounding this topic?

Formally defined, **circumcision** is the surgical removal of some of or the entire **prepuce**, also known as the **foreskin**. The foreskin is an expansion of tissue that covers the *glans* penis, more commonly referred to as the "head" or "tip" of the penis (Brown-Trask et al., 2009; Gray, Wawer, Kigozi, & Serwadda, 2008). Most, if not all, baby boys are born with a foreskin; however, coverage of the head can vary.

Myth: The vast majority of males in the world are circumcised from birth.

Fact: Only 15%–20% of the world's population of males is circumcised. A cultural bias may exist in the United States, where rates are considerably higher (approximately 56%), leading many people to assume validity in this myth (Brown-Trask, van Sell, Carter, & Kindred, 2009).

Reasons and History

There are numerous reasons why people opt for circumcision and probably just as many for opting not to have the procedure done. Historical, cultural, religious, and personal reasons all underpin the common but evolving practice of neonatal circumcision.

The history of circumcision dates back millennia, with some of the earliest historical records garnered from hieroglyphs from ancient Egyptian culture from the sixth dynasty (circa 2345–2181 BCE). In these pieces of tomb art, images show young men (likely adolescents or preadolescents) having their penises cut in a ritualistic practice by priests (Darby, 2005). It is of note here that circumcision was depicted in young men versus infant boys. As history progressed, most civilizations outside of Egypt did not practice this ritual (Darby, 2005). The ancient Greeks and Romans viewed circumcision as mutilation of a perfect aesthetic of the male human form. Most Greek artwork depicted the male form with **intact** (and in some cases, accentuated) foreskins and depicted satyrs and barbarians as having circumcised penises to demean them. During these times only the priestly caste in Egypt, Jews, Proselytes, Nabatean Arabs, and some tribes performed this ritual (Hodges, 2001). Practices expanded to Christians; it has been said that Jesus Christ was circumcised as a Jew and that it served as a covenant between God and his chosen people. In fact, accounts of circumcision appear in the Old Testament of the Bible, when God exclaims to Abraham, "Every male among you shall be circumcised. You are to undergo circumcision, and it will be the sign of the covenant between me and you" (Gen. 17, NIV). Therefore, Christians, particularly orthodox sects, routinely practiced circumcision from a religious perspective. In the medieval and Renaissance periods, most people in Europe, with the exception of Jews, did not practice circumcision. In fact, in 1442 CE, a papal bull was issued that prohibited the practice of circumcision for all Christians (Darby, 2005; Hodges, 2001).

Circumcision in Europe in the eighteenth century was viewed with repulsion and as a mutilation of the human form (Darby, 2003). As such, most men were not circumcised during this time period. It was during the late 1800s and early 1900s that circumcision began to be viewed as useful and practical as a treatment for the supposed social ill of **masturbation** and sexual gratification in boys and young men (Moscucci, 1996). Masturbation was seen as a form of self-abuse and immorality; therefore, circumcision was viewed as a means to desensitize the glans of the penis and lessen the allure of masturbation (Darby, 2003; Moscucci, 1996). This led to approximately 30% of males being circumcised in the United States around 1900, many in adolescence and young adulthood. The practice grew more prevalent, especially in the United States, during World War I and World War II, mainly due to hygienic practices for soldiers who could not regularly bathe. As such, soldiers returning home from war expected their own sons to be like them; therefore, the rates of postwar circumcisions reached its height around 1950 (Darby, 2003). Outside of religious practices and considerations, fathers typically want their sons to identify with them as they grow and develop; therefore a man who is circumcised is likely to have his son circumcised, with the opposite holding true for uncircumcised men.

Many tribes in eastern sub-Saharan Africa practice circumcision as a rite of passage for boys to signify their coming of age into manhood (adulthood). With circumcision comes induction into a warrior class with all of its rights and privileges, such as marriage and acceptance into a fraternal brotherhood. Conversely, those who are uncircumcised often are ridiculed and viewed by tribe members as immature and little boys (Darby, 2003).

Social acceptance and tradition is another common issue pertaining to circumcision. Tradition strongly influences the practice of male circumcision, which is evidenced in different ethnicities. For example, it is estimated that 81% of whites, 65% of blacks, and roughly 54% of Hispanics circumcised their males (Buie, 2005; Laumann, Masi, & Zuckerman, 1997). At its height in the 1950s through the late 1970s, men who were uncircumcised were seen as odd and outside the norm. Ironically, the deviation from the norm in terms of male anatomy *is* a circumcised penis. The issue extends beyond men and involves relationships with other women and men. Generationally, some women have never encountered an uncircumcised penis, thereby possibly creating awkward moments when and if she does have a partner who is uncircumcised. Equity also plays a role in the decision to circumcise. For example, when performed in the first couple of weeks as an infant, charges run approximately $196 USD, whereas costs rise to approximately $1,800 USD if performed later in an operating room setting. Annually in the United States, circumcisions, which are not covered by all insurance policies, cost between $150 million and $270 million USD (Buie, 2005; Van Ryzin, 2000). The latter fact creates a social disparity for those who have health insurance coverage and those who do not, or those who can afford to have the procedure performed and those who cannot. Circumcision involves a confluence of personal, religious, and traditional values.

Statistics

According to recent statistics from the United States, neonatal circumcision (also known as *routine infant circumcision*) is one of the most commonly performed medical procedures, with approximately 56% of all baby boys undergoing the procedure. Previous historical data show a peak in national trends in 1950, with approximately 72% of boys being circumcised. This trend held steady until the late 1990s and early 2000s, with a decrease in 2001–2003 as rates dropped from 63% to their present 56%. Strong regional differences exist as well and are largely based on cultural norms and values. For example, nearly 80% of newborn boys are circumcised in the Midwest and parts of the South, whereas only 33%–37% undergo the procedure in the West and Southwest (Circumcision Information Resource Pages [CIRP], n.d.; Brown-Trask et al., 2009; Laumann et al., 1997). The latter fact is likely due to increasing birth rates in these regions of Hispanic/Latino populations, who typically do not practice routine infant circumcision. Rates of infant circumcision are in stark contrast to most other parts of the globe, where lower rates prevail. For example, Canada reports less than 14%, Australia 10%–20%, Great Britain 12%, and New Zealand 5%. Other countries, such as India and China, with the world's largest populations, are largely uncircumcised (CIRP, n.d.).

Other countries tend to have higher rates of circumcision because of the predominance of certain religious rites, beliefs, and practices, such as among Muslims and Jews. Rates in Arab-speaking and Jewish countries, such as Saudi Arabia, Iran, Iraq, Jordan, Syria, Israel, and several other countries, have some of the highest rates of male circumcision in the population (CIRP, n.d.). Rates and other statistics likely will continue to evolve over time due to changes in cultural beliefs and values, medical evidence, population dispersion, and many other sociocultural variables.

Methods

A variety of methods and surgical techniques for circumcision have been practiced over time. Some of the earliest references to ritual circumcision involved the use of **excising** (removing) the foreskin with sharp objects such as knives and flint rock (Darby, 2003; Moscucci, 1996). More recent methods are the most widely used Plastibell technique, followed by the Mogen clamp and the Gomco clamp (Brown-Trask et al., 2009). Other methods include the Tara Klamp and the Smart Klamp, although freehand methods using a scalpel are still practiced by some physicians.

The first freehand method is known as the *guided freehand technique.* The freehand scalpel method with a shield is generally used in the Jewish rite of *bris,* whereas a forceps guided and scalpel method is preferred in adult circumcisions. The shield is inserted under the foreskin and around the glans, which helps to separate the tissue layers; next a scalpel is used to cut away the skin, leaving a fairly uniform scar when it heals. The *forceps guided scalpel method* is used in many adult circumcisions, when the foreskin is pulled away from the glans and a scalpel is used to cut away the tissue. With the latter method, there are possibilities of more tissue being removed, greater likelihood of uneven scarring, and possibly the use of **sutures** to close the surgical site, again possibly leading to greater scarring.

Occlusion methods include the Plastibell technique, Tara Klamp, Smart Klamp, and Zhenxi Rings. These methods essentially occlude or cut off the blood supply to the foreskin using a clamp, ligature, or a combination of the two. These methods have been routinely used because of the ease of training, acceptable cosmetic results, and low risk of infection. Specifically, the Plastibell method inserts a plastic bell around the glans beneath the foreskin, and a ligature (string) is tightened. The lack of blood causes the foreskin tissue to die, and it usually falls off in 7–10 days after the procedure. The Tara Klamp and Smart Klamp methods are very similar to the Plastibell;

however these methods do not use a string to cut off the blood supply; rather the layer of foreskin is trapped between two sections of the clamp and the same 7–10 day process occurs (Brown-Trask et al., 2009). The Zhenxi Rings use a method similar to the Plastibell and Tara and Smart Klamp designs, which also preserve the integrity of the *frenulum,* which is a sensitive band of tissue on the under surface of the glans and penile shaft.

Other guided methods that involve more of a crushing technique are the Gomco method and Mogen clamp. The Gomco clamp involves both tension applied to the foreskin and cutting any excess skin away from the device. This approach increases the chance for excessive bleeding and is more difficult to learn than the other methods. The Mogen clamp is fast to use, but it also comes with the risk of excess bleeding and possibly infection.

Other less common methods of circumcision include use of a laser, sleeve resections, and partial circumcisions. Lasers have greater risks for burns and ablation (damage) to the penile tissues; not much literature concerning acceptable results is available at this time. Sleeve resections slide the foreskin back on the shaft and a freehand cut is made around the shaft as far back as the scar line is desired. The foreskin is returned to cover the glans, and another cut is made around the shaft at the same position along its length as the first. A longitudinal cut is made between the two circumferential ones, and the strip of skin removed. The edges are pulled together and sutured. The success of this technique is largely dependent on the skill of the surgeon and is more commonly perform in older populations rather than infants. Last, partial circumcision, also known as dorsal slits, involves making a longitudinal incision along the dorsum (top side) of the foreskin to alleviate restrictive pressure, but little to no skin is removed (American Academy of Pediatrics [AAP], 1999; Brown-Trask et al., 2009).

Benefits

The benefits and value of circumcision have been studied for years, and findings continue to shed light in support of this procedure. One of the more obvious benefits of circumcision has to do with **hygiene** and general care of the penis. Some of the first **observational studies** in this area were conducted with men in the U.S. military during World War II, when debris such as sand or dirt would cause inflammation under the foreskin. Soldiers often were circumcised for preventative purposes prior to deployment. Overall results showed lower rates of infection related to poor hygiene (McDermott, Wilson, & Marty, 1982).

Poor hygiene can lead to several problems if not appropriately addressed or taught to a boy growing up. The foreskin acts as a natural protective cover of the glans; however, if it is not maintained and properly cared for through hygiene, infections and secondary infections may result (Brown-Trask et al., 2009). For example, males who are circumcised have a lower incidence of urinary tract infections (UTIs) and balanoposthitis (Brown-Trask et al., 2009).

First, UTIs affect the urethral orifices and main tube, the urinary bladder, and may even travel up the ureter and into the kidneys. This is likely due to the collection of bacteria and other natural debris from the penis, such as smegma (dead cells and tissue that is periodically sloughed off). It has been found that infants and younger males who are uncircumcised are more likely to experience UTIs than are circumcised males of the same age (Brown-Trask et al., 2009). Rates of **uropathic** bacteria also are higher from birth until the first year of life and gradually decrease over time. Of course, proper parental education as to how to wash and maintain excellent hygiene likely solves the issue, but evidence does show circumcision to be beneficial (Gilgal Society, 2004).

A second condition related to hygiene is called **balanoposthitis,** which is an inflammation of the foreskin and glans of the penis. Again, the main cause is poor hygiene with typical signs and symptoms being redness and pain along with a foul-smelling discharge. Treatment involves controlling the infection and inflammation with topical and oral antibiotics and teaching good hygiene (Brown-Trask et al., 2009). The role of the health educator is critical in helping parents who choose not to circumcise their boys in understanding and following good hygiene practices (Buie, 2005). Based on all available evidence, it is unquestionable that circumcision improves overall penile hygiene and lessens the chance for infection.

Two other relatively common issues that circumcision helps attenuate are phimosis and paraphimosis. For most boys (approximately 95%), by the age of four years the foreskin can be fully retracted behind the glans. However, in some males, the foreskin is tight and retracts with difficulty and pain or it does not retract at all; this is referred to as *phimosis* (Brown-Trask et al., 2009). The major issues with phimosis are possible tearing with forceful retraction and inadequate hygiene due to accessibility issues to the glans. The result may be yeast infections, skin irritation (due to urine), and balanoposthitis (Brown-Trask et al., 2009). A related condition to phimosis is *paraphimosis.* In this condition an already tight foreskin may be forcefully retracted over the glans and then cannot be appropriately repositioned. This may occur when a parent or caregiver is attempting to clean the penis. The foreskin forms a tight band and occludes the glans and related tissues, which can result in edema and **ischemic** tissue death to the foreskin and glans (AAP, 1999; Brown-Trask et al., 2009; Gilgal Society, 2004). Paraphimosis constitutes a urologic emergency and needs to be immediately treated if suspected. A common treatment (and prevention) for these conditions is circumcision or a dorsal slit down the foreskin, which allows for more room to accommodate the glans.

Penile cancer is a relatively rare occurrence in males; however, nearly all cases (750–1,000 cases annually in the United States) or 0.9–1.0 per 100,000 men occur in uncircumcised men. The mortality rate for this type of cancer is high at 25%. Additional support for this finding is validated by higher incidence and mortality rates in countries that traditionally have low rates of circumcision, such as Great Britain, Brazil, and India. Additionally, men who were circumcised later in life had higher rates of penile cancer, suggesting that infant circumcision may serve as a protective factor for avoiding later penile cancer and related conditions (Buie, 2005).

More recently, several studies have turned their attention to whether and how circumcision moderates the development of human immunodeficiency virus and acquired immune deficiency syndrome (HIV/AIDS), sexually transmitted infections such as human papilloma virus (HPV), and cervical cancer in females (Ridings & Amaya, 2007; Bailey et al., 2007; Moses, Bailey, & Ronald, 1998; Lane, 2002). The main premise for how this procedure affects these diseases is based on the type of skin that covers the glans region of the penis. The outer surface of the skin is not unlike other skin cells throughout the surface of the body; however, the inner layer of the foreskin is more like mucousal tissues' (Gordon, 2009). The mucousal layers have more viral receptors than the outside skin layers, which may predispose a person to greater exposure to viruses such as HIV and other STIs. Additionally, the inner part of the foreskin is usually a moist, dark environment, which usually is optimal for bacteria, fungi, and viruses to reside and grow in if proper hygiene is not followed (Gordon, 2009). By circumcising the penis and exposing the inner layer of the glans, the skin cells become tougher and more resilient, thus making it more difficult for viruses and bacteria to gain access into the body. This process is referred to as *keratinization* (Buie, 2005). Other theories as to how circumcision lowers one's risk of HIV and other STIs include that the foreskin may experience trauma during sexual activity, causing microabrasions; the foreskin may harbor microorganisms longer enhancing the likelihood for infection; and uncircumcised men may experience more inflammation (*balanitis*), thereby causing the skin cells to be more susceptible (Buie, 2005; Gordon, 2009). For many years it was believed that circumcision played a strong role in explaining why Jewish women had very low rates of cervical cancer, which was linked to their partners' circumcision status. Recent reports have suggested that sociocultural factors play a strong role and not whether or not a man is circumcised. For example, Jewish women who follow traditional practices of Judaism (including sexual practices and hygiene) have lower rates of cervical cancer, but Jewish women who report deviating from traditional practices have higher rates of cervical cancer regardless of their partner's' circumcision status (Menczer, 2003).

Several epidemiological studies have supported the practice of circumcision as a positive public health measure similar to that of routine infant vaccinations (Brown-Trask et al., 2009; Moses et al., 1994; Moses et al., 1998). Most of the research suggesting the positive aspects of circumcision has been conducted in Africa, thereby possibly skewing the interpretability of the data; however, the evidence in the strength of correlation for circumcision status and lower rates of STIs is compelling.

Probably one of the weaker arguments for a pro-circumcision stance has to do with aesthetics and cultural norms. Some cultures and traditions advocate (either directly or indirectly) that males be circumcised. For example, a boy begins to develop his sense of self and identity typically with a male role model, such as his father. Looking different (uncircumcised) may provoke feelings of inadequacy or confusion as he tries to identify with norms in his world (Buie, 2005). Some people simply prefer the look of a circumcised penis; however there are many people for whom it does not matter. If a person has grown up in a society that accepts circumcision, promotes circumcision (directly or indirectly) through media such as pornography or seductive advertisements, and establishes it as the norm, anyone deviating from that norm may experience feelings of isolation, estrangement, or even ridicule. Feeling accepted by a group is critical in one's psychosocial development.

Tradition and religion cannot be ignored as major factors and influences concerning the practice of circumcision. Circumcision is viewed favorably when it attends to religious expectations and rites. For example, Judaic rituals of the ***bris (b'rit) milah*** (ritual circumcision) account for a significant number of circumcisions performed in the United States each year.

VIGNETTE

Six of us, two men and four women, were sitting in a trendy martini bar in Soho in New York City. It was a cool but pleasant November evening. Wendy was pregnant with her first child. One of the other women exclaimed, "Oh my gosh Wendy . . . when are you due?" We all joined in the conversation as our appetizers were brought out. The expected question finally was brought up by my buddy Stephen. "Do you know if it is a boy or a girl?" Wendy responded by saying, "Actually, it's a girl." The look on Stephen's face went from excitement to a "That's nice" look. Wendy noticed his look, burst into laughter, and said, "I am just kidding, Stephen. I am having a boy!" We all laughed, mostly at the expense of Stephen. As dinner rolled along, the conversation mainly centered on baby talk: names, toys, and room décor. We discussed whether everything should be blue.

When Cheryl asked, "Are you having him circumcised?," the group got really quiet as Wendy pondered her response. "Well, my husband Aaron is Jewish you know, but I am not, so I guess we will have to cross that bridge when we come to it." I said it should be something that is carefully thought about. The other women laughed and said, "Ah, it is just a little flap of skin; he won't even remember it!" Stephen looked at me with that "Let's get out of Dodge" look, and I winked to indicate my affirmation. Circumcision and martinis just do not mix!

Risks

As with most medical procedures, there is risk to the patient. Do the benefits of a procedure like circumcision outweigh the risks? There are many national and international organizations that aim to educate and change people's views on routine circumcision due to its inherent health risks and that question its necessity.

One of the first issues adamantly voiced by opponents of circumcision is the introduction of unnecessary physical and emotional pain during the first days of life. One reference details the assertion that circumcision is overwhelmingly painful and traumatic with behavioral changes occurring in the infant male for up to six months post-procedure (Goldman, 1999). It was once believed that neonates did not experience the intensity of pain or would not remember the pain and discomfort, as would older individuals undergoing the same procedure. Recent evidence shows that infants circumcised without **analgesia** experience changes in heart rate, blood pressure, oxygen saturation, and **cortisol** levels indicating markers of pain and physiological distress (Brown-Trask, et al., 2009). The experience of pain in the first moments of life has been suggested to carry lasting psychological complications ranging from repressed emotional pain (Boyle, Goldman, Svoboda, & Fernandez, 2002) to schizophrenia (Flaherty, 1980). Early pain in childhood also has been suggested to provoke greater instances of maladaptive behaviors in adolescents (Kennedy, 1986). As adults, many men express a sense of loss, both in a physical and psychological sense. Since many men did not have a choice in their circumcision status, some express that having something very personal taken away from them (including choice) has led to regret. This can be seen with different devices and techniques proposed to restore one's foreskin using remaining skin and tissue on the shaft of the penis.

Of course, these theories are controversial and somewhat speculative in
nature; therefore one should gather as much information as possible before
entertaining many of the assertions made by opponents of the procedure.
There also have been advances in controlling for the pain and discomfort
associated with circumcision, largely due to the efforts of research that has
dispelled the notion that pain was minimal in neonates (Geyer et al., 2002).
For example, the American Academy of Pediatrics (AAP) made several recommendations regarding the use of analgesics and pain relief methods for
neonatal circumcisions. Additionally, eutectic mixture of local anesthetic,
also known as EMLA, has been used as a topical anesthetic. The cream
mixture is 2.5% lidocaine and 2.5% prilocaine and is typically applied 30
to 90 minutes prior to the procedure. There are other procedures that have
been effective in reducing neonatal pain, discomfort, and behavioral changes,
such as the dorsal penile nerve block and the subcutaneous ring block (AAP,
1999; Brown-Trask et al., 2009).

Procedurally, the process of circumcision involves cutting into tissue and
removing it, which can result in excessive bleeding. Hemorrhage leads in the
category of rates of complications, with 0.2% to 5% of surgeries resulting
in reported complications (Hiss, Horowitz, & Kahana, 2000). Hemorrhage
also constitutes the most frequently reported cause of morbidity, such as
tissue damage, penile deformation, and edema, related to circumcision
(Williams & Kapila, 1993). Additionally, infants generally are not routinely
tested for blood disorders such as hemophilia or other clotting conditions.
These are most likely established only during the procedure, which can have
deleterious consequences for the infant. Bleeding post-circumcision also can
lead to excessive blood loss and result in **hypovolemic shock** and even death
if not recognized early on (Hiss et al., 2000).

After bleeding, infection is another concern post-circumcision. As with
any surgical procedure, there always is the inherent risk of infection and
subsequent effects. Staphylococcal infections are becoming more prevalent,
particularly in medical settings, which call into question the necessity to
perform the procedure according to the AAP (1999). Other infections from
circumcisions have been documented, such as tuberculosis, diphtheria,
staphylococcal pyoderma, impetigo, and in some cases **septicemia** and septic

shock. Infection in particular calls into question the notion of **iatrogenic** disease, when medical procedures meant to help do the opposite and hurt people (Van Howe & Robson, 2007). "Do no harm," from the **Hippocratic Oath**, is one of the cornerstones of medicine, and opponents of circumcision often quote this as a reason circumcision should be curtailed.

Once the healing process begins, individuals will develop varying levels of scarring where the foreskin was excised from the penis. The level of scarring largely depends on two criteria: first, the type of technique used by the surgeon, and second, the skill and experience of the surgeon. For example, freehand circumcisions using a scalpel and forceps may produce a noticeable circumcision scar line, whereas occlusive methods such as the Gomco clamp typically produce a characteristic brown scar or "halo ring" around the penis. For some, scarring is a non-issue; however, for others, the scarring related to circumcision can be excessive and may even interfere with normal function. Excessive scarring can leave skin tags or may even result in *keloids,* which are scar tissue, thus creating excess tissue along the scar site.

Aside from being cosmetically unacceptable, keloids and excessive scarring can impair function both urologically and sexually. As the excessive tissue grows, it can occlude the *urethral meatus* (opening of urethra at the head of the penis), cause bending or curvature of the penis, and impede sexual function later in life. People with a family history of keloids should take this into consideration before having their sons circumcised. Additionally, some racial/ethnic groups, such as blacks and darker-pigmented individuals, are more prone to keloid formation; therefore it is important to take this into consideration as well. Uneven scarring also is possible and again reflects back to the skill and experience of the surgeon. In neonatal procedures, it may be difficult to ascertain how much skin is to be removed; therefore, scarring may vary and produce unacceptable results. Unevenness also may result in excessive removal of skin, leaving what is referred to as a "high" circumcision. Having a high circumcision may limit mobility of the penile skin on the shaft, making intercourse or sexual pleasure difficult. In some instances if a circumcision is high and tight, tearing of the skin may result. In other cases, adhesions may develop as the circumcision site heals. Adhesions form when new tissue attempts to **proliferate** the area where skin was removed during the procedure and sticks to other areas of the penile shaft and glans. Adhesions may result in limited tissue mobility and unacceptable cosmetic results. In some cases the adhesions are so prolific the glans may appear to be partially covered by the scarred skin. Other forms of adhesions from circumcision can pull the penile shaft to one side and can result in deformation and disfigurement. Also, pulling tissue to one side may cause fibrotic tissue (tough scar tissue) to develop within the penile cavities, thus limiting blood flow and possibly causing erectile dysfunction (ED). Last, skin bridges also can develop between the surgical site and the glans of the penis. These pieces of skin can impede sexual functioning because they may limit tissue mobility or even tear in the process of sexual activity. Moreover, skin bridges are cosmetically undesirable and may require additional surgery to correct. Most of the conditions related to scarring, unevenness, skin tags, adhesions, and skin bridges require some form of surgery or treatment depending on the level of severity (Gerharz & Haarmann, 2000; Stromps, Kolios, & Cedidi, 2009).

In some instances, depending on the skill of the practitioner not enough skin is removed during the initial procedure. In this case, a circumcision revision may be desired or even warranted. Revised circumcisions are risky in that there is less skin to work with and additional scarring may occur, not to mention the child is exposed to another less-than-optimal experience early in his life. Opponents of circumcision are very quick to point out that all of these complications are avoidable if the circumcision procedure is not performed.

Removal of the foreskin leads to keratinization of the glans and may desensitize the penis. Keratinization causes skin cells to become thickened and more resilient to outside influences (Fink, Carson, & DeVellis, 2002; Sorrells et al., 2007). This process can be likened to the development of a callus on one's foot due to stress patterns. As the tissue continues to be exposed to the environment (such as friction in underwear) and is no longer protected by the foreskin, cellular changes result. The main issue of keratinization is the loss of sensation and sensitivity in the glans of the penis, thereby possibly diminishing sexual pleasure (Sorrells et al., 2007).

Research is conflicting as to whether or not keratinization causes a decrease in sensitivity of the penis and a reduction in sexual pleasure (Fink et al., 2002). Because pleasure is a subjective concept, research is limited to self-reports. However, recent clinical research has shed new light on sensitivity ratings, supporting that circumcision does in fact diminish sensitivity in select men (Sorrells et al., 2007). Certainly men who have experienced a portion of their lives uncircumcised and have the procedure performed later in life may have a justifiable and reliable comparison, but because many men do not experience this, results are conflicting and controversial. One study from the *British Medical Journal* examined the glans from seven circumcised men and six uncircumcised men; results showed equal keratinization of the glans in both groups (Szabo & Short, 2000). This type of study however, does not account for the subjectivity of sexual pleasure. Other research has looked at men who experienced erectile dysfunction and their circumcision status. Findings revealed higher rates of ED in circumcised men than uncircumcised men. These findings may be limited or confounded in that a higher percentage of the samples of men with ED were circumcised. Moreover, the men who reported ED were from the United States and were born 1950s and early 1960s, when the practice of routine infant circumcision was nearly ubiquitous (Fink et al., 2002). The jury appears to still be out on the topic of whether or not circumcision affects penile sensitivity.

One of the more concerning complications possible with circumcision is physical damage to or loss of the penis. Rates of complications associated with neonatal circumcision range from 2% to 10% and vary in severity (Williams & Kapila, 1993). *Ablation,* which is the removal by destruction of tissue from a body part or surface, can cause damage to the glans, urethral anatomy, or any other part of the penile shaft. This is more likely in neonatal procedures when of the penis is much smaller than that of an adult; thereby making estimation of tissue removal a challenge for the skill of the surgeon. There have been cases where various methods, such as electrocautery, have led to ablative damage to the penis. Penile reconstructive surgery or gender reassignment from male to female have been reported (Gearhart & Rock, 1989). Risk of severe complications is low, particularly in the United States, but parents of newborn boys should be made aware of these potential issues before having the procedure performed.

Amputation of the penis due to circumcision is uncommon, but the possibility does exist, especially as rates of circumcision change throughout the United States and abroad. Again, all risks and complications should be clearly outlined for expectant parents by trained personnel, such as health educators, well before the procedure (Buie, 2005). One of the more prominent cases of penile ablation and resultant amputation was David Reimer (born as Bruce Reimer in 1965). David and his twin brother Brian were born in Canada as healthy baby boys. After six months, the boys' parents noticed they were having difficulty urinating, which was subsequently diagnosed as phimosis or a tight foreskin. Circumcision was recommended to treat the phimosis and the boys were scheduled for the procedure two months later. Bruce (David) was the first in the operating room where electrocauterization, a fairly uncommon method, was used. The procedure did not go as planned and Bruce's penis was burned beyond repair and was then amputated. His twin brother did not undergo the procedure. Bruce was sexually reassigned but never identified as being female. Later in his life, Bruce who was living as "Brenda" decided to change back to a male and became David. After several reconstructive surgeries and hormone therapy, David Reimer married and became a step father to his wife's three sons. Sadly, after years of emotional and physical conflict, depression, and medication interventions, David Reimer committed suicide in 2004 at the age of 38. His story is documented in a book by John Colapinto titled *As Nature Made Him: The Boy Who Was Raised as a Girl* (Colapinto, 2001) Stories like David Reimer's call into question the efficacy of circumcision even when used as a medical treatment for a condition such as phimosis. It should be stressed that instances like David Reimer's are rare occurrences, but issues such as this need to be presented to parents before a decision to circumcise their son is rendered.

Death resulting from circumcision has been documented, but again it is a rare occurrence, with fewer than 1% of complications ending in death (Gerharz & Haarmann, 2000; Kapila & Williams, 1993). However, in a medical world in which physicians abide by the principle of "Do no harm," one death may be considered too many. One of the primary issues surrounding the tracking of deaths due to circumcision is quality of the data. For example, if an infant dies from blood loss, acute infection, cardiac arrest, or any other complication, the cause is typically not listed as "circumcision." So, do people die from circumcision? The direct answer is No; however, if we redefine this in terms of "complications of or related to" then the answer becomes Yes.

Historically, circumcision prior to medical advances in hygiene may have led to far more deaths resulting from complications of the procedure than we know because of lack of documentation in public health. It is documented that male **infant mortality** is higher than that of females (Baker 1979). Does circumcision play a role in this? What about procedures performed in other areas of the world that lack appropriate facilities, trained medical personnel, and minimal antiseptic practices? The bottom line is that many more deaths caused by complications resultant from circumcision may be occurring than once thought. Simply because rates and statistics do not show a problem does not mean problems are not occurring. Answers to these questions largely rest with how we track and classify complications due to circumcision procedures.

A Question of Ethics

A discussion of the value of *paternity* is frequently brought up in the discussion of circumcision practices. Essentially, the value of paternity assumes that others will protect children from danger and harm because children cannot protect themselves (Buie, 2005). In the case of circumcision, the value of protecting a newborn boy from possible physiologic problems later in life has to be weighed against immediate complications due to the surgery itself. Another common debate centers on the intent of the procedure in and of itself. For example, many opponents of circumcision charge those who perform such procedures with the intent to make financial gains for a medically unnecessary procedure (AAP, 1999). There are numerous medical and legal implications surrounding circumcision as well (Gerharz & Haarmann, 2000). For example, use of foreskin **fibroblasts** in medical research (Rabenberg, Ingersoll, Sandrey, & Johnson, 2002) and commercial products has stirred ethical debates. Human foreskin fibroblasts are used in all kinds of medical procedures, from growing skin for burn victims and eyelid replacements to growing skin for people with diabetic ulcers (who need replacement skin to cover ulcers that won't heal) to making creams and collagens in the cosmetics industry (Euringer, 2007). The value of this tissue may become more coveted due to decreasing rates of circumcisions over past decade (CIRP, n.d.). Proponents of using foreskin fibroblasts argue that in the past the tissue was simply discarded; therefore, why not make use of the tissue for beneficial health purposes? Others argue that this is a misuse of medical practices and technology and discredits the rights of the families and individuals who undergo the procedure (Euringer, 2007). Most parents would not even think about what happens to their son's foreskin once a circumcision procedure is complete, but maybe they should. Others place blame on parents for not fully understanding the reasons for having their sons circumcised.

The jury is still out regarding circumcision, especially routine infant circumcisions on neonatal infant boys. In 1999, the American Academy of Pediatrics issued a policy statement that says the benefits aren't strong enough to recommend routine circumcision for all male newborns and is considered an **elective surgery** in most cases (AAP, 1999; Buie, 2005). Today, the AAP leaves the decision up to parents and supports use of pain relief for infants who have the procedure. Routine infant circumcision is not a medical necessity and should not be routinely performed unless it has been presented to the parents so they can make an informed decision on behalf of their son.

Role of Health Educators

The role of health educators provides ample opportunity to help parents make informed decisions concerning their sons' health. Health educators should be prepared to provide unbiased information and consultation for both the pros and cons of circumcision, while taking into consideration the individual, family, social, religious, and cultural influences surrounding the procedure. Informed decision making concerning this issue should not first be presented and discussed once a baby is born; rather, a planned and timely approach is strongly advocated for new and expecting parents. Population-based education concerning the benefits and consequences of circumcision fall within the professional duties and realm of health educators and public health workers and should be handled in such a manner that promotes optimal health decision making for the individual and the greater good of society (Buie, 2005).

Public Health and Circumcision

How does public health view the practice of male circumcision? The practice of circumcision has demonstrated beneficial results across the world in reducing STIs such as HIV/AIDS. Lower rates of STIs obviously affect women as much as males. Does circumcision curb the spread of HIV and other STIs? In a word, no. Circumcision changes the physiologic structure of penile tissue, which may lower the chances of contracting and thus spreading STIs such as HIV (Bailey et al., 2007). What must be strongly considered it that personal safety behaviors, such as using condoms and safer sexual practices, are the most effective practices in reducing the contraction and transmission of STIs.

Mandating policy change is a tough road to navigate, particularly concerning one's personal rights about one's body. There are, however, instances in which public health policy has been introduced for the good of the population, as with childhood immunizations and vaccinations. The Centers for Disease Control and Prevention (CDC) may formally recommend infant circumcision as a means to advance public health in this area (sexual health), which is in contrast to the American Academy of Pediatrics' statement detailing that in most cases circumcision is not medically necessary (AAP, 1999). So, perhaps circumcision is not a medical necessity, and it may be viewed as health-additive in many instances. Additionally, the CDC may set forth a series of recommendations that target men who are at a higher risk for STIs, such as men who have sex with men (MSM). Much of the evidence for the benefits of circumcision come from studies performed in Africa. These studies have asserted that circumcised men were less likely to become infected with the herpes virus and the human papilloma virus, which can cause cervical cancer in women. These facts may help drive future public health campaigns (Kotz, 2009).

The science tracking the medical benefits of circumcision does not necessarily translate to public health practice in the United States and the rest of the world. For example, Europeans have never really embraced the practice and are not likely to do so in the near future. Cultural expectations and sexual practices of people in Africa do not necessarily equate to those of Americans. With the world opening up more than ever before, people will continually be exposed to different cultures, people, and practices. Perhaps the public health of men and of the world does not rest with a controversial "magic bullet" procedure performed in infancy but rather with education on best practice medicine and health education to help people make better-informed decisions concerning their sexual health.

SUMMARY

The focus of the chapter was on health issues affecting males from conception through the first year. There are several sociobiological factors that affect male health during these early years, ranging from simply surviving to biomedical and ethical issues. The worldwide impact of being born male was explored through a thorough analysis of morbidity and mortality rates culminating in a presentation and discussion of what factors are controllable versus ones that are not. The first section took a closer look at what it means to be born male and the sociobiological influences that come along with it. A section explores the impact of single-parent families and the sociocultural impact of families with and without male role models. Biological and sociocultural perspectives were discussed in terms of how they guide male health in today's society. The historical, cultural, medical, and ethical bases for male circumcision was presented and discussed from benefits and risks perspectives.

KEY TERMS

Analgesia   *Bris (b'rit) milah*   Circumcision

Balanoposthitis   Chromosomes   Coping mechanism

Cortisol	Hypovolemic shock	Occlusion
Disparity	Iatrogenic	Prepuce (foreskin)
Elective surgery	Industrialized nations	Proliferate
Encultured	Infant mortality	Resilient
Excised	Intact	Septicemia
Fibroblasts	Ischemic	Stillborn
Gender studies	Masturbation	Sutures
Health promotion	Miscarried	Uropathic
Hippocratic Oath	Neonatal	
Hygiene	Observational studies	

DISCUSSION QUESTIONS

1. Why do you think most cultures use blue to represent boys and pink for girls? Are there other cultures that go against this notion? If so, describe how they are different.

2. How does having a male role model present in a boy's life contribute to his overall health?

3. Describe the specific and unique challenges that a female single parent may experience. How do these factors affect the health of the family as a whole, the children, and specifically male children? Justify your comments.

4. What initiatives are being planned and implemented to enhance male health from birth through infancy? That is, what programs have been established at various levels that address this topic?

5. Does the practice of routine male circumcision set a negative precedent? Does this routine procedure devalue the utility of circumcision as a treatment approach for several public health issues?

6. What role does aesthetics play in the circumcision debate? Discuss how this issue can affect one's health from both physiologic and psychological perspectives.

7. Does one method of circumcision seem like the best option? Take into account health risks and benefits, cosmetic efficacy, and any other points that you would like to consider.

8. Should human foreskins be available to grow more human cells, used for research practices, or used in cosmetics? Should there be costs associated with this market? For example, should parents be compensated if they elect circumcision for their son? Should males be able to "sell" their foreskins?

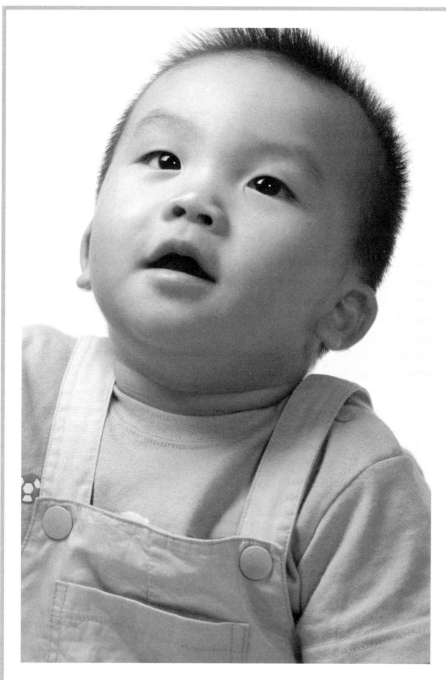

3

Early Childhood

LEARNING OBJECTIVES

- Explain the overall role of parents early in life, in particular father figures or other male role models
- Describe sociocultural influences on male nutrition and how these can influence healthy behaviors
- Describe how sexuality affects young males and identify expected sexual behaviors as well as unexpected ones in boys
- Analyze the role of physical and emotional disparities in determining male health outcomes

DO WE TREAT boys and girls differently, even at ages one to three? What underpins how men and women treat children in general and boys in particular? What are the innate qualities of boys during the early stages of life that may carry positive or negative consequences for their lifetimes? This chapter explores some of the early experiences and exposures in a boy's life that may help shape his future path of health and quality of life.

THE JOURNEY BEGINS

Early on in a boy's life, the groundwork or foundation for a healthier life is being laid each day. Unfortunately, so too are negative influences that can **confound** health-related quality of life. How does a boy form who he is? How are his character and personality shaped and who does the shaping? Are qualities of boys at these ages a result of nature, nurture, or both? Do we need a book such as *The Complete Idiot's Guide to Raising Boys*? (Helgoe & Helgoe, 2008).

Biologically, boys are different than girls. This may seem obvious, but only if we are thinking of physical appearance. Boys are wired differently than girls, which may explain why their behaviors are usually markedly different. For example, girls often develop the capacity for language and reasoning sooner than do boys (Schmithorst, Holland, & Dardzinski, 2008). Lise Eliot, author of *Pink Brain Blue Brain* (2009), asserts that brain research has clearly identified differences in how boys and girls are programmed. Eliot details how our assumptions and values get placed on the developing boy or girl and further guide these natural biological differences. Parental and other social assumptions crystallize into children's **self-perceptions** and possibly self-fulfilling prophecies, reinforcing expected behavior (for example, boys play with trucks and not dolls) and hardly challenging the opposite notion (Bazelon, 2009; Eliot, 2009). Boys also seem more reactive and lacking the capacity to focus on a task such as sitting quietly in a classroom or learning setting. These factors may seem like a challenge for any one- to three-year-old, but they are particularly evident in male behavior.

BOYS WILL BE BOYS? THE ROLE OF PARENTS

Boys look to role models for assistance in their sociocultural development. The influence (or lack) of male role models is vitally important as a boy becomes a **toddler.** Social learning theory explicitly states that people look to others in their sociocultural groups for strategies by which to model their life choices (Bandura, 1977). Boys look to other boys and men unless males are simply not present in their lives. If boys do not encounter male role models, often they will resort to other groups later in life to fulfill this need. For example, boys who become involved in gangs may have lacked strong male role models earlier in their lives and therefore fulfill a social need for solidarity and acceptance.

Myth: Boys will be boys.

Fact: Yes, boys will tend to act more like boys, but sociocultural influences in what defines a male (masculinity) also greatly affect tendencies and behavior. Research has consistently shown that boys gravitate toward more aggressive and rough activities because of hormonal influences (testosterone) but their behaviors are also influenced by what is deemed acceptable.

Those boys who do have male role models in their lives, such as fathers, may benefit in several ways; however, interactions that promote healthy behaviors are only as efficacious as the male role model himself. That is, men who are ill equipped to make positive health choices in their own lives are much less likely to positively influence the health of their sons. We need to be careful with health promotion concepts in families who adhere to the "Do as I say, not as I do" mentality.

Fathers are spending more time with their children than did previous generations. Fathers are hands-on and are a part of many boys' lives, much more so than the provider stereotype from yesteryear (Chiarella, 2006). But, are boys getting what they need from these interactions? The answers may go beyond that of just a father's role in his son's life. A boy needs to see and interact with all types of men and other boys to understand himself and his own position in life, even at the age of one, two, or three. Unfortunately, boys may not bear witness to this diverse community of men. Instead, media outlets may fill that vacuum, often inaccurately depicting what a man is. Over-glorified images and statistics that tell boys that men speed in cars, do not wear seatbelts, get drunk, or get girls pregnant are inaccurate but are present in **culturalia.** These aspects of being male need to be understood by parents so that social interactions can be encouraged in some respects and contained in others.

VIGNETTE

Fully satisfied from a bountiful lunch at the local mall, my mother, sister, and I embarked on a journey to a place where controlled chaos reigns supreme, bodies are constantly in motion, some defying Newton's laws and axioms of physics, and the decibel level competes with a modern-day rock concert. Give up? We arrived at the children's play zone. This space was engineered with a Boston colonial theme, complete with a pseudo–duck pond, baseball park, climbing wall, and Boston Tea Party ship. Children of all ages were rushing from attraction to attraction, often ignoring others in their way. Parents tried to show displays of mutual respect, sharing, and at times discipline. The entirety of the experience was summed up in one word in my mind: *sociology*. We arrived with my niece, a three-year-old dynamo, and my one-and-a-half-year-old nephew. Both kids were eager to get involved with all of the attractions, while I expected to wait and prevent any collisions or arguments among the children. I did not expect to be involved in a sociological study of how pre-toddler boys interact, but I did!

My niece was curious yet reserved in her approach toward the other children. My nephew seemed to do what he pleased, often with the consequence of colliding into other children. He seemed to have very little fear or reservation. Naturally, as a student of the sciences, I began to analyze my own observations and bias. Maybe it was just him, maybe my niece was just shy, maybe . . . maybe I should look around more. Upon observing the approximately forty other children, both boys and girls, I surmised a definitive trend in how the boys and girls were going about conducting their business. The boys were more physical, taking more risks, engaging in more arguments and physical altercations, reacting to others, and doing what they pleased. The girls were doing much of the same, but in a different way.

I shifted my attention to the parents. First and foremost, approximately 95% of the parents were women; only a few awkwardly positioned men graced the space. The men were disengaged and frequently checked their cell phones and watches. Also, the men seemed to discipline their children less often than did the women. I wondered if it would be a different story if more men were there at the time. Additionally, the women seemed more critical of the boys than they were girls; essentially they were protective of the girls and much more liberal in their approaches with the boys. I overheard a couple of women saying, "Oh he is just being a boy, he's just like his father, I can't get anything through to either of them!" I bit my tongue, carried on my sociological work, and dug into my pockets for some money to buy ice cream at the next stop in the mall.

Social interaction among boys lays a foundation for how they interact as adults. For example, a parent who limits the risks a boy may take may influence his ability to develop various forms of **self-esteem** and **self-confidence.** A common example is how parents react to a young boy when he falls down. If a boy falls down and a parent ignores him or tells him to get up, he may develop a sense that he is to endure pain or injury. Male stoicism is not an innate quality boys are born with; rather, it is a learned behavior and response to social stimuli and interactions (Parsons, 2009). Conversely, a boy who is nurtured or given excessive attention due to a mishap may become reliant on others and may not develop a strong sense of independence or self-reliance.

These points of course are the subject of controversy, particularly in parenting circles. The facts may lie within the individual and not what happens later in life. Some boys are simply more sensitive and respond well to attention, whereas others resist it and strive for independence. Parents and guardians need to be more in tune with the factors that guide boys to negative health behaviors rather than enculture them with emotional qualities that promote these inequities. Men have to be willing to care about how boys are treated and taught through cooperative understanding and advocacy (Chiarella, 2006).

NUTRITION AND DIET

Nearly two-thirds of premature deaths in the United States are due to poor nutrition, physical inactivity, and tobacco use (Singh-Manoux et al., 2008). Little is done to combat **obesity** and poor nutritional outcomes, although efforts by the federal government have been increasing during recent years (Men's Health Network [MHN], 2009). One of the first decisions that guide a lifetime of health promotion in children is what foods parents give them. Nutrition for children is largely based on the same health principles as for adults. A quality balance of **macronutrients,** such as carbohydrates, proteins, and fats, along with minerals and vitamins, should underpin a healthy diet in early childhood and beyond. Developing baby boys need quality foods that contain essential nutrients to help their bodies grow and develop in an optimal way. This latter point may seem obvious and certainly applies to both boys and girls; however, do we feed our children differently based on their sex? People have their own food preferences that evolve and develop throughout their lifetimes; however, how, what, and how much a boy eats may not entirely be based on individual intrinsic choices and personal tastes. We often grow up with family nutritional values and principles.

For example, a Japanese family will eat differently than an Italian family. Do boys eat differently than girls? At earlier ages, the answer may be No. As boys interact and experience more male culture in their family structures, nutritional considerations may change. Role modeling again is a factor in what and how much boys will eat. For example, in the United States, it is a sociocultural phenomenon that boys are encouraged to eat more food, whereas girls are encouraged to exercise nutritional restraint (Wardle, Haase, Steptoe, Nillapun, Jonwutiwes, & Bellisle, 2004). One only needs to watch popular television shows and other forms of media that stereotype a man-sized appetite and males gorging on high-calorie non-nutritious food sources. Women are stereotyped as modest eaters who order more reasonable food choices such as salads.

Essentially, a boy who views other males in his family, such as a father, brothers, and uncles, engaging in their dietary practices may begin to adopt their eating patterns even before he knows what he is eating. Fast, processed, fat-laden foods and foods high in sodium content unfortunately have become a staple of the American diet (Singh-Manoux et al., 2008).

Men consume more **calories** from processed foods than from healthful sources of nutrients. Parents typically select foods that the entire family will consume, which sets the tone for a lifetime of food decisions. That is, a father who routinely eats at a fast-food establishment is more likely to introduce his son (and other children) to the same food choices. This begins a slippery slope that makes it difficult for boys to make good food selections in the future. Coupled with a culture that encourages boys to consume high numbers of calories because they are "growing boys," we are seeing higher rates of childhood obesity at even the youngest of ages (Singh-Manoux et al., 2008).

Similar to young girls developing eating disorders such as **anorexia nervosa** and **bulimia nervosa,** young boys are experiencing rates of morbid obesity that have prompted health warnings, particularly in the United States (Kraemer, 2000; Singh-Manoux et al., 2008).

Health consequences resulting from poor dietary choices range far beyond obesity. A lifetime of physical and emotional problems is imminent. High cholesterol, heart disease, colorectal cancers, diabetes, joint diseases, and many other physical problems partner with social stigma, stereotypes, and depression, perhaps leading even to premature death. Exercise will help combat this growing **epidemic,** but with less physical activity time in schools and in general, boys' waistlines will continue to grow. Boys from the ages of one to three years need to be taught how to balance good nutrition and physical activity.

Diet and nutritional principles lay the groundwork for a lifetime of healthy eating habits and choices; however, the odds are stacked against boys. Culture tells them one thing while research says another. Parents are confused as to what boys should do; that is, eat heartily or exercise restraint. Balance needs to be stressed even at these early ages. Boys are not natural overeaters, and parents need to help their developing sons to view food as something that will promote their health and not their masculinity. Nutrition and diet is a modifiable factor that we can use to enhance the health status of developing boys. The best source for promoting this healthy shift is leading by example, especially for the men in their lives. Starting early is essential.

SEXUAL HEALTH

Sexual health may not be on the minds of many new parents of baby boys; however, boys during early childhood and beyond may begin to explore their bodies, including their **sexuality.** Parents report that their sons experience frequent **erections** from the earliest of ages, and they often question whether this is a normal response or not. Other parents express concern that their boy is self-stimulating or masturbating. Is this normal male behavior? The answer is Yes to both questions. Erections at young ages are completely normal and should be expected; there is no harm in erections. The topics of self-pleasure, stimulation, and masturbation are a bit different. Boys typically begin noticing and touching their genitals around six months of age, but they may pay particular attention between the ages of one and three years. In fact, some research using **in utero ultrasonography** depicts babies touching their genitals (WebMD, n.d.a). This demonstrates that we are sexual creatures from birth until death.

So, how should parents handle erections and self-stimulation in boys of this age? This can be a tricky, sensitive, and awkward topic to approach, since the young boy will not entirely understand his own behavior. The boy may be better able to understand the context of his actions better than the actions themselves. For example, if parents reproach the boy and essentially shut down the behavior, he may grow up believing he has done something wrong or that masturbation is a negative behavior. This also may lead to feelings of sexual repression that can cause issues later in life, such as with intimate relationships. Conversely, if a parent accepts the behavior as a normal part and expression of gender identity and formation and sexual expression, this may ease the tension between parent and child. For example, informing the child that what he is doing is normal or even ignoring the behavior altogether may allow for self-acceptance. However, informing and educating on the context in which he is performing these behaviors also is important. Boys need to be taught that behaviors involving self-exploration need to be conducted discreetly and in private settings. Parents need to stress that there is a time and place for everything, including masturbation. Parents who pathologize the behaviors of normal growth and sexual development are only setting the boy up for issues to be dealt with later in life.

Perhaps one of the major concerns for a parent concerning a boy's expression of his sexuality is that there may be something else going on in his life. Certainly emotional issues and maybe even trauma may provoke boys (and children overall) to pursue behaviors that soothe and provide a pleasurable escape. Parents and health professionals need to be aware of an excessive preoccupation with this behavior. Is something amiss? Is a parent absent? Is there a newborn baby in the home? Is the boy using this behavior to gain attention? Is he lacking something in his life, such as attention or love? Is there the possibility he is experiencing some form of **sexual abuse**? All of these are important questions to be considered. Sexual abuse in boys is an issue, with approximately 1 in 6 boys experiencing some form of abuse in their lives before the age of sixteen; however, it is less commonly discussed or even advocated and likely is under-reported (Watkins & Bentovim, 1992). One of the main issues with recognizing and understanding sexual abuse in males is the secrecy and stigma that goes along with it; therefore, parents and practitioners need to be aware and vigilant in trying to understand a boy's behavior.

Boys are more likely to externalize their emotions, whereas girls tend to internalize (Watkins & Bentovim, 1992). That is, boys will tend to act out, especially at younger ages, because they may not know how to express their feelings otherwise. This becomes a common fact of male behavior throughout the life span, abuse or not. Not recognizing sexual abuse in boys has been linked to a lifetime of consequences, including but not limited to becoming sexual predators themselves, sexual identity confusion, lower self-esteem, greater instances of sexual dysfunction, higher instances of hypersexuality, higher occurrences of depression, and more relationship issues, anxiety, and suicidal tendencies (Holmes & Slap, 1998; Watkins & Bentovim, 1992). Understanding boys even at this young age is important and highly relevant for raising a well-adjusted young man.

DISPARITIES IN MALE HEALTH OUTCOMES

Physical Disparities

Males may be born with health issues that carry with them a lifetime of consequences, both physically and emotionally. Some issues are common, but short-lived, such as **hernias** and **asthma.** For example, boys are more than eight times more likely than girls to be born with hernias due to a lengthened inguinal canal where the testicles descend. Asthma is more common in boys at birth and the first couple of years of life, but it gradually attenuates, likely due to the influence of increases in systemic testosterone, which relaxes the smooth muscle of the airways. Many health and physical issues are not so short-lived, however. While many early childhood issues may not become evident until later in life, it is never too soon to begin understanding ways in which to promote healthier strategies to manage such issues in a boy's life.

Some issues result from how boys are taught to handle physical issues early in childhood. We explore common physical issues affecting boys in early childhood, explain how racial and ethnic status disproportionately affects negative health outcomes, discuss how social modeling perpetuates physical stereotypes and male health disparities later in life, and last, how to focus on modifiable variables in younger childhood so that boys will have a fighting chance as they grow and develop.

Research has linked the influence of paternal age, smoking, and alcohol consumption with the development of congenital abnormalities in male offspring (Savitz, Schwingl, & Keel, 1991). Fathers of advanced age had offspring with greater instances of birth deformities and defects such as nasal aplasia (abnormal development of the nasal bones), cleft palate, hydrocephalus (fluid accumulation in the cranium), pulmonic **stenosis** (narrowing of lung tissues), urethral stenosis (smaller, shorter urethra), epispadias and hypospadias (abnormal placement of the urethra relative to the penile shaft), and hemangiomas (blood tumors). Cigarette smoking was highly correlated to boys born with cleft lips (some with cleft palates) and ventricular defects of the heart, in addition to the stenotic conditions previously described.

Many of these early-childhood physical health defects also can be traced to a man's exposure to environmental toxins, often due to his occupation (Savitz et al., 1991). Men are more likely to work in occupations that expose their systems to chemicals and noxious agents (for example, coal miners and dust particles, farmers and pesticides, and military personnel and chemical agents used in war, such as nerve gas).

Men are more likely than women to work in hazardous occupations that can affect their children's health.

©iStockphoto.com/Taylor Hinton

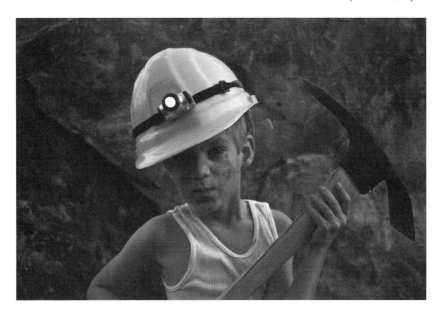

Boys whose fathers were in the military were found to be diagnosed with childhood leukemia before the age of two years at a rate of 4.6 times more often than controls in which fathers were in nonmilitary professions (Wan-Qing et al., 2000). Physical defects also disproportionately affect children of color more than any other group, often due in part to the lack of access to consistent quality health care (Jack, 2005). (Black and Hispanic men are the least likely groups to carry health care coverage in the United States.) Moreover, black men traditionally have been underserved and marginalized in the medical community, which in turn has led to distrust and paternal stoicism regarding their health care. Black men also disproportionately have manual labor jobs that often lead to negative physical health consequences and outcomes. A baby boy of color born into these social conditions may start out "behind the eight-ball" before he even learns how to say his own name (Braithwaite, Taylor, & Treadwell, 2009).

Male attitudes toward their own physical health have existed in a dichotomous world for centuries. **Sex role strain** may influence health care and attention even between the ages of one and three years. At three years old, a boy may be told to "get up and tough it out," or "be a big boy." How does this change as a man ages? If a man in middle adulthood experiences chest pain, he may choose to ignore it, rationalizing to himself that it is just indigestion. Males have been socialized from the earliest of ages to ignore and minimize physical signs and symptoms of their bodies (Jack, 2005; MHN, 2009). Giving in to pain often is viewed as a weakness not only of a man's physical stature, but also of his mental toughness and fortitude. Research has suggested that men often ask themselves some basic questions before they decide to ask for help, participate in health-related activities, or seek medical treatment for a condition or pathology. These four primary questions center around (1) normality, (2) reactions, (3) status, and (4) control (Addis & Mahalik, 2003).

> *Normality.* Males ask themselves if they are acting like other males would in the same or similar given situation. This can be seen at the earliest of ages in boys as they socially interact. A boy may choose to cry when he is hurt if he sees other boys crying, or he may choose the opposite. Parental influence heavily weighs in as well. Males look at their experiences based on a whole set of factors, including age, race, education level, socioeconomic status, location, and several other criteria. Because males in early childhood lack life exposures and experiences, often they will look only to their paternal influence and other boys of their age. Essentially, negative reactions or those that appear to be abnormal according to gender expectations predispose a young boy to potential positive or negative views concerning his health management.

Reactions. Males socially compare themselves to others like themselves. How will others react or respond to me if I seek help? This question plagues males deciding whether to cry or show pain if they fall down while playing as young children all the way to deciding whether or not to ask for directions as they age. Bear in mind that these are more than just gender stereotypes. Health research consistently demonstrates that males are less likely than females to seek medical care for prevention or treatment of illness and injury (Addis & Mahalik, 2003; Jack, 2005).

Status. Status is another factor that heavily weighs in as males decide to pursue or not pursue health positive behaviors. What will I lose if I ask for help or seek assistance? Answers are less clear in early childhood, but it does factor into decisions made by young boys. Will other boys look at me differently if I go to Mommy or Daddy for something? Do other boys do the same thing? Am I normal? These thoughts and decisions carry with them a lifetime of possible biases that may positively or negatively affect a man's health.

Control. Boys and men value a sense of control in their lives. What happens if I give up that toy or my position on the jungle gym to that other child? Will I be viewed as weak or deficient? Again, these thoughts and feelings may not be expressed between the ages of one to three years; however, even young boys tend to value a sense of control in their worlds (Jack, 2005; Meryn & Jadad, 2001).

How do we instill a sense of responsibility and control in young males when they are learning how to pursue health and manage their options as they grow in society? The answers are not clear-cut, nor are they as simple as advocating for education and change. We are talking here about a social **paradigm** change in the way we raise our boys. Shifting the value system many males have grown up with and continue to perpetuate in their own sons will add to the advancement of future generations in their health and personal health beliefs. A sense of empowerment when communicating their health needs and seeking positive health behaviors needs to replace the traditional male stoicism and "tough it out" mentality (Parsons, 2009).

Addressing physical health disparities in males across the life span begins in early childhood and needs to be promoted by all people in the community, male role models in particular.

Perhaps one of the more concerning issues for this topic is the disparate position in health outcomes men of color occupy in the United States. Black males suffer from some of the worst social and physical outcomes of health. Lack of access to quality health care and medical services, distrust for the health care system, stoic attitudes toward the concept of pain and dysfunction, single-parent families, and many other sociocultural determinants have only increased the health care disparity gap in men of color in the United States. Helping young men understand this cycle of social and health-related disparities using culturally sensitive and relevant strategies will begin to address this glaring gap in early childhood (Braithwaite et al., 2009).

Emotional Disparities

The common fears of boyhood seem ubiquitous, yet what about emotional and learning issues that disproportionately affect boys? At this age, children are able to think and reason, manage their feelings, command a workable vocabulary, and socially interact with others in meaningful ways. What happens when a boy is lagging behind in one or all of these categories? What constitutes "normal," and how can a parent or health practitioner know whether a boy is emotionally behind others?

Boy are generally considered to be *late bloomers,* meaning that relative to girls, growth and emotional development generally occur later rather than sooner. For example, at eighteen months girls command approximately ninety words, compared with just forty for boys of the same age. Of course, there is great variability among children, but a key point is to compare boys to boys. Autism, for example, affects nearly four times as many boys as girls, with ratios of nearly 10 to 1 for the entirety of the spectrum of autistic disorders. The latter also includes Asperger's syndrome, which is a milder form of autism (Brun et al., 2009). Why do boys have a greater likelihood for developing these emotional disorders? The answer is not simple and often is linked to both physical and social factors. Imbalances of certain minerals, such as calcium, in a boy's brain may predispose him to these disorders. Boys are three times more likely than girls to be diagnosed with attention deficit hyperactivity disorder (ADHD) and are more prone to dyslexia and delayed speech (Brun et al., 2009).

Early recognition and diagnosis of these emotional issues may help a boy to adjust and receive the best-quality care. Unfortunately, many boys do not have access to quality health care because of socioeconomic disparities. This is particularly evident in black and Hispanic populations in the United States (Davis, Kilburn & Schultz, 2009). One needs only to walk through many public school classrooms to bear witness to this fact. Most boys are not formally diagnosed until later in life when they already have begun school, leaving them behind in social development and education. The first step in helping boys overcome emotional issues and learning disabilities at this young age is to be aware of the spectrum of issues that are possible. Because many of these issues will not become evident until a child has begun his schooling, parents and health practitioners need to look for specific behaviors and signs (Kemp, Segal & Cutter, 2009), including:

- Difficulty expressing feelings and emotions
- Inability to calm oneself down
- Excessive hyperactivity or lack of focus (research suggests most boys are naturally more physically active and explore their world more through experiential learning; this should not be viewed as pathological development)
- Withdrawn from other children or displaying antisocial behavior
- Lack of desire or interest in activities
- Difficulty reading other people's **body language**
- Inability to verbalize or make consistent eye contact with others

It is critically important to weigh these factors with other evidence that leads a parent or practitioner to suspect an emotional issue. There are many support groups and organizations that are free of cost and highly available to new parents; however, lack of knowledge about seeking assistance is a common barrier to receiving quality care.

Costs of Not Preventing Disparities in Early Childhood

It has been said that "you cannot effectively weed half of a garden" (MHN, 2009). The time is past due for addressing male health. Men experience poorer health and health outcomes than women (Williams, 2003). Men of color and other minority groups are disproportionately represented in negative health consequences and outcomes, such as obesity, diabetes, cancers, cardiovascular disease, and die sooner than women (Braithwaite et al., 2009; Treadwell & Ro, 2003). Social positioning and economic and political environments can help systematically determine the course of male health (Jack, 2005).

It is clear that men need to increase their knowledge as to how their behaviors early in life and attitudes toward health can either promote good health in the future or condemn their minds and bodies to illness and dysfunction.

If society continues to perpetuate the notion of "boys being boys," and advocate for the "tough it out" mentality, boys and eventually men will do just that. With this approach come social and physical dues to be paid in the form of health consequences. Boys who are told to "tough it out" or "suck it up" often receive a very clear message: ignore pain and be stoic in terms of your health. Will a three-year-old boy who falls down and scrapes his knee be given attention from his parents or will he be socially trained to "act like a man"? This is not to say we need to coddle our boys or address their every need; independence needs to be replaced, however, with a new paradigm of **interdependence**. Boys and men need to see their overall value in society beyond that of functionality. Ignoring health issues, however minor, sets a wrong precedent for young boys. Gender-based medicine often assumes males will address health issues as they arise, and sometimes they do. However, research indicates males are greatly underserved and even avoid the health care system.

Males are a disparate group in and of themselves. It is and will be a difficult task to change a paradigm of male health that has existed for centuries. Tradition and culture muddle the waters of advancing health advocacy efforts for males. The blending of medical aspects, gender factors such as defining and redefining masculinity and gender roles, racial and cultural perspectives, and many other contributing factors make setting an active agenda a challenge. What is positive and sheds a healthier perspective is that males are becoming involved in their children's lives more so than ever before. This cultural shift is fertile ground for advocating healthier perspectives and behaviors in forthcoming generations of males. Education, reestablishing trust in the medical system, developing gender-based medicine, changing fatalistic thinking, viewing males as inherently valuable from a humanistic perspective, and changing how we define *masculinity* are some great starting points for closing the gap of male health disparities.

Addressing male health issues is critical in building a complete and inclusive health care system. Some advocates have suggested including a medical specialty similar to gynecology, aptly named *andrology*. If society continues to prescribe how a male is to interact in his world, we are doomed to the same abysmal health outcomes for generations to come. If we embrace what a male can be and teach him at an early age how to embark on a life journey that completes him as a healthy individual through self-determination, we will likely see a stronger and more socially productive citizen of the world.

SUMMARY

This chapter addressed health issues common to males in early childhood, between the ages of one and three years. Many of the issues affecting males during these years of life set the stage for health problems later in adolescence and adulthood. Similarly, positive health messages and examples modeled to boys during early childhood may lead to a better overall health-related quality of life as boys advance in age. Sociocultural aspects of how boys interact and develop a male perspective were presented and discussed in detail. The role of parents and parental modeling were discussed.

Next, nutrition and diet perspectives were discussed. Understanding what underpins how males eat and the sociocultural influences that guide eating patterns and exercise behaviors were presented. Sexual health explored issues in developing male sexuality from the earliest of ages. Why and how boys exhibit sexuality and their developing gender roles was presented, with frank discussion on sexual expression as well as self-pleasuring behavior and masturbation. Issues of sexual abuse and its indicators were brought to the reader's attention.

Physical and emotional issues that disproportionately affect males were discussed, along with some emphasis on racial and ethnic disparities. The chapter presented emotional disorders and learning problems, such as dyslexia, autism, Asperger's syndrome, and attention deficit hyperactivity disorder, in young boys from a gender-based disparity perspective. Last, the costs of not paying attention and advocating for closing the disparity gap in male gender health issues was discussed at length.

KEY TERMS

Anorexia nervosa

Asthma

Body language

Bulimia nervosa

Calories

Confound

Culturalia

Epidemic

Erection

Hernia

Interdependence

In utero

Macronutrients

Masculinity

Myelin

Obesity

Paradigm

Self-confidence

Self-esteem

Self-perception

Sexuality

Sex role strain

Sexual abuse

Stenosis

Toddler

Ultrasonography

DISCUSSION QUESTIONS

1. Describe the central role of a father or male caregiver and how his presence or absence promotes health or increases the likelihood for a boy's health disparities.

2. Provide scientific and sociologic evidence for why males tend to act the way they do. For example, why do males act more aggressively than girls even at these young ages? Choose three primary areas in which to focus in your answer.

3. What are the main physical, social, and intellectual differences between one- to three-year-old girls and boys? Be sure to provide specific evidence to accompany your points.

4. What would you say is the biggest myth concerning boys between the ages of one and three years? Where do you think this myth originated? What would be strategies to help educate people and dispel this inaccurate information? Be specific.

5. Why do you think males tend to overeat? Where did these behaviors develop and from whom? What are the long-term health ramifications?

6. What is the role of sexuality in males between the ages of one and three years? That is, what function does sexuality have in boys during this period of time for their overall development?

7. Describe the role of self-stimulation in young boys (one to three years). How may it affect their sexual development? Pick a side of this topic, and advocate for the behavior or argue against it. Discuss the topic in its entirety and don't just respond with your feelings or emotions toward the issue.

8. Find research discussing why boys are more likely than girls to be diagnosed with autism, Asperger's syndrome, and attention deficit hyperactivity disorder, and comment on the researchers' findings and conclusions. Do you support these findings? Can you offer any alternatives to what was found in the research? What are some challenges in diagnosing boys between the ages of one and three?

9. You have been given a $1 million grant to develop a community outreach program aimed at decreasing health disparities in the black and Hispanic/Latino communities in your county. First, choose what your top three issues would be, based on scientific data. Next, briefly detail your primary strategies for each topic you chose to address.

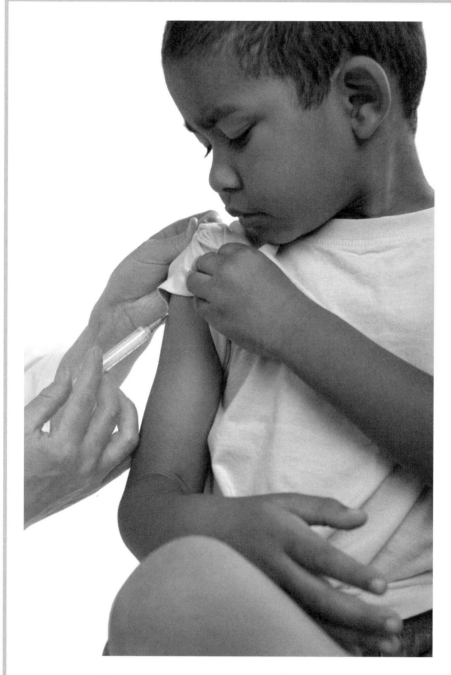

©iStockphoto.com/Alexander Raths

4

Toddler Years and Young Childhood

LEARNING OBJECTIVES

- Name common vaccinations used as forms of primary prevention for toddlers and young children
- Identify the common physical and emotional challenges of male toddlers and young children
- Explain why male toddlers are apt to experience unintentional injuries, identify safety measures for male toddlers, and define curiosity and understand its role in boys' safety
- Outline the broad spectrum of learning abilities and disabilities many male toddlers and young children and their families face
- Explain differences in behavior between male and female toddlers and young children

AS A MALE toddler becomes more aware of his ever-expanding world, health challenges and risks increase exponentially. How does one keep a male toddler or young child healthy, happy, and safe? How do parents, caregivers, and health practitioners handle unexpected emotions, unusual behaviors, learning problems, social issues, and physical health problems during this age? This chapter addresses issues ranging from how a male toddler expresses his emotions to what parents can do to keep him healthy and safe as he grows in his environment.

DEFINING THE TODDLER AND YOUNG CHILD

Generally speaking, a *toddler* is a child between the ages of one and three-plus years, while a *young child* is between three and five-plus years old (American Academy of Pediatrics [AAP], 2009b). Physically, toddlers and young children reach several milestones as they grow and develop. Toddlers begin walking, the spine and abdominal muscles take form, the brain develops to approximately 90% of its adult size, bowel and bladder control advance, the immune system further develops, and height and weight gain occurs (AAP, 2009b). Mentally, a workable vocabulary develops, meaning and value becomes apparent in the child's life, and imaginative play continues. Emotionally, a sense of independence and **self-reliance** often presents during this age. For example, boys may mimic their parents' behaviors (particularly their fathers or male role models), while retaining a sense of accomplishing things on their own. **Tantrums** are common early in a toddler's life, but these generally attenuate as the boy realizes value and right from wrong (Erwin, 2006; Kindlon & Thompson, 2000). Preference for foods, games, and entertainment options become readily apparent during this stage (Erwin, 2006).

VACCINATIONS

Some of the first ways by which to improve a child's health is through routine **immunizations.** Many immunizations and **vaccinations** are administered shortly after a child is born; however, other vaccinations are required or strongly recommended in toddlers and young children. For example, diph-

Table 4.1   Recommended Immunization Schedule for Persons Ages 0–6 Years

Source: Centers for Disease Control and Prevention (2009).

Vaccine ▼ Age ▶	Birth	1 month	2 months	4 months	6 months	12 months	15 months	18 months	19–23 months	2–3 years	4–6 years
Hepatitis B[1]	HepB	HepB				HepB					
Rotavirus[2]			RV	RV	RV[2]						
Diphtheria, Tetanus, Pertussis[3]			DTaP	DTaP	DTaP	see footnote[3]	DTaP				DTaP
Haemophilus influenzae type b[4]			Hib	Hib	Hib[4]	Hib					
Pneumococcal[5]			PCV	PCV	PCV	PCV				PPSV	
Inactivated Poliovirus[6]			IPV	IPV	IPV						IPV
Influenza[7]					Influenza (Yearly)						
Measles, Mumps, Rubella[8]						MMR		see footnote[8]			MMR
Varicella[9]						Varicella		see footnote[9]			Varicella
Hepatitis A[10]						HepA (2 doses)				HepA Series	
Meningococcal[11]										MCV4	

Range of recommended ages for all children

Range of recommended ages for certain high-risk groups

theria and tetanus toxoids and acellular pertussis vaccine (DTaP), pneumo-coccal conjugate vaccine (PCV) and pneumococcal polysaccharide vaccine (PPSV), inactivated polio vaccine, influenza, measles, mumps, and rubella (MMR), varicella, hepatitis A series vaccine, and meningococcal vaccine all are recommended at this age (Centers for Disease Control and Prevention [CDC], 2009). It is important to ensure that all younger children receive all scheduled immunizations at the appropriate ages for a lifetime of good health. The CDC provides a concise immunization schedule for children 0–6 years old, shown in Table 4.1.

Advocacy efforts to assure that all children are routinely vaccinated have led to positive results in toddler and young child health in the United States. However, vaccinations and primary prevention only work if they are acces-sible and consistently administered. Socioeconomic status (SES) is a strong predictor of many health-related outcomes (Jack, 2005). Minority families and families with low SES in the United States may not seek preventative health care such as vaccinations due to several factors, including lack of education and awareness, financial constraints, distrust of the medical system, and lack of accessibility (Braithwaite, Taylor, & Treadwell, 2009; Jack, 2005). Moreover, many developing nations pale in comparison to the United States; this unfortunately may lead to higher incidence of morbidity and mortality in these countries. Coupled with the fact that boys are typi-cally born with weaker immune systems than are girls, primary prevention efforts such as routine vaccinations are critically important in assuring that a boy can grow up strong and healthy (Legato, 2006).

PHYSICAL HEALTH

Male Genitourinary Health Concerns

Most boys are born with normal, healthy genitalia, which include the penis, testes, and scrotum. From time to time, however, there may be an abnormality affecting a boy's testes. An undescended testicle (also referred to as *cryptorchidism*) occurs in approximately 2% to 5% of the population (up to 30% of premature births are affected) and may affect one or both testes (Mathers, Sperling, Rübben, & Roth, 2009). Cryptorchidism is the most common genital abnormality in boys. The condition is generally accounted for within the first year of life; however, some cases may go undetected until the toddler years. Developmentally, each testis migrates down the *inguinal canal* (which is also referred to as the *inguinal ligament*) in the groin during the first few months after birth. Boys who develop cryptorchidism experience a delay of this process, which may persist as they grow. The cause of this condition is not well known; however, research suggests that several factors, such as maternal health, environmental conditions such as pollutants, genetics, hormonal fluctuations, and nerve activity that affect the testes, may influence the development of cryptorchidism. Low birth weight, a family history of males with undescended testicles, **Down syndrome,** alcohol and cigarette use, and diabetes of the mother also have been suggested to affect this condition (Mayo Clinic, n.d.a).

Another common condition that develops as the boy ages is a "retractile testicle" and an "ascending testicle," which migrates back and forth from the scrotum and the inguinal canal. Symptoms are typically vague and may not present as an issue to the boy. For example, pain is not frequently associated with this condition, and it is mainly noticed by a parent or caretaker when changing a diaper or during bathing (Mayo Clinic, n.d.a).

Cryptorchidism generally is not a significant pathological condition; however, it does warrant consultation and attention of a physician to rule out any other abnormalities, such as inguinal hernias and a twisted testicle (testicular torsion). If the testicle does not eventually descend into its proper placement in the scrotum, it can enhance the likelihood for developing testicular cancer and may affect fertility in the future (Hadziselimovic, 2002; Mayo Clinic, n.d.a). The testes need specific temperatures to properly function when producing testosterone and sperm. If the testicle is undescended, it raises the temperature, which negatively affects its ability to function (Mathers et al., 2009).

If an undescended testicle is suspected, it is recommended that the boy be seen by a physician, who may attempt to manually guide the testis into its rightful position in the scrotum. In some cases, this is successful; however, the testis may retract or ascend again. If the problem persists, the physician may recommend seeing a pediatric urologist who can guide further testing. In some cases (roughly 20%), the testis is unpalpable; therefore imaging studies, such as ultrasonography and magnetic resonance imaging (MRI) may be indicated to confirm the location and position of the testis. If the testis is unable to be guided by the physician, a **laparoscopic** procedure or open surgical procedure may be warranted to physically move the testis into the scrotum. The use of **human chorionic gonadotropin (HCG)** is sometimes used to promote a natural migration of the testis. In rare cases, a testis may need to be removed in its entirety (called an *orchidectomy*) (Mathers et al., 2009; Mayo Clinic, n.d.a).

Once corrected, it is important to periodically check that each testicle is in its proper position. As the boy grows and develops, he should be informed that he should routinely check his testes for any abnormalities. All males need to be aware and taught to inspect their testes for signs of tumors or growths that may indicate testicular cancer.

Middle Ear Infections

Middle ear infections, also known as *otitis media,* are a fairly common physical disorder in younger children (Mills, Henley, Barnes, Carreiro, & Degenhardt, 2003). Middle ear infections are more common in boys than in girls (Slowik, 2009; Yano et al., 2009). Infections occur behind the eardrum (tympanic membrane) usually after a common cold and occur more

Figure 4.1   Schematic Diagram of the Inner and Outer Ear

©iStockphoto.com/Dorling_Kindersley

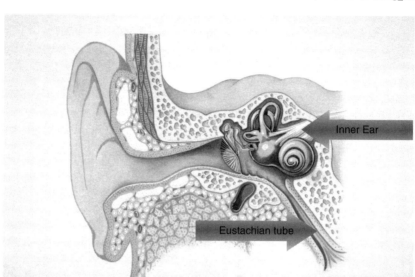

often in younger children ages two to six years, although infections can occur at any time. Inner ear infections are common in younger children due to many factors, including more exposure to new environments, developing immune systems, and shorter Eustachian tubes. Symptoms consistent with middle ear infections include pain, pressure, headaches, nausea, balance disturbances, possible fever, and several other **maladies.** A schematic diagram of the ear is presented in Figure 4.1.

One of the main reasons for these types of infections is that children have shorter Eustachian tubes, which help drain fluid from the middle ear to the throat. These tubes help equalize pressure in the middle ear as well as protect the middle ear from germs. Half of all children will likely have a middle ear infection before the age of three, and those who do are more likely to have future infections (AAP & American Academy of Family Physicians [AAFP], 2004; Mills et al., 2003). There are several theories concerning this phenomenon; however, one of the more plausible ones relates to boys having weaker immune systems and T-cell resistance capabilities than girls (Legato, 2006). Because boys may become sick more frequently than girls with common colds and infections, the incidence of middle ear infection becomes more likely. Bacteria and some viruses infiltrate the **upper respiratory tract** and throat, causing a primary infection. As the child begins to recover, he may start to complain of pressure and pain in his ear or head. The bacteria and/or virus have a shorter distance to travel in the Eustachian tubes to the throat of a child than to that of an older person, therefore infection is more likely (O'Brien et al., 2009). Although common, middle ear infections need to be appropriately addressed to prevent damage to the inner ear structures or worse, such as brain infections and deafness.

Generally, treatment is based on observed symptoms, age of the child, number of infections, relative health of the child, and clinical findings. Identifying the source of infection also can help guide treatment options. For example, inner ear infections caused by a bacterial source often are treated with antibiotics, whereas viral infections typically have to run their course within the body (AAP & AAFP, 2004). In more severe cases, the physician or pediatrician may recommend surgery to aid the Eustachian tubes in their draining of fluid and debris from the inner ear. Tubes are placed from the inner ear to the throat and allow for better drainage and also help keep pressure equalized, which helps to limit pain (Ruohola et al., 2006).

Indicators of potential ear infections in young children include family history of previous inner ear disturbances. Also, consider these facts:

- Babies who are breast fed for at least six months have a lower incidence of inner ear infections, most likely due to an augmented immune system.

- Children exposed to smoking (Hinton & Buckley, 1988; Slowik, 2009) are more likely to develop infections.

- Most children by age five or six outgrow chronic ear infections.

- Middle ear infections tend to occur more frequently in children who attend day care centers than those who do not.

- Infections are more likely to occur in the winter than other seasons.

• Middle ear infections tend to occur more frequently in specific ethnic groups, such as American Indians, Alaskan Natives, Canadian Eskimos, and Australian Aborigines (Slowik, 2009).

Hygiene

Little boys are made of "snips and snails and puppy dog tails," while little girls are made of "sugar and spice and everything nice," says the nursery rhyme from the eighteenth and nineteenth centuries (Opie & Opie, 1997). Are little boys dirtier than girls? One needs only to look at children at play to surmise that this assertion is false and is probably a stereotype of the time period in which the nursery rhyme was composed. In the pre-Victorian and **Victorian eras,** women were expected to adhere to a social code of ladies, while men were viewed more as a functional, utilitarian part of society. Men did the work (oftentimes labor intensive and dirty) while women were caretakers and protectors of social morality.

Learning good hygiene habits at a young age is crucial in promoting a lifetime of good health, regardless of the sex of the child. Personal hygiene needs to be modeled and enforced by parents and caregivers of young children. It is normal behavior for a boy to put up a fuss when bathing. Parents and caregivers can focus attention toward fun aspects of bathing and hygiene. Reward systems also work well. Age-appropriate discussions on germs and bacteria can help a young boy understand that keeping clean will help prevent him from getting sick. Helping a boy place value on his health at this early age will allow him to understand how staying up to date and in tune with his health throughout his lifetime will allow him to be a healthier man.

Oral Health

Another challenge in the toddler and young child years is oral health and hygiene. Several preventable health issues and diseases, such as dental caries (cavities) and head and neck infections, can be addressed by teaching a child good oral hygiene. The American Academy of Pediatrics recommends that all infants receive oral **health risk assessments (HRAs)** by six months of age, which should be continued with regular dental checkups, a balanced diet, **fluoride,** injury prevention, habit control, and brushing and flossing for healthy teeth. Teaching proper brushing technique and habits while explaining why it is important will help a boy understand that he needs to keep up with his oral health as he grows and develops.

Diet is very important throughout the life span, but specifically during this age. Calcium, vitamins, and fluoride all can help augment oral health. Additionally, children need to be taught how certain foods may affect their teeth and oral health (AAP, 2009a).

Baby teeth eventually fall out as the boy ages. Parents, caregivers, and health practitioners should explain the functional importance of teeth (chewing, smiling) and that not taking good care of them can lead to getting sick.

Other topics related to teeth and oral health include discoloration and accidental tooth loss. There are several causes of tooth discoloration, including poor hygiene and cleaning habits, exposure to certain vitamins (such as iron), and some germs, eating certain foods, early tooth decay, injury, and use of some medications, (such as antibiotics) (AAP, 2009a; Lochary, Lockhart, & Williams, 1998). The good news is most of these conditions are preventable and treatable. Oral injuries may result in trauma or loss of teeth. Boys are highly active and may sustain greater instances of injury and trauma at this age than other periods of life. Their normal and natural curiosity may predispose them to falls, bumps, scrapes, and bruises. If teeth are damaged or dislocated, it is important to discern whether the teeth were baby teeth or permanent. If it is a baby tooth, practitioners should assure that no other damage to the gums and root of the tooth socket has occurred. If it is a permanent tooth, action needs to be taken to help preserve the tooth for possible relocation or reconstruction. If a tooth is damaged, a dentist should attend to the tooth within 30 minutes of the injury (Trope, 2002). Other structures in addition to the tooth may be at risk for complications.

The practice of routine hand washing can have a significant, positive effect on a boy's health. Proper and frequent hand-washing practices can eliminate many of the **communicable diseases** in our daily lives, such as the common cold (rhinovirus), influenza virus, such as the H1N1 strain (swine flu), and gastrointestinal infections like those caused by *E. coli*. Research suggests that males are less likely than females to wash their hands after using the restroom. For example, hand-washing rates at the Minnesota State Fair were 64%, 65%, and 75% in three separate female restroom facilities; whereas rates in male restrooms were significantly lower, at 30%, 39%, and 51% respectively (Allwood, 2004). Even in professions like health care that routinely require good sanitary practices, it was found that male physicians washed their hands *less* frequently than female nurses (van de Mortel et al., 2001). One can promote this healthy practice to a boy at a young age by employing an age-appropriate strategy, for example, a game or competition for hand washing.

Potty Training

Potty training is another challenge for toddler boys. Are boys easier or more difficult than girls to train? In a general sense, girls pick up on the practice of using the toilet faster than do boys (Erwin, 2006; Schum, Kolb, McAuliffe, Simms, Underhill, & Lewis, 2002). Many boys will begin to adopt toilet habits around the age of three to four years; however, there is great variability during this age. Potty training depends on a boy's physical awareness of his body signals and his exercising of self-control. A child intuitively knows that potty training is an important milestone in his or her life, simply based on a parent's or caregiver's reaction (Erwin, 2006). The reaction may be one of joy and praise when it is going well or frustration and admonishment when it is not going as planned. Boys may resist potty training for several reasons beyond that of maturational development (Erwin, 2006; Schum et al., 2002). For example, some children may use their ability (or inability) to control a situation with a parent. If he senses that he can get a reaction out of a parent or caregiver, whether positive or negative, he may choose to comply with potty training or rebel. This obviously can and will lead to frustration on the parent's end.

Reasons for resistance to training include stress and lack of a parent, especially a father figure, in his life. Some younger boys also experience difficulty urinating when others are around. Typically referred to as "stage fright," a boy may become sensitive to this at an early age, which can affect him as he matures. Parents and caregivers are advised to question the boy about why he is reacting the way he does and model appropriate, healthy behaviors and habits. They can let him know what it feels like right before he has to urinate; read him a book, such as *Everyone Poops* (Stinchecum, 1993) that presents the issue; assure a diet rich in fluids and fiber to keep waste appropriately moving through his digestive system; and most important . . . be patient. Encouragement and dedication will help him be confident in his abilities to master potty training.

VIGNETTE

A young couple has decided the time is right to begin potty training their three-year-old son. It is a Saturday morning at home and Manny's mom notices that he keeps squeezing his groin area. She asks him if he needs to go to the bathroom, and he nods his head indicating yes. She escorts him into the bathroom and shakes a couple of Cheerios into the toilet to serve as targets for Manny as he tries to "be a big boy."

MOM: He won't go!

DAD: Well give him a couple of minutes!

MOM: A couple of minutes to pee? Wait, wait . . . there he goes. . . . *Ahhhhhhh* . . . all over the floor and toilet seat! So much for using the Cheerios as a target for him!

DAD: Well . . . what did you expect, potty training a boy is gonna have its challenges honey! With Liesl we just popped her on the toilet and said, "Go for it!"

MOM: So, why is it any different with Manny? Why can't he just sit down like Liesl? It would make our job much easier and cleaner!

DAD: Because he is not a girl, dear! Manny is not going to sit down when he goes pee! He is a boy, and that is what boys do!

MOM: Are we really going to continue arguing over this? [laughs]

DAD: Well, no, but what about using urinals when he gets a little older?

MOM: Good point, but for now he is gonna sit until my back recovers from cleaning this urine up from the toilet seat and floor. . . .

(Continued)

DAD: What? Why didn't you put the seat up?

MOM: Because you boys will never put it back down! [laughs] Actually, honey I recently heard of a study that talked about how some toddler boys are being injured when the heavy toilet seat falls and crushes their penis!

DAD: C'mon . . . really? Well, he can sit for now, but . . .

MOM: But . . . when you get down and clean the urine off of the floor all of the time, then he can stand as you wish!

DAD: Well, you can explain to him why all the other boys use the urinals at school when he starts. [laughs]

MOM: Not an issue with me! [laughs]

A related topic to potty training that often affects little boys is bedwetting, also known as *nocturnal enuresis* (Byrd, Weitzman, Lanphear, & Auinger, 1996). Bedwetting is normal at this age; the frequency with which it happens is the greater concerned. Most boys by about age five or six will develop control and will sense the impulse to use the bathroom when urinary urgency occurs (Erwin, 2006). Others may lag behind due to various reasons, including developmental disorders, stress, and physical problems.

Sleep

How much or little sleep is required is a common question concerning boys or girls, but boys seem to be more unpredictable than girls at this age. This may be due to the fact that more boys are affected by disorders, such as attention deficit hyperactivity disorder (ADHD), autism, and Asperger's syndrome than are girls. Hormone levels also play a role in sleep patterns; that is, little boys may be more hyper and harder to settle down than girls (Shang, Shur-Fen Gau, & Soong, 2006). Inconsistent sleep is frustrating for both the parent and child.

Dyssomnias affect the amount, type, and quality of sleep and include insomnia, sleep apnea, restless leg syndrome, narcolepsy, and periodic limb twitching. *Parasomnias* involve abnormal behaviors or physiological events during sleep such as sleep walking, night terrors, sleep talking, nightmares, grinding of the teeth (*bruxism*), and bedwetting (Shang et al., 2006). All of these disturbances can affect sleep. Sleep walking in particular affects more boys than girls during this age and usually attenuates by preadolescence. The main culprit of sleep issues in children is typically poor or inconsistent behaviors, such as excessive daytime napping, going to bed too early, excessive stress and anxiety, food and beverages that contain sugar and caffeine, some medications, obesity or asthma, or environments that provoke arousal. A pediatrician can diagnose a more serious sleep disorder.

Safety Considerations

There is a considerable amount of research that suggests boys are active learners who value experiencing their worlds, which may place them at higher risk than girls for injuries. Additionally, how we treat boys compared to girls may affect the relative safety of children. Being male carries with it sociocultural expectations and norms that may affect the safety of a boy.

Among male toddlers and young children, falls, bumps, scrapes, and bruises will occur on a near-daily basis. It is important for parents and caregivers to protect young boys and also to be acutely aware not to shelter them in the process. Encouraging a boy's innate curiosity in a meaningful way will help him grow and further understand his world.

There are issues that may compromise a boy's safety aside from how we impart expectations and norms to him. One such instance is crush injuries to the penis by falling of toilet seats. Epidemiologic reports and trends suggest this is a point of concern for parents and caretakers (Bicha, Mamood, Sorur, Ananthakrishnan, & Irwin, 2008; Gazi, Ankem, Pantuck, Han, Firoozi, & Barone, 2001).

It is common for little boys to show their caregivers that they can be independent and use the potty on their own. In Great Britain in 2008, a toddler boy was using the toilet on his own; when he lifted the toilet seat to urinate, the seat fell back down, causing trauma to his penis. Luckily, there was little damage to the **urethra** and the condition resolved in a couple of weeks after swelling and pain subsided (Bicha et al., 2008).

There are several strategies that parents and caregivers can follow to reduce the risk of penile injuries in their toddlers. Heavier toilet seats, such as those made from wood or ornamental porcelain, are more likely than lighter ones to cause damage to young boys (Bicha et al., 2008). Installing lighter toilet seats and those that raise and fall in a controlled and slowed manner can be useful. Households with young boys may leave toilet seats up. Teaching young boys to hold the seat up with one hand while passing urine may decrease the incidence of injury (Gazi et al., 2001).

Curiosity

"In this age of video games and cell phones, there must still be a place for knots, tree houses, and stories of incredible courage." This quote, from the popular book *The Dangerous Book for Boys* (Iggulden & Iggulden, 2007, p. xi), exemplifies a boy's quest for exploration and knowledge. Children are naturally curious as they attempt to interact, experience, and make meaningful connections with their external worlds. Their worldviews are largely based on the quality and quantity of these experiences. As boys grow and have the ability to physically interact with their environment, the element of curiosity takes center stage.

Are boys more curious than girls? Many would agree with this assertion; however, it is likely a mute point. Rather, *how* boys express their curiosity is often more important. Boys, particularly in the toddler and early childhood years, are mainly kinesthetic learners; they learn through physical experiences with less emphasis on thought and reasoning. They touch things, engage in physical roughhousing, and sometimes let their natural curiosity get the best of them. Natural curiosity coupled with extreme energy levels imminently puts most male toddlers in harm's way. Keeping boys safe can be a challenge for any parent or caregiver. Should parents and caregivers childproof the entire house? Keep the boy on a short leash? Punish him for taking risks? The answer to each of these points is No.

Like any child, a boy needs to explore his world to learn about it and himself in the process. Most children up through the age of three or four years can understand boundaries. For example, a boy may try climbing on something and fall down several times before he realizes that he just might not be successful. Streets and other busy thoroughfares establish other environmental and physical boundaries. Children learn by exploring their boundaries and sometime pushing them.

Exploration involves a certain degree of risk and challenge. In addition to appropriate and reasonable boundaries, children need to learn discipline and experience love. Punishment is not the same as discipline. Discipline is a positive way of communicating. It establishes rules and guidelines. Discipline, love, and encouragement can help nurture and foster a boy's curiosity and give him reasonable limits and boundaries to keep him safe (Erwin, 2006). Striking a fine balance between curiosity and safety will help a boy learn what he needs to develop into a healthy young man.

SOCIAL HEALTH

Social development is essential for a well-rounded man. Those who grow up lacking social boundaries and skills often experience more difficult life situations and consequences than those who learn them. Research has consistently shown that boys who are well adjusted, feel value and social worth, are less likely to be involved in violent activities, less likely to use drugs and alcohol, and less likely to engage in promiscuous sexual activity (Ginsburg, 2007). However, in Western culture, even though most people would acknowledge that all people must value their emotional health to be well adjusted, emotional health carries with it feminine connotations. Emotional health in males goes well beyond the common **stereotypes** of men who are in touch with their emotions and cry at the drop of a dime. *Emotional health* refers to the stability and ability to process meaningful life experiences in a context that enhances one's overall health-related quality of life (Baraff, 1991; Kindlon & Thompson, 2000).

Boys often are delayed in their development of speech and other communication skills (Nelson, Nygren, Walker, & Panoscha, 2006). The operative term here is *communication*. Little boys may not possess the capacity to verbalize their needs at this age, but they certainly know how to communicate what they want. Contrary to popular belief that males are inherently stoic and less social than females, little boys are highly social creatures (Erwin, 2006). One needs only to look at preschool classrooms, gymnasiums, or recess to see how young boys socialize and interact. Even in the early years, boys are more likely to cry, be fussy, and harder to soothe than are girls (Erwin, 2006; Kindlon & Thompson, 2000). Understanding how a boy communicates will allow for growth and learning in his social arena.

When a boy lacks verbal communication skills, he is set to act out what he needs and what he wants. He possesses enough skills to get by, but he does not communicate as an adult, nor should he be expected to. Pulling a toy out of another child's hands, pushing another child down, temper tantrums, and other forms of acting out are simply ways for a boy to learn by experiencing his world and establishing boundaries. The parents' role is to help guide him through this learning experience. The quality and consistency of parents' and caregivers' interactions with a growing boy will help guide his success. Boys need good examples to develop socially in an appropriate manner. Stereotypical notions that boys are inherently aggressive, violent, and seek trouble must be eliminated. Replacing these stereotypes with a true understanding of what drives and motivates young boys is much more productive for both the boy and his caregivers. Last, social development occurs throughout the life span, but the foundation for positive developmental experiences begins as soon as a boy recognizes his position in the family and in the world.

Learning, Language, and Social Skills

Children begin learning as soon as development inside the womb occurs. They are incredible data-processing machines; they take in inordinate amounts of information, process it, and associate meaning with nearly everything they encounter. People in general learn in all types of ways, for example, some people are kinesthetic or hands on, while others may be more cognitive learners who learn best by reading and thinking about concepts (Cassidy, 2004). We are built and hard-wired to learn. There is no difference between males and females in the capacity and need to learn, grow, and establish meaning in our lives. Rather, how males and females seek experiences and what we do with them greatly differ. Unless a learning or emotional disability is present (refer to Chapter Three), such as autism, **dyslexia,** or Asperger's syndrome, most boys will learn at their own pace. Again, research has confirmed that little boys are typically delayed in the ability to develop verbal and fine motor skills compared to little girls (Bazelon, 2009). Therefore, boys find alternatives to communicate, often by exerting their physical presence. Because a boy's language abilities may be slower to develop, parents, caregivers, and health practitioners need to recognize this and attempt to understand why the boy acts the way he does. This is a great opportunity to help him learn to speak with meaning and develop his **emotional intelligence**. Affirming statements such as "You are acting sad" or "You are being very silly today" can help a boy connect his learning experiences and social interactions with his own emotions (Kindlon & Thompson, 2001).

Expressive Language Delays

Difficulty expressing one's thoughts through language, writing, or other forms of expressive language characterizes an expressive language delay (ELD). A form of learning disability, ELD has a higher prevalence in boys than girls. Different parts of the brain, such as the prefrontal cortex and frontal lobe, may not adequately distinguish between what is taken in and processed versus what is expressed (Nelson et al., 2006; Scarborough & Dobrich, 1990). For example, stuttering is a common ELD in boys, which can plague a boy as he grows into adulthood if it is not addressed earlier in life. The inability to express oneself often leads to frustration and shame, which may further perpetuate inappropriate behaviors and emotions. With an ELD, it is important for parents and other people involved in the child's life to understand that he likely understands and comprehends much of what is communicated to him; however, he may not be able to appropriately communicate back without assistance. Boys with ELDs should be tested for other disabilities and conditions, such as autism, Asperger's syndrome, and dyslexia (Silva, Williams, & McGee, 1987).

How is an ELD treated? Language therapy that focuses on vocabulary development, rehearsal, and practical use of language in context or social specific scenarios can greatly assist the boy in overcoming (or at least improving) his difficulties in communication (Law, Garrett, & Nye, 2003). As he grows and begins to attend school, he may need to work closely with learning support services to develop an individualized education plan or IEP.

Specific signs of an ELD include family history of ELDs or learning disabilities (LDs); parental substance use or abuse, exposure to environmental toxins, and poor or lack of prenatal care; brain injuries; and developmental delays in fine and gross motor skills (Law et al., 2003).

TEMPERAMENT, EMOTIONAL DEVELOPMENT, AND DISCIPLINE

Toddlers are an enigma to many parents and families. They can go from cherubic little angels to demons incarnate in a matter of seconds. The good news is that research knows why it generally happens; the bad news is that little can be done to prevent it from happening because it is part of normal toddler development. One of the strongest influences on behavior is **hormones** and their fluctuations (Biddulph, 2008). Just as adults experience hormonal fluctuations throughout the day, so do children. For example, testosterone in a toddler or young boy may be highest in the morning and later afternoon; therefore, parents and caregivers may notice more combative or aggressive behavior during these times. Hunger and the influence of hormones such as insulin may spark crankiness. Another issue that affects a boy's temperament is emotional development and communication skills. He may become overly aggressive toward a playmate or sibling simply because he does not know of any other way to express himself. Acting out is a form of communication. Some toddlers even bite when they have exhausted ways to express themselves (Molland, n.d.). Self-restraint and appropriate behavior are definitely challenges for a young boy, but with practice, he will develop these skills.

Every boy is different, although society tends to lump boys into a social fishbowl, just as we do girls. Yes, boys show typical behavior that can be classified as commonly male (aggression, for example), but if we lose sight of the fact that boys are all individuals and should be treated as such, they are doomed to face stereotypes and social standards that they may not be adequately prepared to meet. Some toddler boys are rough and tough, some are sensitive and cry often, some are quiet and keep to themselves, and others cannot stop talking. The great variation in boy behavior presents unique challenges and opportunities for parents, caregivers, and health practitioners alike. Boys are highly emotional beings who react to all sorts of stimuli (Erwin, 2006; Bazelon, 2009). Mothers, fathers, siblings, and peers all exert a tremendous influence over a boy's behavior. If he sees warmth, love, and respect, he is likely to embrace those values as he gets older; conversely, if he witnesses isolation, disrespect, and violence, he is likely to react the same way in any given instance. Parenting styles vary, but one truth holds true: boys need love, discipline, warmth, embrace, restraint, values, morals, and many other life skills from parents and other family members. Embracing a boy's uniqueness and harnessing his energy will allow for better adjustment than simply adopting a "boys will be boys" attitude.

Unusual Behaviors

You have noticed that a boy does not seem like himself; or maybe you notice bizarre behaviors and outbursts. Is this normal, or should you be concerned? The question is, what may be driving these emotions and behaviors? Sexual abuse in boys is more common than most people like to think. Boys are as vulnerable if not more so than girls to sexual abuse, mainly because of how society views boys (Holmes & Slap, 1998). Boys are expected to be stoic, strong, and protectors (stereotypically of girls and women); therefore, sexual abuse of young boys may go under the radar. Acting out of character may simply be chalked up to a boy being a boy. Being unable to adequately and appropriately express himself may lead to further shame and isolation.

Myth: Boys are not likely to be victims of sexual abuse.

Fact: While it is true that many victims of sexual abuse are female, estimates of 1 in 6 (17%) of males have reportedly been sexually abused as children. In fact, these numbers are likely grossly *underestimated* due to sociocultural stereotypes and stigma that make the reporting of crimes like this less likely (Holmes & Slap, 1998).

It is important when helping flesh out what is troubling a boy to help him to communicate and develop his emotional vocabulary and intelligence.

Using "I feel" statements are better than a direct line of questioning (Erwin, 2006). If a boy is comfortable and feels less threatened when expressing himself, he is more likely to expose his feelings and troubles. Some behavior, such as emotional withdrawal, moodiness, and possibly an overactive imagination, is simply odd behavior. Maybe he is stressed about something occurring in the household, such as arguments, loss of a pet, moving to a new home, or divorce. Boys are highly sensitive to change and may take longer to adapt and adjust to new experiences than girls. Learning about the driving forces behind a boy's behavior will go a long way in helping him stay physically and emotionally healthy.

SUMMARY

This chapter discussed some of the common health issues pertaining to growth and development, physical and emotional development, hygiene, primary prevention initiatives, safety, social health, learning and language development, temperament and discipline, and abnormal behaviors of male toddlers and young boys. Boys of this age need to be raised with love, direction, and discipline; all of which they crave as they explore their worlds. The most well-adjusted boys and eventually men are ones who can make sense of their world through the love and value experienced as a young child.

KEY TERMS

Communicable diseases

Down syndrome

Dyslexia

Emotional intelligence

Enamel

Fluoride

Human chorionic gonadotropin (HCG)

Health risk assessment (HRA)

Hormones

Immunizations

Laparoscopic

Maladies

Potty training

Self-reliance

Stereotypes

Tantrums

Upper respiratory tract

Urethra

Vaccinations

Victorian Era

DISCUSSION QUESTIONS

1. Nature or nurture? Take a side on whether boys are innately attracted to risk taking or if it is formed through sociocultural nurturing by parents and other role models. Choose a side even though there most likely is middle ground concerning the topic.

2. Explain the differences in the types and number of immunizations and vaccinations that were offered in 1970 as compared to today. What has changed? Do you think children need all of these immunizations and vaccinations? What have you heard about some conditions being association with immunizing or vaccinating a child?

3. What is the greatest safety concern for male toddlers? Why do you think this? Justify your answers using injury data from national registries, such as those provided by the Centers for Disease Control and Prevention.

4. What types of learning strategies would be most beneficial to boys between three and five years old in settings such as preschool? Comment on current educational research pertaining to this topic.

5. List the five most common stereotypes about toddler boys. From where did these stereotypes originate? Advise on these stereotypes with accurate information that you find in your research.

6. A normally charismatic four-year-old boy suddenly becomes very quiet and withdrawn. When asked what is wrong, he declines to answer. Formulate a list of plausible explanations for his sudden change of character. What would you suggest to his parents and caregivers in the interim?

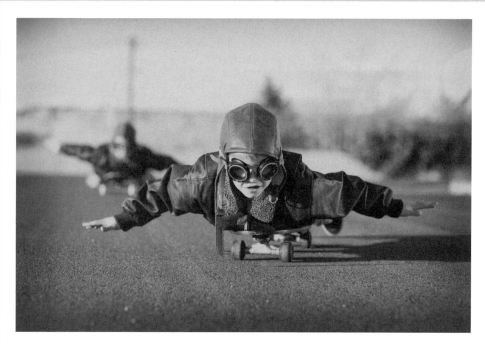

©iStockphoto.com/Andrew Rich

5

School Age

LEARNING OBJECTIVES

- Identify some of the more common physical and emotional health issues that present in boys between the ages of five and nine, including obesity, food allergies, and enuresis; understand the role nutrition plays in a boy's health

- Understand why boys sometimes have trouble in school and describe learning disabilities and developmental issues that often affect boys

- Describe the role and function that sports and competition play in the psychosocial development of boys

- Identify health disparities experienced by school-age boys

W HAT DOES THE phrase "school-age boy" mean? In this book, *school age* refers the age of five to nine years. This marks a milestone in a boy's development because of his growing independence and his interdependence with his family. There are several physical, emotional, and social challenges that a boy will encounter during this stage of life. This chapter covers common health and health-related issues based on epidemiological data and trends. Physical and emotional health, nutrition (including childhood obesity), social health, learning and education, and world health disparities are presented and discussed.

PHYSICAL HEALTH

During the ages of five to nine years, boys experience increases in height and body weight as part of their normal development, although at a slower rate than girls. Table 5.1 presents data on boys ages five to nine years who are in the 50% percentile for both height and weight (Centers for Disease Control and Prevention [CDC], 2000).

As shown in Table 5.1, in five years of life, a boy's height and weight increase by approximately 18% and 37%, respectively. This of course is highly variable and depends on the boy's nutritional and health practices. These types of charts are for relative comparisons and are not final verdicts on whether a boy is "normal" or not. Some boys are taller, shorter, or weigh

Table 5.1   Normal Growth and Development for Boys 5–9 Years

Note: Based on 50th percentiles.
Source: Centers for Disease Control and Prevention (2000).

Age (in years)	Height (in inches)	Weight (in pounds)
5	43	39
6	45	45
7	48	50
8	50	56
9	52	62

more or less. Body mass index (BMI) is important to consider as a boy grows. Simple biometric information (height in meters and weight in kilograms) can be used to note risk for underweight, overweight, and obesity. Although BMI is calculated similarly to adults, the relative comparisons are made to children in similar categories of height and weight.

Nutrition greatly affects height and obviously weight. Diets that are high in quality nutrients and meaningful calories allow a boy to optimally grow and develop. Conversely, diets that are laden with sugars, fats, and otherwise empty calories ultimately lead to poor health and possible **morbid obesity.**

Good health practices and routines remain important during this stage of life and development. Yearly physical examinations and biannual dental visits are strongly recommended. Immunizations and good hygiene practices are good primary prevention measures against disease and illness. A family doctor or **pediatrician** can provide immunization schedules; they are also available on the CDC website (www.cdc.gov/vaccines/). At this age a boy will likely be screened for a variety of physical issues in school or prior to beginning school. Visual exams, hearing tests, dental checks, and postural exams are common in school settings. These are simple screenings aimed at identifying a condition or potential condition and preventing it from getting worse. Prevention is key.

Some physical issues and disabilities are connected with emotional and learning disabilities. Many adult men ignore health issues simply because they were never taught how to express concern, address concerns, or shed the stereotype of invulnerability (Addis & Mahalik, 2003; Baraff, 1991). It may seem rudimentary, but boys need to learn how to take charge of their own health.

Bedwetting

Many boys (and parents) struggle with the issue of bedwetting, also known as **enuresis,** well past the potty training stage (Robson, 2009). Accidents can be traumatic and embarrassing for both the child and the parent. For example, a young boy may decline attending a friend's sleepover party because he fears an accident, thus limiting his social health and overall confidence. Why do boys sometimes struggle with bedwetting? There are several theories, including sleep issues, stress, hormonal imbalances, smaller bladder, slower development of the central nervous system, family genetics, abnormalities in the urinary system, and infections or disease (Family Doctor, 2009; Robson, 2009).

Some children, particularly boys, are referred to as "deep sleepers." They seem to sleep through anything and often are difficult to wake up. Being such a deep sleeper sometimes causes the inability to discern visceral responses, such as nerves that cause the bladder to contract when urination is needed (Family Doctor, 2009). Stress also has been implicated in bedwetting. Stress comes in many forms (Family Doctor, 2009; Robson, 2009). A boy may be stressed about schoolwork or relationship problems at home, or maybe he is being bullied at school.

Family stressors, such as divorce or a loss in the family, can affect a boy. Some theorists suggest that, in particular, stress between a father (or lack of) and a boy may cause bedwetting (Family Doctor, 2009). Next, hormonal imbalances, as with vasopressin, which regulates how much fluid is shunted from the kidneys to the bladder, may cause too much fluid to be retained in the bladder. Developmentally, some boys may have smaller or less well-developed bladders than other children. Some boys have slower developing nervous systems, which may or may not be pathological in nature. Over-excited nerves or sometimes under-excited nerves may cause mixed signals to the bladder, causing involuntary urination (Robson, 2009). Family genetics have been suggested as a cause of bedwetting (Family Doctor, 2009; Robson, 2009). If siblings or parents have experienced issues and challenges with bedwetting, the likelihood increases for other children and family members. In some boys, abnormalities in the urinary system go unrecognized until bedwetting becomes a recurrent, severe problem for him and his family. Last, infection and disease may be the cause of bedwetting episodes. In particular, urinary tract infections (UTIs), often caused by bacterial agents in the tract, may cause pain and nerves to misfire, causing involuntary urination (Family Doctor, 2009; Robson, 2009). Though less common in boys than girls, UTIs should be suspected and ruled out if chronic bedwetting persists.

Boys who experience enuresis are not lazy, and it is not that they do not want to get out of bed. Connection and reassurance are perhaps the most effective means to help a boy through this issue. Parents should not limit fluid intake but try to understand his normal behaviors and patterns (Family Doctor, 2009).

What can be done to address the issue and at the same time protect the emotional status of the boy? Depending on the cause of the bedwetting, behavioral treatments and/or medicine may be warranted if he does not seem to gain control of his urinary mishaps. Such methods may include limiting fluids immediately before bedtime; establishing a routine of urinating right before bed; investing in an alarm system that rings when the bed becomes wet during the night, which will help him recognize when wetting occurs; praise and reward systems when dry nights happen; involving the child in changing the bed and laundering when an accident occurs; and practicing bladder training (a form of **biofeedback**) so he knows what a full and not so full bladder feels like while he is awake and alert. If behavioral methods do not seem to work, medications can limit urine production. Most doctors only prescribe medications to children over age seven, and there may be side effects such as thirst, dry mouth, and thermoregulatory problems. If there is an infection causing issues, a simple round of antibiotics may do the trick (Family Doctor, 2009).

Eczema and Skin Rashes

Some boys may be sensitive to environmental agents or may have autoimmune dysfunction that causes conditions such as **eczema.** There are no definitive statistics that suggest boys have a more difficult time with eczema and skin rashes than girls.

What is eczema? The epidermis (outer layer of the skin) can become inflamed and irritated for a number of reasons, such as pollutants, environmental irritants like pollen or mold, and dryness of the air. The irritants cause a chronic reaction of the skin, which forms itchy, scaly rashes and patches, which may form cracks, blisters, oozing, and bleeding. The term *eczema* has been broadly applied to a multitude of skin disorders, and the exact causes are currently unknown, although many models and theories exist. When the irritants cause itching, the child may scratch the skin, causing more irritation and itching. This cycle continues until it is broken via removing the irritant or the introduction of medications into the system (Odhiambo, Williams, Clayton, Robertson, & Asher, 2009). Some people have autoimmune disorders that provoke the inflammation as well, which can be brought on by certain foods.

What can parents, caregivers, and health practitioners do to address eczema in boys? Because no one specific cause has been attributed to eczema or random skin rashes, investigations into the child's environmental exposures and dietary habits are warranted. Environmental irritants and pollutants are common and difficult to avoid. Some children may react to shampoos, body washes and soap, fragrances, and even laundry detergent. Often, allergies and skin problems may not become apparent until the child enters school (Odhiambo et al., 2009). School introduces a completely new environment. Moreover, school lunches and other types of foods, such as wheat, milk, or nuts, can cause internal, systemic reactions as well. A dermatologist or other specialist can prescribe treatments, including dietary modifications and medications such corticosteroid creams, to alleviate most symptoms and address the chronic cycle of eczema.

NUTRITION

Nutrition is of great concern and rightfully so since it sets a benchmark in a boy's dietary habits that will likely stay with him throughout his lifetime. Good eating habits are becoming more of the exception than the rule in today's world. Rates of childhood obesity are skyrocketing and have topped the agenda in public health for a number of years (Wang & Lobstein, 2006). Recent reports from the CDC suggest that unless aggressive control measures are adopted soon, 1 in 5 school-age children will likely succumb to morbid obesity. The United States has adopted a new term to describe this phenomenon: *obesogenic* (Doak, Heitmann, Summerbell, & Lissner, 2009). A recent study out of Sweden (Doak et al., 2009) demonstrated that males who meet obesity criteria by age twenty have roughly a double mortality rate than men who are normal weight. These data show that for every 1 point increase in BMI, a 10% increase in the likelihood of death occurs. Data also shed light on disparities in obesity rates in low- and lower-income children, who have a 14% higher rate of being morbidly obese than children at baseline values (Doak et al., 2009). A decline in vigorous physical activity, such as playing active games and simple free play with other children, also contributes to the increase in boys' waistlines as they grow. Increasing obesity also has caught the attention of the U.S. military. Many males who are of the age to serve in the military would not meet the physical criteria to do so. This latter point designates obesity as even a threat to our national security in the United States.

A paradoxical world seems to exist in which boys are full of energy and are active learners yet also seem to be at-risk eaters. How is this so and what can be done about it? Modern conveniences, such as transportation options, video games, fast food, and media, as well as legislation on physical activity all have converged to affect children in general. Children have more choices because parents have more choices to offer them. We may think we are doing a child a service by offering him many options and choices; however, research strongly suggests that children look for, need, and even desire structure and minimal options (Erwin, 2006; Kindlon & Thompson, 2000). When people, especially children, are overwhelmed, they usually will default to the easiest option, which may not always be the healthiest.

Boys may be picky eaters who seem to eat everything in sight one moment and barely touch a crumb the next. One of the "vegetables" children most widely consume is French fries (Lorson, Melgar-Quinonez, & Taylor, 2009). Maybe a boy only eats macaroni and cheese for a month straight or refuses anything that is green or ends in *-occoli*. Most child experts, dieticians, and nutritionists alike agree that unusual food choices in younger boys is perfectly normal (Erwin, 2006). As long as the boy gets food and drink into his system and there do not appear to be any other signs of difficulties, such as digestive disturbances or **allergies,** he will be fine. Food and choice play both a role in nourishing his body as well as providing him with a **visceral** experience.

Aside from offering specific choices and patterns of eating for a boy, parents' and caregivers' modeling of good eating behaviors is paramount in setting a lifetime of good eating practices and habits. Most boys will defer to fathers or other male role models (Jack, 2005). A man who eats fast food, stacks his plate with meat and heavy starches, drinks soda and alcohol, and has barely anything of green color on his plate is clearly communicating a message to a young boy. Adult males have to be acutely aware of how they represent and teach things to boys. Passive teaching occurs when one least expects it. Children *are* listening and they *do* notice everything.

Boys often defer to their male role models in food choice and eating behavior

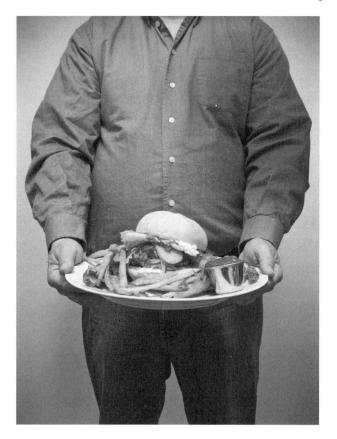

Another common topic of concern is food allergies. Allergies, particularly to food products, can range in severity from mild irritation to potentially severe health consequences, such as rashes and asthma and even death. Data suggest that food allergies are on the rise in all children, with a reported increase in emergency department visits from 116,000 to nearly 317,000 in years 2003 to 2006 (American Academy of Pediatrics [AAP], 2009; Branum & Lukacs, 2009). In particular, peanut allergies are one of the most common problems in younger children. Researchers also found that in 2005–2006, 9% of U.S. children one to seventeen years of age had positive serum immunoglobulin E antibodies to peanuts (AAP, 2009). With more public awareness concerning allergies and children, parents have become more vigilant in reporting and seeking care for their kids.

Black younger males appear to be at the highest risk for allergies, which often go unrecognized or under-diagnosed. The latter may be caused by several factors, including disparity in quality health care in various U.S. populations as well as environmental determinants (Braithwaite et al., 2009). For minority families who suffer from disparities in access to quality health care, allergies may go untreated or mismanaged. Black boys in particular are affected by **lactose** intolerance, which is sensitivity to milk and milk products, and also eggs, shellfish, and peanuts (Branum & Lukacs, 2009). Health risks associated with food allergies need to be recognized and addressed at an early age so that a boy can optimally grow and adjust his dietary habits to his needs.

While constipation is prevalent in both boys and girls at younger ages, boys tend to experience more extended difficulties with the issue than girls (Biggs & Dery, 2006). Constipation may occur for many reasons, some physical and some emotional. Constipation involves the difficulty in evacuating stool (feces) from the body. This may involve pain, cramping, gas, bloating, and loose stool accidents, among other complications. Emotionally, some children voluntarily withhold their stools and defecation because doing so gives them a sense of control. This is not uncommon when boys are potty training and want to exert control against their parents' wishes (Erwin, 2006). School-age boys are not likely to withhold stool for defiance but to avoid accidents and resultant shame. A condition called **encopresis** may result as a complication of chronic constipation and is more common in boys than girls. Voluntary control of their bowels may be less developed than girls; therefore, accidents are more likely in a younger boy, causing shame and embarrassment (Hardy, 2009). A cycle may develop in that a boy may be constipated, which causes discomfort and pain; defecation may cause an increase in pain as he attempts to evacuate his bowels, so he may withhold his bowels, leading to longer constipation. Conversely, if the boy loses bowel control, he may force himself to control his bowels to avoid another mishap, which may prompt constipation as well. The result can be pain, discomfort, irritability, and in more progressed cases, impacted bowel and bowel distention, which may require medications or even surgery (Hardy, 2009).

What can be done to prevent and treat this? A solid diet that involves natural dietary **fiber** and positive fluid balance is optimal. Plenty of water, fruits, and vegetables should allow for enough fiber to do the trick. Some foods, such as milk (including soy), cheese, yogurt, cooked carrots, and bananas, may be binding up his system. Limiting the consumption of these foods can alleviate bouts of constipation (Biggs & Dery, 2006). Physical activity can prevent and alleviate symptoms as well. In more progressive instances, stool softeners may be warranted to avoid complications.

EMOTIONAL HEALTH

Most parents, caregivers, and health professionals agree that there is quite a difference between a five-year-old boy and a nine-year-old. Parallel to his physical growth and development, a boy encounters tremendous emotional growth and development during this period. His young brain is continually developing new **schemas, cognitions,** and **emotions** via a multitude of life experiences (Kindlon & Thompson, 2000). He is able to reason more and distinguish between right and wrong, morals, and values. As he enters school, he establishes peer and social groups that challenge his way of thinking. He may become more resistant or defiant (Erwin, 2006). Most researchers agree that this is a normal part of emotional development.

Emotions are often viewed as superfluous by males. Don't they just get in the way of rational decision making and logic? Research suggests the opposite may hold true. People use and need emotions to help connect the decisions they make in their efforts to remain safe and secure. Emotions typically provoke action; therefore it is critical that people understand what their emotions mean and how they can maximize their use (Bayram, Fahridin,

& Britt, 2009; Kindlon & Thompson, 2000). For example, if a boy is experiencing the emotion of anger, he needs to figure out why he is experiencing it versus simply reacting to it, which may involve harmful, risky behavior. Famed psychologist Erik Erikson described eight stages of emotional development in humans. Among boys of school age, most are well into stage 2, learning autonomy and establishing their own will; stage 3, learning initiative and purpose, such as with play, roles, and fantasy; and stage 4, development of competence, which involves mastering various educational and social skills (Erikson, 1959). If emotions are inherent to all human experiences, why then do many men shirk them, consider them to be a female attribute, and ignore them altogether?

A male who embraces emotions or is classified as "emotional" often has been considered to be less of a man (Baraff, 1991; Bayram et al., 2009; Becker, Kendrick, Neuberg, Blackwell, & Smith, 2007). Those who experience or let their emotions "get the better of them" traditionally have been viewed as weak or incompetent. Science tells us that emotions are experienced by most people and serve to integrate our experiences so that physiological senses work together and help establish meaning in our worlds (Erwin, 2006). Failure to adequately experience emotions leads to less meaningful experiences in life and more emotional dissonance. Emotions *do* count (perhaps more heavily) for boys because of boys' propensity to repress them or inappropriately express them.

Dr. Adam Cox, in his book *Boys of Few Words* (2006), presents various physical and developmental reasons why boys may not master expression and other forms of communication. He discusses emotional and social reasons that boys often choose other ways in which to express themselves, such as physicality or even aggression. The emotional vulnerability of boys is explored as a precipitating factor to why many boys are emotionally "silent."

Dan Kindlon and Michael Thompson, in their book *Raising Cain* (2000), present some general strategies for helping school-age boys learn to deal with their emotions in healthy ways. For example, a boy can recognize that he has an internal life and can experience the full range of human emotions. There are no female or male emotions, simply emotions. Teaching a boy to use self-affirming "I" statements can help a boy develop his emotional vocabulary and emotional intelligence. Additionally, Kindlon and Thompson recommend acknowledging boys' high level of activity and energy and helping them to use words, feelings, and emotions to complement their behaviors.

SCHOOL AND LEARNING AND SOCIAL HEALTH

Upon entering school, some boys who enjoyed reading as toddlers and young children become less inclined to voluntarily read or may complain about reading assignments. They consider reading "boring" and "stupid."

Do boys simply lack interest in reading? Are they more inclined to be physical and learn actively? Do books and reading have a role in the learning and development of boys? Most parents and educators agree that reading is essential to the learning and development process. What is the issue with school-age boys and reading?

When a boy is, say, age four, parents usually are thrilled to introduce him to books of varying themes, such as animals, trucks, adventures, science, and color. They read to him and then read with him as he becomes able to command language, vocabulary, and expression. Then the boy enters kindergarten, and his interest in reading may begin to wane. The end result may be a man who is disenfranchised from reading altogether.

Boys' interests may be stifled by reading and literature that are chosen for them from a prescribed list. They cannot connect with the material, and their interest in the process is limited. Some boys view the activity of reading as something that girls do or that it is "feminine." The latter point creates a slippery slope of academic disinterest that may lead to subsequent failures and dropout rates.

According to an article by Tom Chiarella (2006), boys are more likely to drop out of school. Thirty-seven percent of twelfth-grade boys score lower on basic writing skills tests and score lower on basic reading tests; 35% of boys are more likely to be held back in grades; 16% of school-age boys have been diagnosed with attention deficit hyperactivity disorder or learning disabilities, twice the rate of girls; and other issues manifest because of social and educational factors (Chiarella, 2006). Are boys inherently slower and less capable than girls? Likely, the answer is a resounding No. Boys do learn differently than girls; therefore a change in the environment and approach we take with boys' education needs be instituted (Bazelon, 2009). Are schools set up to encourage boys to learn or do they counter most boys' interests and learning abilities? According to an article by Jill Parkin (2007), schools tend to cater to the learning needs and styles of girls, often at the expense of 50% of the other part of the classroom. **Learning styles** and preferences in educational engagement are crucial for optimal learning environments. Are school curricula and discipline policies geared in favor of girls? Are boys outcasts in one of the most important experiences of their lifetimes?

Myth: There are few differences in how boys and girls learn.

Fact: Research shows that not only do boys learn differently and at a slower pace (early on) than girls, but the environment matters as well. For example, boys learn better in cooler classrooms as compared to girls in warmer ones (Bazelon, 2009).

Men are certainly as capable as women of teaching young children, yet few preschool and primary school teachers are men. Teaching youngsters has traditionally been the role and responsibility of women, while men function more as advanced educators and disciplinarians. The reason for this phenomenon may lie, at least partially, in how society perceives men and what they do as professions. Men who teach children at younger ages may be viewed as odd or even feminine. These stereotypes and social stigma may keep capable and interested men out of teaching younger children.

Men also teach differently than women (Parkin, 2007). Children need the teaching and learning styles of *both* men and women to fully appreciate what education has to offer. All educators can help boys learn best through a variety of methodological strategies for engagement. Curricula that encourage restraint, discipline, and fondness of reading and literature may well suit girls but may exclude boys from learning (Parkin, 2007).

As Robert Baden-Powell, founder of the Scout Movement, once said, "The spirit is there in every boy; it has to be discovered and brought to light." Primarily, fathers can read and show that they like to read to their sons at an early age (Chiarella, 2006). How men embrace reading, learning, and education goes a long way in positively influencing future generations of boys. Curricula should be analyzed and restructured if necessary if it caters only to girls or even to the teacher's style of teaching. Methods need to be as varied as the learners who receive the education and material. Teachers need to closely gauge what interests all students in their classrooms and adjust if learning is not happening.

Boys and their motivation for learning need to be better understood. Selwyn Duke, in his article titled "Banning Boyhood," argues that being a boy and learning the world as a boy has been pathologized by many schools and educators (Duke, 2007). Boys tend to learn more through experiential learning and active learning than structured educational environments (Fillion, 2008). The current climate of schools, according to Duke, perpetuates the notion that schools need to function to "civilize" children, particularly boys. This paradigm inherently sets up boys to grow disenfranchised with school and learning and may cause them to rebel and even drop out later in life (Duke, 2007). Some boys just "get through" day after day of school. If a boy consistently gets in trouble because he appears to not want to learn, he may see school as a place where he consistently fails.

> "For example, a disruptive boy in my son's primary class was impossible to deal with until the day his exasperated male teacher challenged him to an arm-wrestling match (yes, it's probably a sackable offence). The boy lost, took it with good grace and became considerably better behaved. There was a male code at work that he recognised. The same teacher also knew when playground fights were serious and when they should just be allowed to run their course. The women teachers, wanting a tidy playground, always stopped them. Such macho attention-grabbing needs to be harnessed, not ignored. Boys need sports, they need exams, competition and recognition. You only have to look at how boys spend their spare time. They shout themselves hoarse at football matches; they knock hell out of each other in the virtual world of the computer. In short, they

compete. Mine does, anyway, even though he devours books, too. It ought to go without saying that boys and girls are different. But today's schools are denying this basic biology. In fact, any society needs both sexes to succeed and to be inspired by their education. Right now, though, the lads are chucking their kit on the floor and asking: 'What's the point?' And, frankly, I don't blame them." (Parkin, 2007)

Other initiatives have been enacted to help bridge the gap between boys and learning. The problem may not be boys at all, but men. Men need to be involved in all aspects of a boy's life. (Chiarella, 2006). Jon Scieszka, a former elementary school teacher and children's book author, developed the Guys Read Project (www.guysread.com), which offers ways to engage boys in reading and learning, as well as lists of books and reading suggestions from other boys. It is not as critical *what* boys are reading as *that* they are reading. Another initiative, called the Boys Project, fosters interest in developing boys' academic skills and learning ambitions through state- and government-funded sources. The Healthy Boys Project and Citizen Schools are efforts to engage more boys in their learning and educational experiences. The Healthy Boys Project (www.edequity.org) studies gender expectations and raises awareness among educators and parents as to how they may be inadvertently limiting boys. The notion of Citizen Schools (www.citizenschools.org) engages students through experiential learning such as apprenticeships and volunteer learning opportunities. These schools are not exclusively male; rather they aim to teach in ways that support the way experiential learners learn (Chiarella, 2006).

There is certainly much work to be done to engage boys in their own educational and learning processes. Simple steps, such as reading and modeling good behaviors and enthusiasm, can be taken on the part of parents, especially fathers, to instill lifelong learning habits in their sons. Other efforts are more difficult and will take time, effort, and advocacy to change for the better. For example, school curricula, reading lists, and discipline statutes that often limit or curtail normal boy behavior in the classroom can be revised. Better educational outcomes have been linked to better overall children's social and physical health in the future, such as with better jobs, more stable families, and lower risk behaviors. Boys will learn and learn to love learning once they feel engaged, vested, and respected in the process.

Other Issues in Learning

Aside from engagement in learning, some boys struggle because there may be underlying pathologies or disorders that preclude them from normal inquiry and emotional development. The major issues that may affect learning and are commonly noted during the early school years are attention deficit disorder with or without hyperactivity (ADD or ADHD), autism, Asperger's syndrome, Tourette's syndrome, and tic disorders. A boy's developmental issues may necessitate a later entrance to school.

Attention Deficit Disorder   What comes to mind when someone mentions ADD or ADHD? There are many forms of ADD, which may or may not include impulsivity and hyperactivity. What is ADD, and how do you know if a boy has it or not?

ADD is reportedly diagnosed nine times more often in boys than in girls, and it may be diagnosed at any point during a person's lifetime. The main signs and symptoms are inattention, inability to focus on tasks, becoming easily distracted, and exhibiting compulsive activity. There are several theories as to what causes ADD, ranging from environmental stimuli to genetic problems (Wodka et al., 2008). Many researchers agree that people with ADD and ADHD often have seemingly limitless talent but manifest it in inappropriate situations. Scientists also argue that it is not an overactive brain that causes ADD, but the exact opposite. People with ADD strive to create activity in their brains and resultant experiences because their brains do not do it at acceptable levels (Barkley, 1997). It seems counterintuitive to think a person with ADD and ADHD is bored and understimulated, but magnetic resonance imaging (MRI) and CAT (computerized axial tomography) and PET (positron emission tomography) scan imaging routinely have shown that the brains of people with suspected ADD and ADHD have consistently lower levels of brain activity in specific regions (Wodka et al., 2008). Medications such as Ritalin are prescribed to stimulate the brain, which will in turn settle down behaviors.

Why are boys diagnosed with this condition nine times more than girls? The answer may rest in two areas: better awareness and screening practices and normal young boy behavior. Unlike other diseases and disorders, ADD is mainly diagnosed through observations and interviews by trained clinical professionals (Erwin, 2006; Wodka et al., 2008). A primary factor in diagnosing ADD is that the behaviors cause problems and are disruptive in nature. If a boy is rambunctious, inattentive, disruptive, bored, or exhibits any other classically inappropriate behaviors, the health professional needs to analyze these behaviors in the context of the boy's environment (Wodka et al., 2008; Fillion, 2008). Would a boy's behavior qualify as ADD if he were playing in preschool? In a play area of the mall? With his group of friends? There are no blood tests (yet) or biological samples that can confirm a diagnosis. This sets up the paradigm of possibly pathologizing normal young male behavior.

School and structured classrooms increase the likelihood of a child being diagnosed with ADD. Better understanding and screening for this disorder has helped many children adjust and lead more productive and healthy lives. Parents and teachers need to closely monitor a boy's behavior and from where it may stem.

Medication can be helpful in calming a boy's behavior, but there also are side effects such as flat affect and excessive **lethargy** and fatigue (Barkley, 1997). Many parents claim ADD medications make their children "zombies" and rob them of their attitude and excitement. Former Boston University student, now entrepreneur, Peter Shankman credits his ADD for inspiring him to have the ability to multitask, create, and support his booming networking technology business (Walsh, 2009). Parents need to be aware of their boy's needs and motivations. Knowing how boys act and respond in various situations can help parents make better decisions and recommendations. Sometimes doctors are even too quick to diagnose ADD in boys.

Autism and Asperger's Syndrome Autism is a developmental brain disorder characterized by social and emotional difficulties in expression and interaction. Asperger's syndrome is similar to autism but involves a less well-defined spectrum of signs and symptoms. Autism usually is noticed and diagnosed by the age of three, whereas an Asperger's diagnosis may be delayed because of the less defined symptoms. What is known is that autism is fairly common, affecting approximately 1 in 163 children and formally diagnosed four times more often in boys than in girls. Genetic and brain differences have been postulated as to why this disparity exists, but future brain research imaging is still forthcoming (Farzin et al., 2006). Recent studies have reported that autism and other **spectrum disorders** (including Asperger's syndrome), may be as high as 1 in 100 children (Johnson, 2009). Similar to ADD, these rates may be affected by better and more sensitive screening options as well as broader definitions of the disorder.

Some school systems have attempted to integrate children with autism spectrum disorders (ASDs) into classrooms with non–ASD children. This has been met with some success, but also with some failure. In 2007, a boy diagnosed with Asperger's syndrome stabbed another boy to death in a suburban town in Massachusetts (Grigsby-Bates, 2007). While this is more the exception than the rule, integration of students with ASDs is routinely called into question in education circles. Many children with ADSs can do quite well, but there always will be challenges. For parents of boys with an ASD, there are support groups and numerous websites, such as that of the Autism Society of America (www.autism-society.org/), that are dedicated to providing the best-quality information.

Tic Disorders and Tourette's Syndrome   Tic disorders are fairly common in children, with 4%–24% of school children affected. These disorders also are three to four times more common in boys than girls (Kurlan et al., 2002). More than 75% of tic disorders begin and become apparent by age eleven.

Tic disorders are characterized by consistent, persistent, involuntary muscular movement, gestures, or sounds. Some are very noticeable, whereas others are subtle. Research suggests that neural connections in the brain are mainly responsible for the tics and that as a child develops, more connections form and misfirings gradually resolve (Kurlan et al., 2002). Most children below the age of ten cannot control the tics, but as they age, they typically can better manage their actions.

Emotional and environmental stresses also are believed to play a role in the development of tics among children. Neurochemical causes also have been postulated to cause dysfunction, as well as brain changes and family (genetic) factors. In fact, in more than 75% of cases there appears to be a genetic basis (Kurlan et al., 2002).

A more severe tic disorder is Tourette's syndrome. To be diagnosed with Tourette's a person must have experienced both multiple motor and one or more vocal tics at some time during the disorder, although they do not have to occur at the same time. Children and adolescents with Tourette's syndrome frequently experience additional problems, including aggressiveness, self-harming behaviors, emotional immaturity, social withdrawal, physical complaints, conduct disorders, affective disorders, anxiety, panic attacks, stuttering, sleep disorders, migraine headaches, and inappropriate sexual behaviors. It has been reported that 50%–80% of children with Tourette's also have ADD or ADHD. Treatments range from minimal to medication and brain surgery (Robertson, 2000). Behavioral and cognitive therapies are effective when used consistently. In some cases, medications such as Haldol, Orap, and Risperdal may be used to control the tics and involuntary movements (Kurlan et al., 2002; Robertson, 2000).

A holistic approach is generally best for the child. When appropriately controlled, boys with tic disorders (even Tourette's) can effectively manage their behaviors or even outgrow their tics and lead healthy, productive lives (Kurlan et al., 2002). Education for parents and caregivers of children with these types of disorders will help them remain patient and effectively manage them.

Additionally, closely working with school personnel can construct a learning environment that is most conducive for the child with a disorder. Children with tic disorders or more severe forms, such as Tourette's, may experience ridicule, hazing, and other forms of bullying and teasing from their peers. Counselors and teachers can minimize problems these children may face by educating students about such disorders. This often takes the fear of the unknown out of the scenario and other students may be less likely to make light of the child with a disorder.

Developmental Concerns

The practice known as "redshirting"—delaying children from beginning school because of developmental issues—has become common. There are no formal statistics validating that children who are held back do better later in school and in life in general. The trend may even seem unfair to parents and children who begin school on time. Children do not learn and develop in predictable, linear patterns; therefore, some children may respond to being held back, whereas others may be better served by starting school on schedule. Leading educators, such as Dr. Ada Beth Cutler, dean of the College of Education and Human Services at Montclair State University, have weighed in on the topic. Cutler said, "I worry about parents making that decision not because the child is not ready, but to give the child a leg up" (Nussbaum, 2003). Additionally, age may simply not be the best indicator for readiness for school; it should be viewed as one of many measures and markers of school readiness. Trends on education come and go; for example, it was popular in the 1980s through the 1990s to send children to preschool and even school earlier rather than later because it would integrate them into the learning system faster, thus giving them an edge up on the next kid. Either way, parents and caregivers need not simply follow trends but evaluate a boy's physical, emotional, educational, and social abilities and readiness for school. Parents and caregivers should consult with school educators and the school system to make the best decision regarding school entrance timing for their young boy.

VIGNETTE

Stephen was born in mid-October, and his parents were unsure if he would be ready to attend kindergarten the following September. He would be slightly younger than his kindergarten cohort, but his mother, Beth (who also happens to be a third grade teacher), was talking with colleagues about a trend concerning delaying entry into school for boys. She claimed that because boys typically develop more slowly than girls, beginning school a year later (closer to six years old) would be more beneficial in terms of his social, cognitive, and learning processes. Beth discussed this issue with her partner Lee. Lee concurred with Beth that boys do indeed develop differently and slower comparatively to girls. Lee had read that boys who are held back by one year are encouraged to attend a development class that focuses on social and group activities to help them integrate into the school environment. Beth and Lee shared many discussions about what to do with their boy. In the long run, they both decided that it would be best to hold Stephen back one year to allow him to fully develop his age-appropriate social and cognitive skills before entering kindergarten. "Great, now we can focus on Stephen's picky eating habits and occasional bedwetting!" exclaimed Lee.

Girls' and Boys' Social Engagement

During this age, relationships between boys and girls are continuously developing. During toddler years, boys hardly know or even care about the differences in their playmates. As boys continue to establish their autonomy and identity and note differences between the sexes, they will likely experience friendships with girls. Unlike the adolescent stage, the school-age boy is more likely to approach girls as friends, playmates, or even not at all. This is not to say boys and girls are not friends; simply how they express their friendships and interests in each other vary. Boys typically socially engage with other boys in larger groups as compared to girls (Erwin, 2006). They play intensely with other boys and sparingly communicate with girls. Healthy social relationships are the key outcome during this stage for boys. As a boy grows and develops in his social world, he will define what (and who) he likes and does not like.

Sports Participation and Competition

An inherent sense of competition drives most boys' behavior. Sports and competition occupy a very important role in many boys' lives; they help them define who they are and what they value in social settings (Chiarella, 2006). For boys five to nine years old, sports fulfill many roles. Sports help boys learn about their bodies and psychomotor capabilities, reinforce values such as sportsmanship and fair competition, teach discipline (mental and physical), forge new social groups and interpersonal relationships, and provide many other benefits.

At this age, engaging in sports can greatly improve overall health of children. Confidence and self-esteem are some of the stronger aspects of health that are positively affected by sports participation, but physical health, as with weight control through physical activity (CDC, 2009; Kindlon & Thompson, 2000), is also improved. The harnessing of boys' natural energy and fidgety behavior is another benefit. Healthy competition needs to be stressed; some boys feel pressured to achieve and to win at all costs. This usually develops because of pressure from parents, coaches, and other adults. Pressure at such a young developmental age often strips the fun and purpose of competition out of boys. Boys like to compete to compete. They enjoy seeing and comparing their abilities with others. Sport is a medium to teach life skills, which should be the major focus during this stage of a boy's development.

In his article, "Banning Boyhood," author Selwyn Duke talks about how normal boyhood competition and inclinations are slowly being questioned and phased out. Some people feel sports foster violence, aggression, and overly competitive attitudes and behaviors. This has prompted some children's sports organizations (Massachusetts Youth Soccer) to ban keeping score, and winners do not get trophies or other traditional forms of recognition for winning. Duke questions what is next: cops and robbers, dodge ball, or musical chairs? He goes on to say, "There are many ways to describe this trend. One might say it's a result of the left's antipathy toward competition, the increasing litigiousness of the day, or the inordinate concern with self-esteem and hurt feelings. Then, if I am to speak only of my feelings, the word stupid comes to mind. Really, though, regardless of whether the motivations are good or ill or the reasoning sound or not, at the end of the day I find a conclusion inescapable. Slowly, incrementally, perversely, boyhood is being banned" (Duke, 2007).

Is boyhood being banned, and if so, why? Is it litigation, sparing of feelings, or a social trend in neutralizing gender and gender roles? Sport is a unisex entity, but boys may value the process differently than do girls. Similar and different lessons are learned by both sexes, which can provide positive lifelong lessons concerning physical and emotional health. Boys love games, competition, hierarchies, and locking horns with each other (Chiarella, 2006; Duke, 2007); if this is discouraged or even taken away, to what do boys turn to express their energy and passions? Boys do value competition, discipline, hierarchies, and winning, all of which are embedded in the very fabric and fiber of sport. What we do with sports and how well we blend sports into the lives of school-age boys is up to each parent, caregiver, and family. Sports and health benefits will become critically important venues and mechanisms in advancing the physical (and emotional) health of boys well into the future.

HEALTH DISPARITIES AMONG SCHOOL-AGE BOYS

A *disparity* is an inequity or "haves and have nots" in groups. The school-age boy has several physical, emotional, and social challenges before him. What about boys who are less fortunate or populate marginalized minority groups? What happens to their health outcomes during this stage?

Not every boy has the chance or consistent opportunity to attend school. Even though the U.S. government mandates schooling for all children, some simply fall through the cracks and experience inconsistent opportunities in school. For those who do make it to school, education may be the last topic on their minds.

Physical health is one of the first indicators of whether a child can succeed in school or not. Children with physical health issues or disparities may not receive adequate opportunity to engage in learning despite advances with the **Americans with Disability Act.** Policy does not always translate to action, leaving some children underserved or even ignored altogether. Emotional health rests with how an individual interacts with others, peers, family, and society in general. Boys from troubled households, single-parent families, or even abusive settings may not integrate well into a school setting. A boy may be distrustful, hostile, introverted, or any other description that characterizes how he may try to protect himself from further harm and insult. Boys who are emotionally abused often become reactive and abusive themselves. Acting out against others is very common among school-age boys. If a boy is frustrated or feels that he cannot make his voice heard, he is likely to take action against others (Kindlon & Thompson, 2000). A period of life defined by learning, exploration, and joyful experiences that is marred with trouble, punishment, and angst needs to be further explored by adults. Angry boys or boys who act out often are dealt with by further punishment and isolation in the school system. This punishment does very little to address the problem and help the boy in the process. Making a bad situation even worse for a boy will likely only yield disappointing results for society as a whole. Appropriate remediation strategies are critical.

Nutritional disparities are another common problem for many children in the United States and abroad (Wang & Lobstein, 2006). Childhood obesity has become rampant in the United States and threatens to become a global issue soon. Disparities in nutrition in the United States mainly exist as a function of family structure and socioeconomic status. Lower-income families often have to decide on foods that will address hunger by being filling, but also cheap enough to allow for the acquisition of other life necessities. These cheaper foods often come at the expense of a boy's waistline, as they are filling but heavy in empty calories. Diets poor in high-quality nutrients often are implicated in overweight and obese children, learning disabilities, type 2 diabetes mellitus, and gastrointestinal issues, among others (Lorson et al., 2009; Wang & Lobstein, 2006). Many minorities and first-generation families have yet to establish solid incomes, and many single-parent families also struggle with costs of living. Unfortunately, food becomes one of the easiest solutions to financial stress because of the vast array of fast-food establishments in many communities.

According to a study in the *Annals of Internal Medicine*, Hispanic men became obese 2.5 times more than white men, and after their early twenties, black men became obese at a rate of 2.2 times that of white men (Hiatt, Riebel, & Friedman, 2007). Children overall need a healthy diet to grow and thrive at optimal levels. Children who are obese risk physical and social consequences that will plague them well into their adult years.

Some children often go without food. In developing nations, children (particularly boys) work to help support their families instead of going to school. Some may go days without an adequate meal and thus fail to thrive. In many developing nations, boys may be of shorter stature not only because of genetics, but because of the quality of nutrients that are available for their consumption. These nutrition-related health disparities are top priority for national organizations and policies, such as *Healthy People 2010* and *2020,* but according to recent data and statistics, there is much left to be done (U.S. Department of Health and Human Services, 2010).

Possibly related to nutrition, black boys were found to be more likely to have food and skin allergies than other groups. They also are more sensitive to foods, such as peanuts, eggs, and milk, thus further linking skin problems with possible dietary factors (Odhiambo et al., 2009). Consider that many foods contain these items and families that are of lower socioeconomic status may not be able to afford substitute foods that are typically higher in cost and less readily available at food stores. The skin shows relative nutritional status, which can be seen in many developing nations where children have issues with eczema, dry skin, rashes, and lesions that can compromise overall health.

Learning and education are critical for the development of life and social skills. Unfortunately, many boys are not only unengaged in classrooms because of unstimulating or perceived unrelated curricula (Parkin, 2007) but also because of fear and unsettled home lives. Children who are distracted by events outside of the classroom, such as violence and domestic abuse, lack of good nutrition, living on the streets or with inconsistent family members, have little room for engaging in learning. In his 1991 book, *Savage Inequalities: Children in America's Schools*, author Jonathan Kozol articulates how the environment of the school only partially predicts the success of its students. Basic safety and nutrition precede learning. Many times, we focus on the behavior of boys instead of investigating and addressing the factors that drive them to behave a certain way. Once we begin to do this, under-served, marginalized boys and children might be positioned for success rather than lumped into a system that has routinely failed them year after year and decade after decade.

Boys enjoy physical activity and organized sports. Marginalized groups may not have the opportunity to partake in certain sports because of the associated costs. Sports like ice hockey, football, and lacrosse are equipment intensive. Equipment costs money that some boys and their families may not have. Even sports such as basketball, track and field, and soccer have costs for shoes, balls, and court access. Sports such as tennis, golf, and ice hockey have more white children participating than non-whites. Sports may be the least of a boy's concerns when his family depends on him to watch other siblings or even work to bring money into the home.

A whole world of opportunities exists to allow boys in the United States and in the world to experience good health during their early years. Social action coupled with advocacy will give a voice to underserved and under-represented minority groups. One way to assure that these efforts continue to improve is through programs at the national level, such as Healthy People initiatives. Grass-roots efforts also are key. A sense of community and ownership in one's own destiny go a long way in sustaining positive social change that will close the gap in gender-based disparities.

SUMMARY

This chapter focused on the school-age boy from the ages of five to nine years. A definition of *school-age* and general developmental and social challenges were presented and discussed in detail. Physical health concerns and considerations, such as normal growth patterns and nutritional considerations as with eczema and skin rashes, were highlighted. Emotional and social health factors were described in addition to challenges of the learning environment. Normal learning patterns as well as developmental learning disorders, such as attention deficit disorder and tics, were presented. The role of physical activity and sports in boys' development was discussed. Inequality and disparities also were discussed in the context of affecting the lives of younger boys and their opportunities.

KEY TERMS

Allergies	Emotions	Lethargy
Americans with Disabilities Act	Encopresis	Morbid obesity
Biofeedback	Enuresis	Pediatrician
Cognition	Fiber	Schemas
Dermatologist	Lactose	Spectrum disorders
Eczema	Learning style	Visceral

DISCUSSION QUESTIONS

1. Look up current theories on why rates of autism and Asperger's syndrome seem to be increasing over the past ten years. Comment on what you find.

2. Do you think school curricula in the United States favors females? Justify your opinion based on educational data that support your assertion.

3. What do you see as being the strongest reasons for holding a boy back from entering kindergarten? How would you educate parents, caregivers, and educators who may not be in favor of this practice? Be sure to cite any research findings in support of your answer.

4. Look up current theories on why rates of autism and Asperger's syndrome seem to be increasing. Comment on what you find.

5. Discuss some long-term outcomes that may result when boys become disengaged with school. What does this mean for male health and public health?

6. What advice would you give school systems to assure all boys stay actively engaged in the curriculum?

7. Do you think sports should *not* focus on scores, outcomes, wins, and intense competition? Discuss how this may or may not affect boys.

8. Why do you think boys are so competitive? In what other areas are boys competitive? What value does this competitive spirit carry as a boy becomes an adult man?

9. Research school graduation and dropout rates for boys in the United States who are black, white, Hispanic/Latino, Asian, and Native American. What trends did you find? You may choose to put the results into a chart for ease of comparison. Interpret what these results and findings mean in the greater context of being male in the United States.

10. Name five major world health disparities affecting boys between the ages of five to nine. Discuss how you think these will or will not change in the near future (approximately ten years).

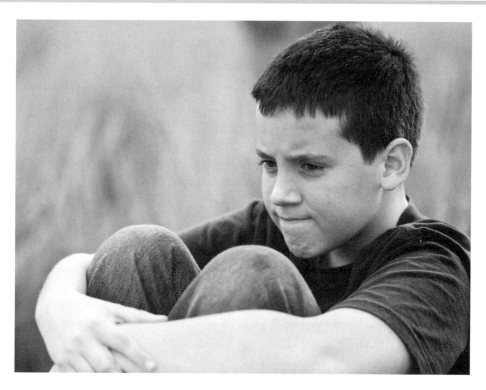

©iStockphoto.com/Juanmonino

6

Preadolescence and "Tween" Years

LEARNING OBJECTIVES

- Identify the physical growth and development challenges of preadolescent males, as well as psychological and social considerations
- Assess risk factors for preadolescent males using national data, and devise strategies to prevent unintentional injuries
- Analyze the role of parental role modeling in helping boys make positive health-related decisions
- Outline ways in which preadolescent males learn how to become men through various rites of passage

WHO IS THE preadolescent or "tween" boy? What challenges does he face and present for those who care for him? What is the difference between an eleven-year-old boy and a fourteen- or fifteen-year-old? Do a couple or a few years really make a big difference? The answer is yes. In this chapter we discuss the preadolescent years and physical, emotional, and social health challenges boys experience during this stage, such as endocrine disorders and rates of depression.

THE PREADOLESCENT YEARS

Physically, a preadolescent boy may be underdeveloped or overdeveloped for his age; either way, he is likely to feel at odds with his physical being until puberty kicks in and he grows or others catch up to him. A boy may be perfectly normal and adequate in a physical sense; however, peer comments can provoke a negative sense of self or even limit self-confidence. Some boys fear they will never get bigger and stronger, whereas others may not know how to function in their **precocious** bodies. Often, adults simply shrug off a boy's worries about his physical development. Some even promote insecurity, remarking that a boy is a "weakling" or a "wimp." Recent research has shown that boys, similarly to girls, *do* take comments about their physical development and body image development seriously, some with negative health consequences (Cohane & Pope, 2001; Jones, Vigfusdottir, & Lee, 2004; Leone, Fetro, Kittleson, Welshimer, Partridge, & Robertson, 2011). Reassurance by parents, caregivers, and health professionals should focus on what a boy's abilities and talents are and what he can become with persistence and effort. Boys left to fend for themselves will do just that, which does not usually correlate to positive decisions concerning their health.

Emotionally, a preadolescent boy may not feel secure or may be confused as to what he should be feeling. Is he a boy? A man? Should he act grown-up, or is it acceptable for him to be boyish? Should he be responsible or can he be carefree? Does he listen to his parents, or is he trying to establish his own sense of identity separate from his parents and family? The emotional development of a tween is varied and complex. Many boys are torn between being the little boy and the awaiting man. They may hold on to the last remains of boyhood one minute and eagerly usher in adolescence in the other.

Socially awkward and possibly unsure of his own capabilities, the preadolescent boy is actively engaged in his world to learn, experience, and eventually define who he will be and who he wants to be. The role of adults and role models is to help a boy successfully navigate this course. Social development and parental expectations are closely related, but social development should result in **autonomy** for the boy and not the expectations of a parent or other adult (Erwin, 2006). Many boys emulate and admire their fathers or other male role models and want to be just like them. They may follow in the same educational paths, occupational routes, or even the same attitudes and health behaviors. Others may reject their fathers' influence and philosophies. Some boys rebel and define their own worlds. Others may not have father figures or male role models. A boy may create and piece together his own expectations and reality. There is no right or wrong way to become a man, simply differences. Forcing a boy to follow in the footsteps of his father or even exerting pressure to do so likely will be met with resistance, and even if he is compliant, he may harbor a lifetime of resentment. It is critically important that parents and caregivers allow a boy the freedom to define his own path but also to be an active parent or caregiver and role model in the process (Erwin, 2006).

The preadolescent boy questions much about life, himself, and his place within it. He experiences tremendous physical, emotional, and social growth and development. The preadolescent or tween years carry with them several implications for a boy's health. If poor health choices, practices, and attitudes are left unattended, a boy is likely to grow into adolescence making decisions based on unhealthy factors. Moreover, health practices that are modeled to him earlier in life carry lasting implications and possibly consequences as he ages (Kindlon & Thompson, 2000). Good decisions pertaining to his health lessen the likelihood that he will consistently make negative health choices. A boy who is taught to value his physical, emotional, and social health will likely take action to make healthy, positive choices. Those who lack knowledge and skills and have negative attitudes toward health and health care providers will encounter numerous health consequences. For example, many boys between the ages of ten and twelve experience pressure to drink alcohol, smoke or use tobacco products, and engage in promiscuous sexual activity.

PHYSICAL HEALTH

Unintentional Injuries

Sometimes, no matter how well prepared or protected a boy is, accidents will happen. Child passenger safety is the greatest public health issue facing children and is the leading cause of death. One out of every 3 injuries due to fireworks occur in males under the age of fifteen. Emergency departments see approximately 200,000 children under age fourteen for playground-related injuries each year. **Traumatic brain injuries (TBIs)** are most frequent in boys up and through fourteen years old. Drowning is the second leading cause of death in children ages fourteen years and younger (National Center for Injury Prevention and Control [NCIPC], 2006).

Intentional injury refers to purposeful injury inflicted on oneself or others, as aggression, violence, or planned attacks like bullying. *Unintentional injury,* often referred to as *accidents,* refers to physical harm incurred without predetermined intent, such as motor vehicle accidents (MVAs), drowning, and falls (Cunningham et al., 2009). Both types may or may not lead to death, but most result in physical consequences that can last well into adulthood. According to the Centers for Disease Control and Prevention (CDC), injury is a serious threat to the health of children. In fact, injury is consistently the number one cause of disability and death in this age group. From ages one to forty-four, unintentional injury is the leading cause of death for all boys and men (Centers for Disease Control and Prevention [CDC], 2006). In boys ages ten to fourteen, motor vehicle traffic accidents were the number one cause of injury and death, followed by homicide and firearms (CDC, 2006). Additionally, falls were the leading cause of emergency department visits in boys ten to fourteen years old, according to CDC data from 2007.

These and similar statistics are enough to trouble any parent of a younger boy. Why do boys seem to get into situations that may result in injury more so than do girls? Boys are more likely to physically experience their worlds as they grow and develop (Bazelon, 2009). The inherent physicality of boys leads to more exposure to dangerous situations. With experience come risk and the possibility of physical injury. Coupled with interpersonal and social pressures preadolescent boys face, unintentional injuries skyrocket. For example, boys typically play on school playgrounds by running, climbing, and bumping into things. When confronted with "dares" and "bets" from other boys, they may be more likely to take greater risks. Socially, boys are praised for taking risks because it is viewed as normal male behavior and supports a "boys will be boys" mentality. Risky behavior is a negative health pattern that carries with it a lifetime of consequences, including premature death.

What can be done to minimize the risk of unintentional injury in boys and promote healthy behaviors? From the earliest of ages, good role modeling will carry positive, healthy messages for boys (Erwin, 2006). Health practitioners can advise parents that simple steps such as wearing seatbelts can reduce harm and likely will encourage positive behaviors well into the future. Because boys tend to roughhouse often, parents can assure their boy that it is okay to stop when he is hurt, report an injury when it happens, and avoid risky behaviors altogether.

Modeling good behaviors likely will translate to boys doing the same
©iStockphoto.com/Andreas Steinhart

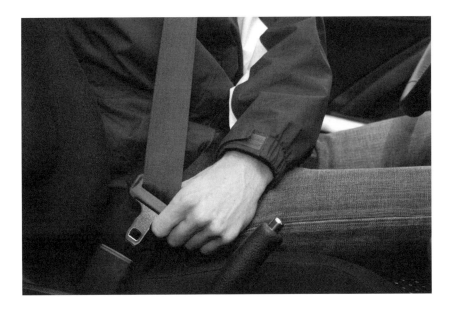

Downplaying safety during a boy's younger life will inherently set him up to undertake the same risky behaviors as he ages. Ignoring an injury when he is younger may create and foster an attitude that he presents with throughout his entire lifetime. "It's just a bruise" may turn into "It's just a concussion," to "It's just chest pain" in middle age (Men's Health Network [MHN], 2009. Minimizing occurrences and severity should be a goal of any parent. Parents, caregivers, and health professionals have to do a better job harnessing natural boyhood tendencies and helping boys process social expectations and reality.

Childhood **concussions** have increased during the past twenty-five years, likely because more children are participating in organized sports. Unintentional injuries such as concussions carry lifetime consequences, such as memory deficits, headaches, depression, and severe conditions such as **chronic traumatic encephalopathy (CTE)** (Kirkwood, Yeates, & Wilson, 2006). Health professionals should educate parents, coaches, peers, and the boys themselves in how to identify injuries, report them, and seek proper treatment.

The ability to process media critically is a key skill that will advance boys' health in avoiding unintentional injury. Media such as television and movies tend to glamorize risky male behavior. Yet movies, television videos, video games, and other media outlets typically do not account for or show the multitude of consequences of risky behavior. "Reality" TV programs morph what and how we view life and social expectations. Boys who only see males being aggressive, physical daredevils, and risk takers, devoid of physical or social consequences, are likely to accept this as normal and part of their own reality. For example, recent discussions have analyzed the role and influence of YouTube videos depicting risk-taking behavior. While there are no confirmatory studies or data to support the contention that boys (or girls) who consistently view so-called real videos are more likely to try out the actions, anecdotal reports support that this is a trend to monitor. Restricting content and viewing may not be the best strategy, because boys will interact with other children and adults and eventually will face challenges and temptation. Parents and caregivers will better serve boys by teaching them skills to process, resist, and model good health behaviors. Developing **resiliency** helps boys remain confident in their own abilities to make good health decisions.

Endocrine Disorders

The endocrine system is a series of glands throughout the body that secrete specific hormones that affect certain tissues and organs that help to regulate the body and its function, such as mood and growth and development (Sherwood, 1997). A key gland in the endocrine system, the *pituitary,* is responsible for the changes associated with puberty. Puberty is a hallmark in growth and development in all humans. During puberty the body prepares to enter into the reproductive years through a series of hormonal actions and interactions (Sherwood, 1997). As with any stage of life, signals can be faulty or pathology may result from injury or other influences, resulting in endocrine disorders. Two of the most common endocrine-related disorders in boys are delayed puberty and advanced puberty, often referred to as *precocious puberty* (Niedziela, 2007). Other terms used are *hypogonadism* for delayed puberty and *hypergonadism* for advanced puberty. Most boys advance into puberty (referred to as *andrenarche*) between the ages of nine and fourteen, with most exhibiting signs by age twelve (Niedziela, 2007). Of course, there is great variability depending on factors such as nutritional status, genetics, environmental influences, drug use, and pathology.

Tanner Stages of Physical Development

For more than forty years, the Tanner scale has been used by physicians and other health care practitioners to document physical development in boys and girls. The scale uses both statistics and graphics to help delineate which stage of physical development a boy may be in and is often used to compare normal versus abnormal development in children. Primary and secondary sex characteristics such as height, weight, genitalia, and hair patterns are documented in each stage of development. Each scale has five specific criteria and explanations, called *stages,* for boys and girls (Marshall & Tanner, 1970).

In boys, there is much overlap in growth patterns. Tanner stage 1, also known as *prepubertal,* is primary marked by increases in height and body weight but little to no growth of the external genitalia (penis, testes, and scrotum) and secondary sex characteristics such as pubic hair (Marshall & Tanner, 1970). Preadolescent boys are likely to be in Tanner stage 2 or beyond, which is characterized by further physical development. Height continues to increase at a rate of 5–6 centimeters per year along with more body weight in the form of lean muscle mass. The testes increase in size and volume, sparse pubic hair develops around the base of the penis and under the arms, and the penis increases in length and width (Marshall & Tanner, 1970). Hormones also influence body shape, which often produces the characteristic "awkward" or "lanky" appearance of many boys in puberty. Vocal cords develop and are influenced by hormonal changes that can produce a "cracking" of the boy's voice. Other physical changes typically occur later as a boy progresses into adolescence and puberty (Tanner stages 3–5).

Physical changes are normal but may be unexpected for some boys. Formerly confident in his body and physical abilities, a boy in the midst of preadolescent growth and development may become distraught over the multitude of changes he is going through. Physical changes may confuse a boy, and some report feeling that they are "losing" something or that their parents and peers view and treat them differently. Conversely, he may be pleasantly surprised by becoming taller, heavier, and stronger. Open discussion and reassurance with good health information will go a long way in helping a boy transition through these natural life stages of growth and development.

It is important to understand the Tanner stages of physical development in boys to be able to identify what is normal and expected versus what can present as an issue or even a disorder. Some boys may experience hypogonadism or hypergonadism. Variables and influences such as genetics, nutrition, and more recently, environmental exposures have been implicated in various growth and developmental disorders in boys (Sherwood, 1997). Plastic chemicals in common, everyday products such as bottles and containers may be altering the brains of baby boys, which in turn may make them more feminized. Chemicals known as *phthalates,* which are in products such as vinyl flooring, shower curtains, packaging, and plastic furniture, seem to be influencing hormonal development in boys. Phthalates may affect developing boys' brains, which can limit the production of testosterone (Doheny, 2009). Some boys are born with genetic predispositions that can influence their normal growth and development as they approach and enter puberty.

Fragile X Syndrome

Also known as Martin-Bell syndrome or FXS, this condition is one of the most common forms of mental **retardation**, and it occurs more in males than in females (Hagerman et al., 2009; Martin & Bell, 1943). The syndrome presents with a spectrum of signs and symptoms that affect physical, emotional, and intellectual health and range in forms from mild to severe retardation (Hagerman et al., 2009; Martin & Bell, 1943). It is caused by is a single protein sequence located on the X chromosome that fails to produce enough or any sequences for gene expression that affects normal neural connections and function. Mutations are more common in females (approximately 1 in every 259 females versus 1 in every 2,000 males); however, males have a higher incidence of active expression than females because they only inherit one X chromosome. Males cannot transmit this genetic disorder to their sons because they contribute only a Y chromosome; however, they can and do transmit it to daughters on their X chromosomes (Hagerman et al., 2009). Most affected boys demonstrate moderate to severe forms of the disorder, whereas females vary from mild to no signs and symptoms at all (Hagerman et al., 2009; Martin & Bell, 1943).

Persons with this disorder typically display elongated faces, large or protruding ears, flat feet, strabismus (lazy eye), and larger than normal testes in males (also known as *macroorchidism*) in addition to psychological and emotion underdevelopment. Boys exhibit poor muscle tone for their age and abnormalities in Tanner stage development criteria (Hagerman et al., 2009; Martin & Bell, 1943). Social impairments also are common, especially pronounced shyness, disengagement, inappropriate gestures, and social **anxiety.** It is fairly common that boys with FXS are confused with boys who have autism or Asperger's syndrome. The key features between autism and Asperger's syndrome and FXS, however, are the marked physical features mentioned.

If a boy seems to present with social and intellectual impairments, he is more likely to do so earlier in life and can be properly diagnosed and helped (Cornish, Turk & Levitas, 2007). Macroorchidism can be picked up during routine physical examinations for school and sports (Hagerman et al., 2009; Martin & Bell, 1943).

If detected early in life, and depending on the severity of the disorder, boys can learn to adapt to this disorder with the help of supportive parents, peers, and medical professionals. Boys with FXS often learn 2.2 times slower than boys without the disorder. Communication and behaviors can be learned over time with repetition and patience on the part of all involved parties. Diagnosis is possible through confirmatory genetic testing but may not provide an accurate picture of how the person will develop because of the variations in social and physical development (Cornish et al., 2007). In vitro testing has been advanced over the past few years; however, there remain no cure or drug therapies for the disorder (Hagerman et al., 2009). Behavioral therapy, special education, and physical treatment for conditions such as eye problems and orthopedic issues continue to be the standard of care for persons with FXS. **Genetic counseling** may be warranted in families with strong FXS traits or family members affected by the disorder (Cornish et al., 2007).

Klinefelter's Syndrome

Similar to fragile X syndrome, Klinefelter's syndrome (KS) or *XXY syndrome*, is a **sex-linked** genetic disorder present in males. Males with this disorder have an extra X chromosome in their genetic code (Klinefelter, 1986). Statistically, KS is the most common sex chromosome disorder, occurring in approximately 1 in every 1,000 males; however, it has been reported that as many as 1 in every 500 males have an extra X chromosome without displaying overt signs and symptoms (Bojesen, Juul, & Gravholt, 2003). First described in medical literature in 1942 by Dr. Henry Klinefelter, KS most commonly leads to abnormal growth stature and reproductive insufficiency in males (Klinefelter, Reifenstein, & Albright, 1942). Some boys with KS have been described as looking more feminine in their body appearance and features. Some boys have undetectable, subclinical signs and symptoms of KS that may only present later in life, when conception of a child is desired. This is because boys with KS have underdeveloped gonads (testes) that produce little to no viable sperm, leaving them infertile (Klinefelter et al., 1942; Klinefelter, 1986).

The exact cause of KS is unknown, but research postulates that genetic mutations cause the retention of an extra X chromosome that fails to incorporate as one (Bojesen et al., 2003). Signs and symptoms of KS may not become apparent until preadolescence and adolescence due to lack of hormonal influence of secondary sex characteristics in younger boys (Klinefelter, 1986). Common signs and symptoms include a youthful facial appearance despite tall stature, lanky limb structure, some intellectual dysfunction, more feminized appearance with rounded hips, narrow shoulders, and breast tissue development (referred to as *gynecomastia*), which is present in approximately 33% of all KS patients. Boys with KS are commonly described as *hypogonadal,* which means the testes do not effectively produce testosterone and other hormones, whereas other hormones such as follicle-stimulating hormone (FSH) and luteinizing hormone (LH) are overly represented in the body. Less testosterone production leads to more feminine characteristics, and underactive testes present as much smaller in size than among developmentally active boys (Klinefelter, et al., 1942; Klinefelter, 1986). The protective function of testosterone is minimized as estrogen, FSH, and LH hormone levels predominate (Bojesen et al., 2003; Klinefelter et al., 1942; Klinefelter, 1986). These developmental challenges can predispose a boy to early osteoporosis, certain types of cancers, pulmonary disease, rheumatoid arthritis, and diabetes mellitus.

So, what can be done to account for KS? Confirmatory testing can be performed by simple blood tests. **Amniocentesis** can determine if there is a marker for KS in utero. Approximately 50% of confirmed cases of KS in a developing fetus are aborted (Bojesen et al., 2003). If a boy is born without previous confirmatory testing, recognition and diagnosis become more tricky, because other than some intellectual deficits, most KS boys

appear normal or within normal variances. As a boy advances into preadolescence and puberty, the Tanner developmental stages may provide critical
clues into this disorder (Klinefelter, 1986). A pediatrician can help diagnose
the disorder and arrive at a salient treatment protocol. Boys with KS may
be advised to undergo testosterone replacement therapy. Other supportive
therapies can include surgery to remove excessive breast tissue development, nutritional supplements to offset the effects of osteoporosis and subsequent bone loss, and consistent monitoring and follow-up to assure other
abnormalities are not present or do not become issues (Mandoki & Sumner,
1991).

Perhaps one of the most important treatments is counseling and support
from family and peers (Rovet, Netley, Keenan, Bailey, & Stewart, 1996).
Preadolescence and adolescence are difficult transitional periods of life for
any boy, let alone one with a genetic disorder such as KS. Social anxiety due
to differences in stature and physique may lead to feelings of isolation, low
self-esteem, and low confidence. Boys who are diagnosed with KS should
routinely follow up with their physicians and counselors, support groups,
or both. Parents or caregivers of boys with KS should plan to initiate these
supportive functions before preadolescence and adolescence to avoid physical and psychosocial consequences and negative health outcomes. Boys with
KS can lead meaningful, enjoyable, and fulfilling lives; however, they likely
will be sterile (Klinefelter, 1986; Rovet et al., 1996). Reproductive counseling and discussion of alternative family planning strategies should be
presented if a family is desired in the future.

Pituitary Disorders

The pituitary gland is a small, pea-sized endocrine gland that extends off
the hypothalamus gland in the brain. The gland sits in the *sella turcica* at
the base of the brain and primarily functions to secrete hormones that regulate **homeostatic** relationships in the body (Hormone Foundation, n.d.).
The pituitary gland plays an important role and function in all body processes to keep people healthy in growth and development.

One of the primary features and responsibilities of the pituitary gland
is the secretion of sex hormones that activate the development of secondary

sex characteristics (Hormone Foundation, n.d.). For most boys, the pituitary gland functions appropriately (Tsigo & Chrousos, 2002). In some cases, the pituitary may not properly function, causing dwarfism (limited growth) or gigantism (excessive growth). Pituitary dysfunction can occur for several reasons, including organic causes such as tumors, damage from concussions or other head trauma, genetic predisposition, or hormonal imbalances (Hormone Foundation, n.d.).

Both dwarfism and gigantism present in both males and females (Hormone Foundation, n.d.). However, Western culture places an inherent value on male height. The average height for a Western full-grown man is approximately 5 feet 9 inches; variance above and below this norm often is scrutinized by society and culture (Tsigo & Chrousos, 2002). Males who are above the norm are typically valued as competent and confident. As one research study suggested, taller men get more in life, from recognition and respect (Judge & Cable, 2004) to choice of mate and financial benefits (Pawlowski, Dunbar, & Lipowicz, 2000). Males who fall below the norm or standard often are viewed as less competent and less successful and are less desirable to the opposite sex for reproductive purposes, as suggest by researchers (Pawlowski et al., 2000). Many males fear not being tall enough, which can affect their psychosocial status and lead to negative overall mental health. Similarly, males who tend to be taller often do not voice their concerns because of the relative benefits society ascribes to them. Regardless of what society ascribes as the norm in male height, endocrine disorders such as dwarfism and gigantism present physical and emotional consequences.

Dwarfism   Although there are many causes of dwarfism, a lack of growth hormone in one's system due to an underactive pituitary gland, called *pituitary dwarfism,* is likely a main cause of this type of disorder (Hormone Foundation, n.d.). People of short stature (also called *little people*), usually have an adult height of 4 feet 10 inches or shorter. Some dwarfs' features, such as hands and fingers, are proportionate to their bodies, and others have disproportionate features, such as longer fingers and toes. *Achondroplasia* is a condition of dwarfism in which the limbs are disproportionately short compared to the trunk (Gollust, Thompson, Gooding, & Biesecker, 2003). Short stature can be addressed with a multifactoral approach. First, the nature and cause of the disorder needs to be ascertained. If there is a family or genetic history of dwarfism, genetic counseling is strongly recommended. If an organic cause of dwarfism, such as a tumor, is suspected, surgery and subsequent treatment with growth hormone may yield successful results. However, growth hormone treatments in many dwarfs will not yield many efficacious results and should be administered on a case-by-case basis (Hormone Foundation, n.d.).

Boys who are of short stature without an obvious family history should be referred to an appropriate specialist, such as an **endocrinologist,** who can determine the nature and cause of the short stature. Many physicians will guide treatment options based on normal growth charts among other supportive therapies, like counseling. Perhaps one of the most critical features concerning short stature in boys is helping them to adjust to a world that typically values height. *Heightism* has been proposed as a form of discrimination in today's society. Parents need to realize that self-esteem, confidence, and positive health decisions may be compromised in boys with dwarfism or who are shorter. Support groups and counseling are strongly advocated by specialists in this field to help a boy adjust to his world (Gollust et al., 2003).

Gigantism   On the other end of spectrum is *gigantism,* or clinical growth in height well above the mean in a population. Gigantism is less well defined due to normal variances in male height (Hormone Foundation, n.d.). Some disorders carry physical complications for taller people. One such condition is *acromegaly,* which is a systemic condition caused by an overproduction of human growth hormone. The condition causes excessive growth hormone to affect all tissues in the body, leading to disproportionate large stature. Physical features such as excessive bone growth, organ tissue growth, and organ enlargement are common in acromegaly. Many people with acromegaly develop cancers and suffer from weakened tissues and degenerative disorders because of excessive body mass. Some people with the disorder do not live past the fourth or fifth decade of life. Other noticeable features include tall stature, a prominent jaw line and brow ridge, large hands and feet, thick, tough skin, and visual problems. Organic causes of acromegaly are generally tumors that influence the pituitary gland; however, some conditions may be genetically linked or caused by damage or injury (Nabarro, 2008).

Another condition related to gigantism is Marfan's syndrome. Marfan's syndrome is an inherited connective tissue disorder that compromises vascular function. People with Marfan's syndrome are typically tall and lean, have visible chest deformities such as *pectus excavatum* (sunken-in chest), visual abnormalities, and an abnormally long arm span double that of their vertical height. Many people with Marfan's syndrome have a heightened risk for aortic **aneurysms** and death because of weakness in their connective tissues (De Paepe, Devereux, Dietz, Hennekam, & Pyeritz, 1996). Boys who are of abnormal height and display other symptoms of Marfan's syndrome or any other growth disorder should be referred to a specialist for further consultation and confirmatory testing.

Pituitary disorders may become apparent during the preadolescent years as a boy transitions into puberty. Dwarfism may be less apparent because many boys experience delayed growth spurts; however, precocious, taller boys may be scrutinized more closely. Parents need to be acutely aware of their own genetics and family history of these and related disorders. If a boy is afflicted with a growth disorder, he will need counseling and support from doctors and specialists as well as family and peers.

Other Disorders

Preadolescent boys may be predisposed to other disorders related to normal growth and development, such as thyroid problems and diabetes. Thyroid disorders involve the thyroid gland, which is located in the lower neck, upper breastbone area of the body. The gland produces hormones (thyroxine and triiodothyronine) that help to control how the body uses energy. *Hyperthyroidism* occurs when the body uses too much energy too quickly, whereas *hypothyroidism* does the exact opposite. Diseases of the thyroid, such as Graves' disease and Addison's disease, are genetically linked; therefore, parents with a family history should be aware of their son's development (WebMd, n.d.c). Boys with hyperthyroidism may display an inability to concentrate, which could lead to an inaccurate diagnosis of attention deficit disorder (ADD) or attention deficit hyperactivity disorder (ADHD). A boy with an overactive thyroid gland may perspire more and lose weight more readily. The problem is that many of these signs and symptoms are consistent with normal activity. The main tell-tale signs include unexplained weight loss despite consumption of more food, excessive sweating, irritability or inability to sleep, and difficulty concentrating (WebMd, n.d.c). Thyroid conditions are difficult to parse out from normal growth and development; therefore, if parents or caregivers have concerns, they should consult with a family physician.

Hypothyroidism, like hyperthyroidism, is a regulatory disorder of the thyroid gland. However, unlike hyperthyroidism, energy metabolism is slowed and less efficient. Common signs and symptoms include fatigue, sluggishness, feeling cold in normal temperatures, and slower heart rate. Skin changes also may become apparent. Boys may experience delayed growth, but this is not a hallmark sign of the disorder because many boys may develop more slowly in height and weight because of normal genetics. Weight gain may be another sign; however, hypothyroidism is not a direct cause of weight gain. Fatigue may lead to less physical activity, thereby promoting weight gain (WebMd, n.d.c). The key in understanding thyroid disorders is the presence of a combination of signs and symptoms and not just one specific manifestation.

Diabetes is a metabolic disorder that carries with it a lifetime of physical health consequences. There are two types of diabetes, DM type I and DM type II. Both involve dysfunction of the pancreas, which regulates carbohydrate metabolism through the secretion of the hormone insulin. Type I DM involves a primary, often genetic dysfunction of the pancreatic cells, thereby limiting regulatory control over blood sugar levels. If left untreated, a person can go into a coma and potentially die if levels rise too high or fall too low. Type I diabetics often present as normal weight and stature and may experience their first signs and symptoms in preadolescence. Treatment involves regular monitoring and administration of insulin injections on a daily basis (Cooke & Plotnick, 2008). Type II DM is a direct result of poor diet, which results in primary insulin resistance. Essentially, the body is unable to effectively control blood sugar and metabolism because of poor dietary choices and their effects on the pancreas over time. Dietary habits and behaviors are forged early in life; therefore, boys who overeat and run the risk of becoming overweight or even morbidly obese often suffer from DM type II (Rother, 2007).

The United States has a marked obesity epidemic, which demonstrates high rates in preteen and teenage boys (Duncan, 2006). States in the Southeast reported 44% of school-age children, either overweight or obese (National Survey of Children's Health, 2007). Obesity and DM type II carries severe health-related consequences that tax the person as well as the health care system. For example, diabetics have dependence on more medications, incur more physician visits, have more hospitalizations, and require more resources overall than do nondiabetics. All of these health consequences can be prevented through good dietary choices along with regular physical activity (Duncan, 2006). Coupled with socially engrained attitudes of how boys and men eat and consume more, diabetes is an inevitable health consequence for many. Until there is a fundamental shift in how boys are taught to make good choices in food selection, and we eradicate the "clean your plate" mentality, diabetes and other metabolic problems will persist.

EMOTIONAL HEALTH

Preadolescent boys experience tremendous growth in emotional status. Physically, a boy may be differentiating from the younger boy that he was, but not all boys emotionally develop at the same pace as their physical changes. Some boys may be nearly 6 feet tall yet still enjoy playing with their toys and friends, whereas others seem more emotionally advanced than they appear physically. These variations are due in part because of hormonal fluctuations within his body and also because of changing social values and structures. He has been in school now approximately seven years and has interacted with many new people (friends, teachers, other parents) and has had many diverse experiences. As the boy grows and develops, he begins to challenge the old with the new. New friends provoke alternative ways of thinking and expose the boy to new adventures. And boys have a natural, inherent curiosity.

VIGNETTE

Having lived in four states and having spent quite a bit of time in my home office writing, I have become very familiar with the neighborhood happenings at each location. Being an academic "voyeur" of sorts has allowed me to witness the growth, development, and interaction of children throughout the days, weeks, months, and years at each location. Two kids in particular stand out in my mind. There could not have been more than two or three years difference in these brothers' ages, but social development differences were quite apparent.

Mason was the older one and Owen the younger. When they were younger, they were inseparable, doing most things younger boys do together, such as play games, sports, fight, ride their bikes, and fight a little more. Their mom, a single woman also raising two daughters, always seemed to encourage her boys to go outside and play, and that they did, and quite frequently. Quite often, the younger boy, Owen, would tag along with his older brother and his group of friends. As Mason got older and began high school, Owen seemed to become more isolated. Often I would see him alone in his backyard kicking a soccer ball, doing yard work and chores, and engaging in other "boy" pursuits. Mason often would rush into the house on his cell phone, barely acknowledging his little brother. Owen soon developed a small group of his own friends and rarely interacted with his brother's friends. Owen replaced his lemonade stand with an eclectic variety of side jobs, including shoveling snow in the winters and raking leaves in the fall. He still played, but he was discovering his own sense of self and independence.

Emotional health often goes underappreciated in boys because society and culture still view emotionality in males as a feminine quality that should be discouraged. Emotional boys often are considered weak; therefore, in a social system in which value is placed on strength, unwavering dominance, and hierarchical order, boys' emotional health suffers (Kindlon & Thompson, 2000). In his book *Men Talk*, Dr. Alvin Baraff (1991) presents accounts of men who disclose the fears they had about women, sex, relationships, themselves, and issues growing up. Many of these accounts were **retrospective** regrets for not having had more outlets to express their emotionality in their younger lives. Many men reported feelings of inadequacy in expressing their feelings when they were younger and observed how these manifested and affected their relationships later in their adult lives.

Authors Dan Kindlon and Michael Thompson offer practical strategies to protect, engage, and encourage the emotional health of boys in their book *Raising Cain* (2000). When we actively attend to both the physical and emotional health of boys, society will be better served by producing men who are not only physically strong and capable but also emotionally competent and resilient. The social stigma of emotional boys tends to keep them away from seeking help and treatment when they are most in need.

Boys and Depression

Boys with depression often go under-recognized. Many boys fear the social stigma of being accused of being feminine if they expose their emotional sides (Shain, 2007). Culture sends boys mixed messages about how they can express themselves. For example, a man or boy who cries because his team just lost the championship usually is more acceptable than a man or boy who cries because he is stressed out. Crying and other expressions of emotion often are replaced by more acceptable male responses such as aggression, anger, and violence. Lack of emotional expression, however, can lead to repressed emotions and unresolved issues that can spiral into full-blown depression (Baraff, 1991). As emotions go unchecked and unresolved, the likelihood for developing depression increases exponentially, regardless of sex.

A closer look at the numbers and statistics concerning boys and depression reveals some startling findings. Boys are better than girls at hiding their emotions and subsequent depression. Anxiety disorders are as likely to occur in boys as girls, according to a report from *Psychology Today* (McGrath, 2002). Anxiety can lead to depressive episodes to which many boys simply do not know how to respond because they have never been encouraged to express themselves and their emotions (Baraff, 1991). Rates of depression also vary based on life stages. For example, in a large sample of more than 60,000 children surveyed, it was found that boys from eight to twelve years old scored higher in depression than did girls (Twenge & Nolen-Hoeksema, 2002).

There are many theories as to why depression is spiking in younger males. Gender role confusion as girls have reached parity with boys in traditional arenas such as sports, parental conflict, absent fathers and lack of strong male role models, and other social pressures and expectations add to the issue (Shain, 2007). Many of the consequences become evident later in life, but they start during a boy's formative years. A study based in Australia identified male depression as the most common reason for consult with a psychiatrist, more than three times the rate of the next issues of insomnia and anxiety (Bayram, Fahridin, & Britt, 2009). Boys are confused and stressed just as girls are, but society typically ignores or looks away from the immediate issue because boys revert to what they know, getting in trouble by inappropriately expressing their emotions through aggression and anger.

The inability to effectively communicate emotion is referred to as *alexithymia*. Not all males experience this disorder; rather, many boys feel and experience their emotions very deeply but express them in covert ways. Boys need to see that other males and people in general do care about their physical and emotional health and status (Kraemer, 2000). Greater value of emotional experiences will help combat the negative consequences of depression.

Boys and Suicide

Depression in males often goes under-recognized and under-diagnosed, which increases the risk for suicide by nearly fourfold (Shain, 2007). Rates of suicide also are higher in boys than among girls, especially among black boys (Xanthos, 2008), and it is well known that depression almost always coincides with suicidal tendencies and attempts (Shain, 2007). Some research suggests that females are more likely to attempt suicide; however, males appear to be successful (NCIPC, 2006). Teenage boys are more than five times more likely than girls to attempt *and* successfully complete suicide. Groups with disproportionately high rates of self-harm and suicide include boys who are consistently in trouble, have emotional and learning disabilities, and who are homosexual in orientation. The results do not get better as males age, with twenty- to twenty-four-year-old men being more than seven times more likely to commit suicide than women of a similar age (NCIPC, 2006).

Suicide in young children is rare (only about 10 per year according to the CDC), but psychological adjustment issues coupled with bullying may send a boy over the edge (CBS News, 2010). Additionally, not being fully able to realize the permanence of death may factor into why these tragedies occur.

Myth: The risk of suicide is uncommon in younger males.

Fact: Because of hormonal changes and new social challenges and pressures, many boys who are in the preadolescent stage may be at a *higher* risk for depression and suicidal ideation. Additionally, boys are less likely to attempt suicide than girls, but when they do, they are more successful at completing it. (Shain, 2007).

Why do rates of suicide stand out so markedly for boys? Boys often fail to express and communicate their feelings because of social norms and expectations. Holding in one's feelings and emotions without proper outlets of release can become a mounting psychological problem (Baraff, 1991). Boys may turn to aggression, violence, and substance abuse to cover their true feelings and emotions. Continued emotional suppression and substance abuse leads to a cyclical pattern of increasing depression and more means to repress emotional pain (Kindlon & Thompson, 2000).

Lower rates of diagnosed depression in males compared to females and high rates of successful suicide strongly suggest that there is a disconnect in how boys are taught emotional intelligence and management. Females are more likely to express how they feel and males are more likely to do something about it. Self-destructive behaviors among males are avoidable or at least can be addressed and minimized. Many males fear weakness and vulnerability and often feel immune or deny emotional problems. To overcome these barriers, parents, caregivers, and health professionals need to communicate **empathy,** compassion, and respect, as well as foster a safe, communicative environment. There is no better time for attacking and being proactive in these issues than the present.

Encouraging Emotional Development and Emotional Intelligence in Boys

The ability, capacity, or skills to identify, assess, and manage one's own emotions is referred to as *emotional intelligence* or simply, EI (Vernon, Petrides, Bratko, & Schermer, 2008). Boys learn this ability as they learn anything else in life; some will learn easily; others will struggle. Some boys will easily embrace emotional expression, some will learn it, some will struggle with it, and others may never fully develop this life skill.

Boys process and display stress differently than do girls. Boys are more likely to deny emotions and distress, play them off as inconsequential, and avoid discussion altogether. Parents, caregivers, and health professionals are advised to introduce emotion and how to process these emotions into a boy's world. Since most boys are experiential learners, parents and educators are advised to provide experiences for boys to explore, process, and express their emotions (Parkin, 2007). Learning experiences can be structured to help boys connect and relate to their emotions. For example, in the classroom, teachers can choose books or media that display boys and males in emotional situations (Parkin, 2007). Students can explain and express how they would help the characters. Clips from movies such as *Stand by Me* and *Lord of the Flies* can be used to show examples of the "stoic male" and the emotional boy. Discussions help to highlight the concepts.

Boys need to know that feelings and emotions are good, positive, and a source of personal empowerment and not an expression of weakness. Boys who hear and see emotions from their fathers and other males will likely embrace them rather than hiding and excluding them from their lives. Other strategies include helping boys develop emotional vocabularies and make regular use of them. Help boys name emotions, such as frustration, anger, happiness, patience, and sadness, as they present in life.

If a boy routinely acts out, parents and caregivers are advised to take immediate control of the situation. Empathy is very useful; the preadolescent boy can understand what it might feel like to be in another person's shoes. Therefore, help him to reflect on what others may or may not be experiencing. Boys are competitive by nature; it is important that they become strong and confident but not at the expense of others. Extrapolate good sportsmanship to other areas of life. Honesty and mutual respect occur early in the formative years of psychosocial life, so parents are advised to emphasize these as he grows, develops, and interacts in his world.

When boys are emotionally threatened, they may detach from the situation as a coping mechanism. Parents and educators can recognize and attempt to reconnect them to the situation. Don't let emotions slide; encourage interaction as with conflict resolution. Boys are likely to become defensive when they don't know how to process their emotions. The closer a boy is to others, the more supported and safe he may feel. Encourage boys to ask for feedback (Erwin, 2006). Boys raised with consistent appraisals and constructive criticism will feel more comfortable when others offer suggestions and advice. Help them take the guesswork out of social interactions. All of these are opportunities to help boys understand what they are feeling, why it may be occurring, and what they can proactively do about the situation.

Boys always will struggle with emotions, positive and negative; the healthy approach is acknowledging that he has a wide range of feelings and reactions and that you are a critical lynchpin in his psychosocial development. With enough consistency, love, support, and an understanding of when to step away, a boy will learn the value of his emotions as a tool for advancing communication and better emotional health outcomes in his life.

BOYS AND "RITES OF MANHOOD"

When do boys become men? What does it mean to become a man? Compare this to the female experience. A hallmark event in most young women's lives is the onset of puberty and the menstrual cycle. Most modern societies and cultures agree that a girl has now become a woman. She is able to conceive a child. Clearly, the onset of menstruation is a well-defined concept and time in a girl's transition to womanhood. What befalls a boy as he becomes a man?

In many cultures across the world, numerous ceremonies commemorate a boy's becoming a man. Males for thousands of years have sought a moment in time that defines them as men. Many of these ceremonies are symbolic in nature and are based on the chronological age of the boy. For example, in Judaic traditions, a boy of the age of thirteen typically celebrates becoming a *bar mitzvah*. This ceremony typically coincides with the onset of puberty, but it is considered the moment a boy becomes responsible for his actions as a man (Oppenheimer, 2005). Some cultures, such as those in Malawi Africa, require boys to go through physical tests and feats of strength. In ancient Native American cultures, vision quests, in which preadolescent boys are left alone in the elements, have been recorded. It is expected that the boy becomes aware of himself apart from his parents and elders, thus making him realize he is a man. Some parents (usually fathers) give their boys a ceremonial welcome to manhood that may encompass a variety of sociocultural norms, rights, and traditions. Some of these ceremonies are dangerous and physically and emotionally exhausting. Boys in the island nation of Vanuatu perform land diving, which requires boys as young as eight years old to jump from 100-foot-tall platforms made out of wood and vines to demonstrate their masculinity. It is desirable for the boy's shoulders to scrape the ground in order to prove himself a man. Some Aboriginal tribes in Australia practice "late circumcision," which welcomes a boy into adulthood. Boys are secluded for a week with tribesmen who perform the circumcision without the use of **anesthetics;** essentially, the boys are supposed to prove their manhood by not reacting to any pain. Algonquin Indian tribes in Quebec, Canada, were known to give their boys a powerful drug called *wysoccan* and then place them in cages. It was believed that these boys would have visions to be able to "see" themselves as men (Gilmore, 1990). From physical bravery to psychological awareness, many of these ceremonies were and are performed to inform others that a boy could now function as a man.

In modern Western society, many boys are unsure as to what makes them men. Is it a first sexual experience? Is it when he begins to notice pubertal changes, such as body hair, more muscle, or greater height? Is it when he gets his first job? Boys in Western society often lack a defined "mark" of adulthood. Many boys lack strong male role models or father figures in their lives; therefore, persons who teach them and help them to transition through this important phase of their life become imperative. Boys who are left to figure things out for themselves may find themselves on the wrong side of the law, emotionally distant from others, apathetic toward their own health status, and even depressed and suicidal. Boys need meaning as they move from one stage of life to another. They need emotional support and guidance to help them understand and process their physical health and changes. Boys who feel lost or lack guidance may engage in their own rites of manhood. For example, a boy may smoke or drink to prove he is of age or that he fits into a peer group; he may do something physically aggressive or violent to gain peer acceptance and prove his toughness; he may engage in sexual activity to show others that he is a man through his actions and conquests. Boys will always be tempted to prove themselves, particularly among peers; however, the health consequences of their actions need to be considered.

There are steps parents, caregivers, and members of the family and community can take to enhance a boy's life positively and ease his transition into adolescence and eventually adulthood. A boy needs someone to help him understand the challenges of becoming a man. This can be anyone who cares about him in life, but a male influence will allow for associative connections. Adults can help him define who he is, what he believes, why he believes what he does, who he wants to be, and what he does well in life. Focus on the positives and minimize the negatives. Planned criticism can be phrased as *opportunities to improve* versus *weaknesses.*

Responsibility will undoubtedly challenge a preadolescent boy. All of a sudden he has to *do* things that previously were done *for* him. Help him understand that this is a positive attribute that will help him value what he does as well as show his value and meaning to others in life. A boy raised with a responsible conscience and a virtue of ethics and morality will likely carry over these qualities to others in life. If boys honor and respect themselves, they likely will do the same for others.

Boys need to mature in economic understanding. A boy may have a part-time job, allowance, or other means of gaining money; it is critical that parents and caregivers instill a sense of duty and responsibility in the handling of money. Boys at this age need to learn the differences between "wants" and "needs."

Parents or caregivers are advised to be the primary teachers about boys' physical and sexual changes, whereas schools should augment what is learned at home. This is difficult because many parents lack the time, understanding, and reliable and valid sources of information to educate their sons. Strategies to lessen the divide in preadolescent boys' physical and sexual maturity can be provided by doctors, nurses, health educators, health education programming offered at community centers such as the YMCA or local Boys & Girls Club, and reliable books and online resources (Erwin, 2006).

Social and emotional guidance will help him become self-efficacious and confident. Confidence may help him become resilient and resist drugs, alcohol, sexual activity, and bullying and violence. A boy who knows who he is should be able to exercise his moral and ethical muscles as he interacts with more and diverse social groups. Peer pressure becomes more easily handled and therefore, better health decisions will be possible. Many boys, adolescents, and men search for what they call "respect." Respect is not an inherent right; rather, it needs to be earned through one's actions and representations of oneself to others.

SUMMARY

This chapter opened with a discussion of preadolescence and the "tween" years of boys. The preadolescent boy was discussed from a physical, emotional, and psychosocial perspective. Unintentional injuries were presented as some of the leading causes of injury and death in this age group, particularly in boys. The types of accidents and predisposing factors, such as competiveness and aggression, were elucidated. Endocrine disorders common to developing boys were discussed at length. Specifically, conditions such as Klinefelter's syndrome, dwarfism, and diabetes were presented as they affect boys during this stage of life. The emotional health of preadolescent boys was discussed. Boys' experience of depression was presented. Rates of suicide among boys were discussed and compared to those of girls and males adolescents and men. Emotional intelligence development was presented as a strategy to offset emotional health risks. Last, a brief discussion concerning the passage into manhood through rites was presented in the context of multiple cultures and examples within cultures.

KEY TERMS

Amniocentesis   Aneurysm   Autonomy

Anesthetics   Anxiety   *Bar mitzvah*

Chronic traumatic
encephalopathy (CTE)

Concussion

Empathy

Endocrinologist

Genetic counseling

Homeostatic

Precocious

Resiliency

Retardation

Retrospective

Self-efficacy

Sex-linked

Traumatic brain injury
(TBI)

DISCUSSION QUESTIONS

1. Why do you think height is a coveted trait or attribute in males, particularly in Western society?

2. Compare and contrast fragile X syndrome and Klinefelter's syndrome in terms of their causes, identification and diagnosis, and treatment and management.

3. Why are boys more likely than girls to be successful at suicide? Justify your answer with statistics.

4. How do you think lack of emotional health, emotional intelligence, and outcomes such as depression affect male health? Give examples.

5. What are the three biggest challenges for parents and caregivers of preadolescent boys when helping them transition to adolescence?

6. Research how schools may or may not assist boys in transitioning into adolescence. For schools that have programs to assist boys, describe what they do; for those that don't, explain how this is handled otherwise.

7. Do you think schools are set up to encourage emotional intelligence in boys? Justify your response.

8. Select five cultures not covered in this chapter and briefly describe how they mark a boy's transition to adulthood (manhood).

9. Do you think younger boys should be required to do community service to develop a sense of responsibility or respect? Should schools mandate this? How might this help a boy transition into adolescence? Justify your responses.

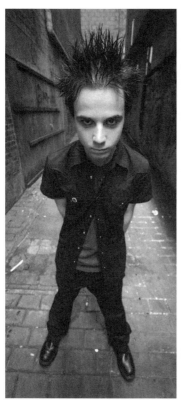

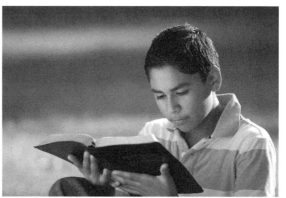

©iStockphoto.com/Aldo Murillo

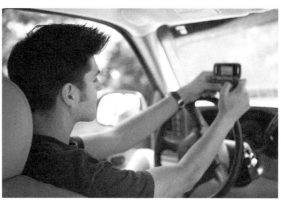

©iStockphoto.com/Jamie Evans

©iStockphoto.com/Pawel Gaul

7

Adolescence

LEARNING OBJECTIVES

- Identify the physical and emotional changes that occur in males during puberty, including the role played by hormones
- Describe the sexual health of adolescent males and apply strategies to stay connected with them
- List the primary signs and symptoms of sexually transmitted infections, rates, trends, and modes of transmission, and preventative strategies
- Evaluate the biology and sociology of homosexuality in males
- Discuss factors that influence adolescent male drug use and abuse and preventative strategies

ADOLESCENCE IS USUALLY defined as the period of time between the onset of puberty and adulthood. Typically, as with any change, it may be difficult for a boy to adjust to this period of life. Body changes bring emotional changes. Socially, boys will join groups, diversify friends and interests, and stray more from the immediate family unit. Those who are well supported and loved may find adolescence to be a welcome time of change that carries with it the wonders of exploration and new journeys. For those left to their own devices, adolescence may be confusing, scary, and a period of time that can make or break their relative health status. There is no specific guide to adolescence, and each person will experience it differently based on his or her culture, society, and background. This chapter presents the physical and emotional changes a boy may experience with adolescence and puberty: sexual and reproductive issues, aggression, violence, and bullying. and social issues.

PHYSICAL CHANGES

Mainly initiated by the influence of hormones, puberty in boys marks the beginning of a cascade of physical changes that prepare a boy to become reproductively viable. The most influential male sex hormone is testosterone, which causes the development of primary and secondary sex characteristics (Marcell, 2007). For example, testosterone causes a boy to develop hair in the pubic and axillary (underarm) regions, on legs and arms, and on the chest. Testosterone also increases lean muscle mass, deepens the voice, and increases sex drive (Bhasin, Woodhouse, & Storer, 2001).

The age at which a boy enters puberty will vary based on his age, family history, and nutritional status, but puberty generally encompasses a range from ages thirteen to nineteen years. Boys typically enter into puberty later than girls by two to three years, which may make a boy feel awkward if he is not on par with a girl. One of the first signs of puberty in boys is the enlargement of his testicles, followed by increases in height, weight, bone mass, shoulder width, and penis growth, among others (Marcell, 2007). Body changes are classified using the Tanner classification stages introduced in Chapter Six. Puberty typically begins in Tanner stage 3 and continues until stage 5. In stage 3, height increases at a rate of 2–3 inches per year, testes increase in size, body hair becomes apparent, the penis increases in length and width, and muscle mass increases along with "cracking" of the voice. In stage 4, height continues to increase at a continued rate of 3 inches or so per year, genitalia become more adult in appearance, and body hair develops in adult patterns throughout the body.

Additionally, due to the strong influence of testosterone and other hormones, **acne** (*acne vulgaris*) may appear on the face and other areas of the body (Bhasin et al., 2001). Acne is perhaps one of the more troubling aspects of puberty because of its visibility, particularly on the face and neck. In Tanner stage 5, peak height is generally attainted by age seventeen, although males may continue to grow in height up until age twenty-five; genitalia are of adult size by age sixteen or seventeen; body and pubic hair are normally dispersed; facial hair is consistent; the physique has an adult appearance; and a male is reproductively viable (Marshall & Tanner, 1970).

PHYSICAL HEALTH

Testicular Exams and Testicular Cancer

Although rates are not very prevalent, the most common periods in life for developing testicular cancer are the teenage years and early adulthood. According to 2009 statistics, there were approximately 8,400 new cases in the United States and 380 deaths as a result. Overall rates were 5.4 per 100,000 according to 2002–2006 statistics. Rates were highest in white/Caucasian males, at rates of 6.3 per 100,000, and lowest in black males, at 1.3 per 100,000. There are two primary types of testicular cancers: seminomas and non-seminomas. *Seminomas* grow inside a testis at a fairly slow rate and often respond well to radiation therapy. *Non-seminomas* grow at a more rapid rate and are less responsive to therapies (National Cancer Institute [NCI], 2009).The exact causes of testicular cancers are not well known; however, genetics and familial patterns, exposure to environmental toxins such as pesticides, and testicular trauma all have been postulated as possible causes (Horner et al., 2008). The main risk factors for developing testicular cancer are *cryptorchidism* (undescended testicle), unusual testicular development, white/Caucasian race, family history, and genetic disorders such as Klinefelter's syndrome (see Chapter Six) (NCI, 2009).

Prevention of testicular cancer (*primary prevention*) is the most desirable strategy. Screening for testicular cancer (*secondary prevention*) is a relatively simple process that can be conducted by the adolescent or young adult himself. Screening is used to identify any abnormalities that may exist and can be managed by a medical professional. Routine physical examinations, such as for sports participation, should assess for the presence of testicular abnormalities. Treatment (also known as *tertiary prevention*) is the least effective outcome due to the fact that the cancer is already present.

Changes of the testes may include acute pain, increase in size or a decrease in size of a testis, a heavy feeling in the scrotum, aching or pain in the groin or lower abdomen (unrelated to other causes), and abnormal fluid collection in the scrotum. Most males have one testicle that hangs lower than the other (usually the left side) and some have dilated (enlarged) veins on one side that may be benign (called a *varicocele*) (NCI, 2009).These factors don't necessarily mean a person has cancer, but they should be checked out by a medical professional.

Diagnosis of testicular cancer and other abnormalities can be conducted by a trained health care professional, such as a physician, physician's assistant, or nurse practitioner. Tests such as blood panels, physical examination, and diagnostic ultrasonography all can confirm the presence of pathologies. Perhaps more effective are consistent self-monitoring practices such as testicular self-exams or TSEs. Health professionals should advise adolescents about this fairly simple process that should be performed at least once per month by males age fourteen or older. The main advantage of performing TSEs monthly is to understand what "normal" feels like so that if something does indeed change, the adolescent can seek medical care by a primary care physician or urologist. For teenage males, discussing sensitive issues like this often is embarrassing, which may preclude identification, diagnosis, and effective treatment of disease. It is very important for health professionals, parents, and caregivers to openly discuss overall health with boys, even sensitive topics such as the genitals.

Gynecomastia

Another fairly common issue in adolescent males is the development of excess breast tissue, called *gynecomastia,* usually around the areola of the nipples. Thirty to 60% of adolescents may experience gynecomastia (Braunstein, 1993). This is a mostly benign condition that may or may not resolve with age. The main reasons for the development of gynecomastia are previous family history, excess hormonal levels, drug use (anabolic steroids and marijuana), and environmental toxins and exposures. Because adolescence involves many shifts in circulating hormone levels, all body tissues can be affected. For example, when estrogen levels are higher, adipose (fat) tissue may increase and deposit in and/or around the breast of a male (Braunstein, 1993).

Some males may develop gynecomastia due to drug use or environmental exposures. Chronic marijuana and anabolic steroid use often lead to the development of gynecomastia. The active drug in marijuana, delta-9-tetrahydrocannabinol or THC promotes the retention of fatty tissue and may cause or exacerbate gynecomastia. Chronic use of anabolic steroids also may cause gynecomastia; because as testosterone breaks down in the body, it is metabolically converted into various forms of estrogen, which in turn promotes fat retention and distribution patterns around the breasts among other areas of the body (Bembo, 2004).

Although gynecomastia is usually not an area of concern, it can be very distressful for the developing teenager. Gynecomastia may prompt issues with self-esteem and confidence. Some males may be teased or ridiculed as being less of a man because of breast tissue development. Gynecomastia in adolescence usually resolves within a couple of years as hormone levels normalize (Braunstein, 1993). Drugs such as tamoxifen and therapies can reduce tissue growth. Compression garments can be worn to make the tissue less obvious to others; in less common instances surgery to remove the excess tissue may be warranted (Bembo, 2004; Braunstein, 1993).

It is important for parents and caregivers to encourage males to discuss their concerns and help them understand what is occurring in their body. Reinforce that these changes are normal and often will pass with time and development.

Breast Cancer

Although breast cancer usually occurs in females, males are affected by it, with rates suggesting that approximately 1% of all breast cancers occur in males. Testosterone helps to suppress breast tissue growth, which is why males are less likely to experience this form of cancer. Various risk factors in men, such as exposure to radiation, higher levels of estrogen, genetics, Klinefelter's syndrome, and exposure to certain drugs and chemicals, are associated with breast cancer (American Cancer Society [ACS], 2010). Adolescent males are encouraged to conduct periodic breast self-exams (BSEs) in addition to TSEs. If any anomalies are found or suspected, the adolescent is advised to consult a primary care physician.

PSYCHOLOGICAL AND EMOTIONAL CHANGES

Males also undergo dramatic changes in their emotional and psychological status accompanying the physical changes associated with puberty (Marcell, 2007). A boy may become withdrawn, moody, or aggressive. Most boys will experience these emotional changes as they attempt to define who they are and what they represent. However, as described in Chapter Six, depression and other emotional problems may go unrecognized because people often judge male inexpressiveness as normal. While it is true that boys will differ in their relative expressiveness and social engagement, parents and health providers need to be acutely aware of pathological emotions that can harm adolescent boys' health (Vernon, Petrides, Bratko, & Schermer, 2008). Avoidance, anger, reactivity to criticism, physical pains, and isolation from specific groups of people are not normal elements of male puberty.

Puberty is confusing because of the physical changes, but the emotional changes that accompany them are equally challenging for a boy to process. Many boys will not express themselves adequately or even appropriately and therefore may act out their emotions. This is where support, love, and encouragement of the development of emotional intelligence will assist him in progressing in a healthy manner.

One of the strongest areas of influence concerning psychological and emotional health lies within the realm of body image. Body image health has been an understudied area in male health for decades, although recent research has made some inroads (Pope, Phillips, & Olivardia, 2000). *Body image* is defined as the internal, subjective representations of physical appearance and bodily experience as well as a multidimensional phenomenon that plays a vital role in dramatically influencing quality of life (Phillips, 1998). Males with positive and healthy body images typically are able to handle life's challenges and experience limited negative consequences, whereas those with a low sense of body image also have lower resiliency skills, self-esteem, and poorer health outcomes. For example, males with a low self-esteem and a negative sense of body image are more likely to bully others, join gangs, use **illicit drugs,** and engage in promiscuous sexual activity (Kanayama, Pope, & Hudson, 2001; Lenehan, 2003). Understanding male body image is important for parents and educators so as to promote good health choices while at the same time being acutely aware of negative factors that reduce health in this population. For example, during puberty, boys usually are highly self-conscious, even though they may not outwardly show it. Because it traditionally has been viewed as unmasculine to worry or express concern about one's looks as a male, boys are caught in a health **paradox.** That is, expressing concern may provoke criticism from others, particularly other males, but holding in one's emotions and feelings may lead to further internal conflict.

VIGNETTE

Claude slowly walked into the guidance counselor's office for the fourth time this week. He was agitated and obviously dejected. Mrs. Creswell greeted Claude in her usual cheerful tone only to get a barely audible grunt out of him. She smiled and asked him to have a seat. Mrs. Creswell certainly knew who she was dealing with, having seen countless adolescent boys in her nearly thirty years of experience at the high school level.

"Claude, how are ya? I'm certainly getting to know a lot about you lately!"

Claude barely made any eye contact with Mrs. Creswell as he uttered, "Yeah. . . ."

Mrs. Creswell knew she somehow had to relate to Claude to get the ball rolling.

"So, how did the Bruins do at Fenway the other day, Claude?"

(Continued)

After looking up and trying to control his laughter, Claude replied, "Huh . . . haha-hahaha. . . . Oh, you mean the Red Sox, right?"

"No, I meant the Bruins, Claude, how are they doing?"

Again Claude smirked and said, "Yeah, okay, the Bruins have been losing bad lately, not sure why, 'cause their effort has been really solid, but the goaltender has been a little weak."

"What would you do with the team or goaltender if you were coach?"

Claude eagerly replied, "Well, for starters, I would have him take more practice time. . . ."

"Yeah, what would you emphasize in practice, Claude?"

"I would drill him with some new stuff, so he knew what other teams bring at him, like a new drill I was reading about online."

At this moment, Mrs. Creswell knew she had Claude; she opened him up through a commonality and something that was relative to him. "Geesh, Claude, you're pretty strict, would he have to be at practice every day and on time?"

"Of course!" Claude responded, "That is how ya get better!" At that very moment, Claude looked at Mrs. Creswell and uttered in his low tone, "Okay, I got it. . . ."

"Excuse me, Claude, what was that you said?"

"I said I got it, I know what you are doing." He smirked at her.

"And what is that?"

"You're trying to make me see that I need to be like the goaltender or coach; I need to be more consistent, focused, and dedicated to school. . . . Like I said, I got it."

"Okay, Claude, well . . . getting it is good. How are you gonna practice it and put it into action?"

"I dunno."

"Well, what would the Boston Braves do?"

"Huh?!"

"You heard me, what would the Braves do?"

"it's the Red Sox, Mrs. Creswell!"

"Is it, Claude? Perhaps you need to dig a bit deeper in your sports history lessons."

"I'm really confused now, is this about my schoolwork, sports, history, or what?!"

"Yes," Mrs. Creswell replied.

"Yes, what, Mrs. Creswell?"

"Yes, you get my point. . . . I think you are able to relate to what I am saying and what I am asking from you Claude."

"So, what should I do, Mrs. Creswell?"

"Help that goaltender be the best he can, Claude!"

"Gotcha. . . Thanks!"

As Claude got up from the chair, Mrs. Creswell knew that she would be seeing him again, but there now was a bond, a connection that might help Claude continue to navigate the world of high school and adolescence.

The onset of puberty presents another area of concern for boys. Feeling as if he is not physically maturing at the pace of his peers may provoke undue distress in a male's psyche. Additionally, a boy's body image may be distorted. A boy who experiences puberty earlier may feel empowered because of his physical prowess relative to others, but he also may feel confused. Conversely, a boy who is late in development may have feelings of inadequacy and anxiety, especially in the presence of his peers. Boys often insult and test each other's limits so as to establish social hierarchies; therefore, a boy who experiences growth and development later versus sooner may undergo teasing and even physical harassment. Teasing, harassment, and bullying can test the psychological limits of a boy, with some becoming so anxious and depressed that suicide becomes a valid option.

SEXUAL HEALTH, SEXUALITY, AND SEXUAL ORIENTATION

Sexual health is a key feature as a boy develops and experiences changes associated with puberty. "Sexual health is a state of physical, emotional, mental and social wellbeing in relation to sexuality; it is not merely the absence of disease, dysfunction or infirmity. Sexual health requires a positive and respectful approach to sexuality and sexual relationships, as well as the possibility of having pleasurable and safe sexual experiences, free of coercion, discrimination and violence" (World Health Organization [WHO], 2002). The effects of hormones, especially testosterone, provoke the development of secondary sex characteristics and also the ability to become reproductively viable. Hormones and other factors create strong physical and emotional feelings, desires, and urges during development. For example, males may experience spontaneous erections, become distracted by someone they are attracted to, and explore and experiment with their sexuality and bodies (Bhasin et al., 2001). Normal sexual health and development involves an awareness of intrapersonal, interpersonal, and social factors that influence health and health-related behavior (Serrant-Green & McLuskey, 2008). Unfortunately, some males don't understand or are not given the proper guidance to appreciate these factors and make errors in judgment. Several factors, such as education and awareness, community health care and programming, and health care services, contribute to sexual health.

Sexually Transmitted Infections

One of the primary topics in the area of sexual health is infectious diseases, their rates, prevalence, transmission, and prevention. Formerly referred to as sexually transmitted diseases (STDs) and venereal diseases (VD), sexually transmitted infections (STIs) are various infections that *cause* disease processes to occur. There are many infections that can cause problems and disease, such as chlamydia, syphilis, gonorrhea, HIV/AIDS, human papilloma virus (HPV), genital herpes, and several others. It is important to realize that STIs can be passed on from anyone to anyone regardless of sex, sexual orientation, age, race/ethnicity, or times of exposure. Even limiting sexual encounters does not guarantee a person will not be infected. Infections can occur in several ways, including skin-to-skin contact, penile-vaginal contact, oral sex, anal sex, and exposures to various bodily fluids (mucous, blood, semen, and vaginal secretions). Each type of infection has its own way of affecting a person and causing signs, symptoms, and disease. Common signs and symptoms of a STI in a male may include discharge from the penis, tenderness of the scrotum and testes, irritation of the penis, difficulty and/or pain while urinating, and flu-like symptoms (U.S. Department of Health and Human Services [USDHHS], 2009).

In the United States, some of the more common infections in males are genital herpes, HPV, gonorrhea, and chlamydia. Females have higher rates for chlamydia and gonorrhea than males; however, males were much higher in rates of syphilis: 11.1 per 100,000 as compared to 1.5 per 100,000 for females as of 2009. Rates also may be higher in women for the other STIs because females are more likely to seek screening, therefore increasing reported rates. Chlamydia infections have been increasing overall, but are twelve times higher in black males than white males. Syphilis rates are five times higher in men than women and are particularly prevalent in men who have sex with men (MSM) (USDHHS, 2009). Worldwide, STIs are a growing problem. The WHO estimates that 340 million new cases of syphilis, gonorrhea, chlamydia, and trichomoniasis occurred throughout the world in 1999 in men and women ages 15–49 years, with newer data showing similar trends. The largest number of new infections occurred in the regions of South and Southeast Asia, followed by sub-Saharan Africa, Latin America, and the Caribbean. The highest rate of new cases per 1,000 population occurred in sub-Saharan Africa (WHO, 2002).

Chlamydia   Chlamydia infections are more common in females than in males, but males are implicated in the spread and transmission of this infection (Weinstock, Berman, & Cates, 2004). Chlamydia is caused by the bacterium *Chlamydia trachomatis* and may cause severe repercussions in females. The infection can be transmitted through vaginal, anal, and oral sex and can be passed on from mother to child during childbirth. Chlamydia infections annually have the highest rates compared to all other STIs in the United States. Additionally, chlamydia rates are higher in men who have sex with men due to the higher incidence of anal and oral sex.

Overall, chlamydia is referred to as the "silent infection" because it typically has very few obvious signs and symptoms, particularly in men, and symptoms often take weeks to appear if they do at all. The primary symptom in males is discharge from the tip of the penis; other symptoms include itching and irritation around the urethral opening and painful urination. Rectal pain, bleeding, and discharge are common with chlamydia in those who have receptive anal intercourse as in MSM (Weinstock et al., 2004).

If unrecognized or left untreated, most males will not experience severe consequences. Many men go unaware of their infection status, which leads to more infections. In rare occasions, the infection can spread to the epididymus and testes, which can cause permanent damage and even sterility in some cases. Identifying the infection can be done through **urinalysis** and site cultures from the penis or infection site. Treatment is fairly effective, with a course of **antibiotics,** such as azithromycin or doxycycline (Weinstock et al., 2004; USDHHS, 2009). The best method of treatment is prevention. Knowing infection risk and status can help curb the spread of the infection.

Syphilis   Caused by the bacterium *Treponema pallidum*, syphilis is more common in males than females, with rates almost six times higher in males. This infection is tricky to distinguish because it shares many common signs and symptoms with other infections, which is why it has earned the nickname of the "great imitator" (Weinstock et al., 2004). Primary and secondary syphilis was noted in 36,000 identified cases in the United States in 2006, with rates increasing in males from 2000 to 2006. As of 2006, nearly 64% of all primary and secondary syphilis was documented in MSM (USDHHS, 2009). Syphilis is transmitted through direct contact with a person who has an active syphilitic sore (a *chancre*) typically found on the genitals, rectum, anus, and even the mouth and lips. In some instances, a pregnant mother can transmit it to her baby. The sores in the primary stage of the disease are typically small and may go unrecognized for months and even years. Many people may not know their infection status because of this, with typical incubation times being between 10 and 90 days with an average of 21 days until the first symptoms appear. The chancre often is painless and resolves in 3 to 6 weeks; therefore, many people assume the infection has left the system and they are healthy again (Weinstock et al., 2004). No symptoms often equals no follow-up with trained medical professionals, thus increasing the chances of passing it on to another person. Additionally, adolescent males may be embarrassed discussing anything about their bodies, especially their genitals, thereby lessening the chance of curtailing the progression and transmission of this infection.

Left untreated, syphilis goes from a primary infection stage to a secondary stage where skin rashes throughout the body and lesions on mucous membranes begin to appear. Rashes vary in severity and are not always apparent and noticeable. A person also may develop flu-like symptoms such as fever, fatigue, sore throat, headaches, and weight loss, which also complicate the recognition, diagnosis, and treatment process. Moreover, the symptoms of secondary syphilis will resolve on their own with time; however, the disease may enter a latent stage in approximately 15% of the population and may take ten to twenty years to manifest. During the latent stages, a person's internal organs, such as the brain, heart, and central nervous system, become affected, which may lead to poor muscle control, coordination, dementia, and even death. Syphilis can be diagnosed by examining the material in a sore or through a blood test for antibodies. Treatment is relatively simple if syphilis is caught in the early stages of the disease, with courses of antibiotics. The disease can recur if it is not appropriately treated or prevented in subsequent exposures (Weinstock et al., 2004).

Education is paramount, particularly because many of the signs and symptoms of this disease are relatively obscure. Additionally, the co-occurrence of syphilis and HIV infection is very high, with a two- to fivefold increase in the likelihood of contracting HIV (USDHHS, 2009). Because syphilis and other STIs can cause open sores, the transmission of HIV is markedly increased with unprotected exposures (Weinstock et al., 2004). Realistic sexuality education that focuses on primary refusal skills as an outcome, and safer sexual practices, such as 100% use of latex condoms and other barrier methods, need to be advocated with adolescent males. Males who engage in sexual activity with other males need to be targeted for reliable and valid quality sexual health information.

Gonorrhea   Another very common bacterial STI is gonorrhea (USDHHS, 2009). This infection is caused by the bacterium *Neisseria gonorrhoeae* and readily thrives in the warm, moist, and dark environments of the reproductive tract, mouth, throat, eyes, and anus (Weinstock et al., 2004). According to Centers for Disease Control and Prevention (CDC) estimates, gonorrheal infections are annually among the most common STIs in the United States, with rates estimated at 120.9 infections per 100,000 persons (USDHHS, 2009). Gonorrhea is primarily transmitted via contact with infected tissues, such as the mouth, anus, vagina, and penis. The most at-risk groups for this STI are sexually active teenagers, young adults, and African American groups.

Many people who are infected with gonorrhea don't know their status because signs and symptoms are typically "silent." The range of symptoms makes recognition and diagnosis a challenge, which can perpetuate subsequent infections. Many males will not experience obvious signs or symptoms; however, some may experience burning with urination, a white, yellow, or green discharge from the tip of the penis, and swelling of the testes. Rectal infections may produce bleeding, itching, and general soreness. If symptoms do occur, they may take upward of 30 days or longer to develop, thereby increasing the likelihood for passing on infection to other people (Weinstock et al., 2004).

Left untreated, gonorrhea can cause serious physical health consequences, such as epididymitis, which inflames the tubules attached to the testes. Long-term infection can lead to sterility or blood and joint infections (Weinstock et al., 2004). People with gonorrhea are more likely to contract HIV as well as transmit it to others because of sores and other open infections (USDHHS, 2009). Gonorrhea can be diagnosed through cultures obtained by swabbing infected areas and through urinalysis if it is present in the urethra. A Gram stain sample can be conducted in a doctor's office or clinic and can be read onsite; these tests generally work better in males than females. Treatment for gonorrhea and other bacterial infections is a course of antibiotics (Weinstock, 2004). Recently, however, resistant strains of gonorrhea have surfaced, making treatment a challenge, particularly for people who have more than one type of STI (Vastag, 2009). The CDC strongly recommends that a person who tests positive for gonorrhea is checked for all other STIs (USDHHS, 2009). Early recognition and treatment of gonorrhea is critical to avoid future consequences; however, prevention is key. As with most other bacterial STIs, education, limiting exposure, and use of protective barrier devices and methods (such as latex condoms and **dental dams**) should be encouraged, especially in adolescent populations who may be more sexually active.

Human Immunodeficiency Virus and Acquired Immunodeficiency Syndrome

One of the more higher-profile STIs is the human immunodeficiency virus (HIV), which causes acquired immunodeficiency syndrome (AIDS) and

AIDS-related complex (ARC). The virus itself gained the attention of the world in the early 1980s with its mysterious symptoms afflicting many gay men. Soon thereafter public health officials recognized that it was more than just a gay man's disease; it infected countless people (Weiss, 1993). The virus invades, manipulates, and eventually destroys the host's T-cells, which enable a person to fight off infection.

When T-cell levels fall too low, a person may become unable to fight off simple bacteria, viruses, and other infections. These infections prey on the compromised immune system, earning the title "opportunistic infections." As the infections increase, the body is gradually unable to recover and begins to systematically shut down as HIV progresses to AIDS. A person dies from complications due to AIDS, such as cancers, dementia, and pneumonia, and not directly from HIV (Centers for Disease Control and Prevention [CDC], National Center for HIV/AIDS, Viral Hepatitis, STD, and TB Prevention [NCHHSTP], 2009). Worldwide, HIV/AIDS has decimated many nations and countries, but in particular the continent of Africa (Worobey et al., 2008). Once viewed as an acute infection that claimed the life of a person usually within one year, in Western society HIV/AIDS is more commonly referred to as a chronic disease like cancer. Advances in medical care, diagnosis, treatment, and medications have made a positive impact in the health of people with HIV/AIDS; however, worldwide, there is much to be done (Bowman, Archin, & Margolis, 2009).

Gay and bisexual males, referred to by the CDC as men who have sex with men, continue to be the highest risk group for HIV/AIDS. All racial groups are affected by this disease; however, MSM HIV/AIDS rates are the only ones in the United States that are rising versus stabilizing. Nearly half of the one million-plus people living with HIV/AIDS in the United States are MSM (48% or 532,000 cases), and more than half (53%) of all new infections (28,700 cases) are MSM (CDC, USDHHS, 2009). Greater educational and prevention efforts need to be targeted to younger male populations, especially among America's gay and bisexual male youth. The age of onset of new infections for HIV/AIDS differs by racial/ethnic categories in the United States. Young black and Hispanic males are infected at younger ages than are white male populations. For example, young black males ages

Table 7.1   New HIV/AIDS Infections by Race/Ethnicity

Source: CDC, NCHHSTP (2009).

Age Grouping	White MSM	Black MSM	Hispanic MSM
13–29 years old	3,330	**5,220***	2,300
30–39 years old	4,670	2,470	1,870
40–49 years old	3,740	1,860	950
50+ years old	1,480	640	270

13–29* have nearly twice the rates of HIV infection of any other group (white or Hispanic). Table 7.1 details estimates of new HIV/AIDS infection in the United States (CDC, NCHHSTP, 2009).

Due to the nature of HIV infections, many of the younger males who have it don't know their status (HIV-positive or HIV-negative). According to one study conducted in five major U.S. cities, nearly 80% of young males (ages 18–24) did not know they were infected with the virus, which partially explains why this disease has been so difficult to control in younger male populations (CDC, 2009).

Advocacy and education targeted at younger male populations, particularly MSM, may help promote safer sexual practices. The simple fact that HIV is so prevalent and that many younger males don't know their infection status calls our current HIV/AIDS educational efforts into question. Knowing level of risk and getting tested once or twice per year (or more often if a person engages in high-risk sexual activity, such as multiple partners or not using protection) will help enhance a person's knowledge of his or her health and thereby may decrease new infections and control present ones. Many younger males are complacent about the risk and damaging effects of HIV/AIDS because many of them were born after the early scares and epidemics of the early 1980s. Moreover, younger people, particularly males, often feel a sense of invincibility about their health, while others believe treatments and even cures are available if they should become sick. Therefore, it must be stressed to younger populations that HIV/AIDS risk *is* real and it is *not* curable at this time. Other younger males may fear the social stigma associated with HIV/AIDS and may not want to reveal their sexual orientations. Delaying diagnosis and care can lead to severe health consequences in the future.

Substance use and abuse is fairly common in younger male populations; therefore, drug advocacy and educational programs need to be tailored and targeted to younger male populations. HIV/AIDS and adolescent risk factors are quite common in heterosexual males as well as homosexuals and bisexuals. All people need to be prepared to handle this potentially life-threatening STI. The CDC (CDC, NCHHSTP, 2009) recommends that health professionals initiate the following concerning HIV/AIDS:

- Give the facts about HIV/AIDS to adolescent males so they know how it is transmitted and how it can be prevented.

- Recommend that adolescent males get tested and know their HIV status.

- Advise younger males to take control and lower their risk status; abstain from sexual activity or remain in a monogamous relationship in which safer sexual practices are used (100% condom use and other barrier methods).

- Suggest that males talk to others about HIV/AIDS; the more knowledge and freedom to discuss this issue, the less stigma and fear will be associated with it.

Human Papilloma Virus   HPV can cause cervical dysplasia (abnormal cells) and possibly cervical cancer in females. In 2008 the American Cancer Society estimated that more than 11,000 women would be diagnosed with cervical cancer in the United States (Dunne et al., 2007). Often, the public's perception of HPV is that it is a female disease and that males are immune. Contrary to this belief, males are equally affected by the disease but may show less severe symptoms and consequences and therefore may never know that they have the virus (USDHHS, 2009). In fact, according to the CDC, most people in the United States will have HPV at some point in their lives, making it one of the most common STIs in the country (CDC, NCHHSTP, 2009). Such high rates of infection (upward of 50% lifetime incidence and approximately 6.2 million new infections per year) indicate that HPV needs to be controlled and prevented (Dunne, Unger, & Sternberg, 2007; Planned Parenthood, n.d.).

Infections mainly are caused by sexual contact with an infected individual. There are more than forty variants of this virus, and the fact that it is a virus versus bacteria make it a challenge to control and suppress because there are currently no cures for viral infections (Weinstock et al., 2004).

Some strains of HPV are known to cause penile and anal cancers, but they are relatively rare, with rates lower than 1% in the population (Koutsky & Kiviat, 1999). Penile cancer affects 1 in 100,000 males in the United States, and anal cancer was reported in 1,900 males in 2007. Obviously HPV is not as damaging and threatening as some other STIs in male populations (USDHHS, 2009). Some populations are more at risk than others for HPV infection. According to the CDC in 2009, HPV rates were markedly higher in gay and bisexual male populations, which increases the chances for developing deadly forms of anal cancer in men (CDC, NCHHSTP, 2009). MSM, as well as males who have compromised immune systems (as caused by HIV/AIDS), have anal and penile HPV rates seventeen times as high as comparative populations (CDC, NCHHSTP, 2009).

Myth: Males cannot get the human papilloma virus.

Fact: This is completely false! The operative word here is human, meaning it affects and infects anyone. Females may develop cervical cancer, whereas males often are asymptomatic, have genital warts, or in some rare cases, develop penile cancer (Castle & Scarinci, 2009).

Many males don't know they are infected because HPV presents few to no symptoms. If symptoms do appear, they are likely to be one or more small bumps (warts) that may appear on the penis, scrotum, groin, thighs, and anus. Warts usually are small and flat and may group together and take on a "cauliflower-like" appearance. They can appear as small bumps or an accumulation of bumps, often referred to as a *condyloma* or *condyloma accumunata*. These grouping of warts often are **benign** but may pose issues with self-esteem. Most warts don't hurt, some may itch, and they may take several weeks to months to develop after sexual contact. Warts in the anus may itch, bleed, discharge fluid, and obstruct bowel movements and **defecation** as well as cause swelling in the groin region and lymph nodes. Some males may mistake anal warts for hemorrhoids, which present with similar signs and symptoms, and thus delay diagnosis and care.

Testing for HPV in males is a challenge as there are no available tests to confirm its presence; therefore, many males may unknowingly pass the virus to another person through sexual contact. The use of white vinegar (acetic acid) can help confirm the presence of flat warts, as it causes them to turn a lighter color relative to the surrounding skin. **Pap tests** of the anal tissue also are suggested in MSM due to the high prevalence of anal cancer in these groups. Some physicians may elect to treat apparent warts with antiviral suppressant medications, freezing, surgical removal, or no treatment at all (USDHHS, 2009).

Prevention of HPV is very difficult even with regular condom use. Areas not covered by a condom may come in contact with the virus and thus become infected; therefore **abstinence** is the only way to prevent and protect oneself from HPV infection. With such a high prevalence of HPV in the general population, monogamy is strongly recommended as well as regular checkups and screenings (Koutsky & Kiviat, 1999). If males don't see symptoms, they may not realize they can pass on a virus that has much more deadly consequences for others, particularly females. Many cervical cancers are caused by HPV strains; therefore, males need to be aware that their actions may not directly affect them but may adversely affect a female at some time (Myers, McCrory, Nanda, Bastian, & Matchar, 2000).

Vaccinations for HPV   Most females appear to contract HPV between the ages of fourteen and twenty-four years old (CDC, 2007), which is why primary prevention efforts in *both* males and females need to be initiated. Since 2006, females have had the option of two vaccinations, Gardasil and Cervarix, which were approved for use in females by the Food and Drug Administration (FDA). With males a common **vector** in the transmission of HPV, prevention such as vaccinations for males is continually discussed in the realm of public health.

In the United Kingdom, Gardasil has been licensed for use in males from ages nine to twenty-six years old, and there is a recommendation to the FDA in the United States to follow suit (Castle & Scarinci, 2009). However, safety and efficacy testing still preclude vaccinations from being recommended for males (CDC, NCHHSTP, 2009).

In a *New York Times* article entitled "Vaccinating Boys for Girls' Sake?" (Hoffman, 2008), the ethical and sociocultural issues of the topic were presented and discussed. Is it ethical to expect males to be vaccinated for the protection of others? Is this **paternalism**? Some people, mainly parents, have stated their opposition to males receiving HPV vaccinations because they view it as an issue of chivalry rather than of public health. Others view male vaccinations as an opportunity to protect both sexes, a win-win situation for public health.

In another study, 115 young males ages eighteen to twenty-three were asked if they would receive an HPV vaccine. Of this sample, 35.7% stated they would not because they were not having penile-vaginal sex, they did not know about HPV, and they lived in rural areas (Crosby, Benitez, & Young, 2008). There is an apparent educational gap concerning HPV: not having penile-vaginal sex does not protect against HPV because it also is transmitted by skin-to-skin contact. Moreover, MSM may interpret this differently because of the term *vaginal,* whereas anal and oral sex may not come to mind. Not knowing about HPV seems to have lessened perceived risk of infection in this sample. Certainly, the infection rates according to the CDC indicate that HPV is common in both sexes (USDHHS, 2009). Living in a rural area may indicate lack of access to education and health care agencies; therefore, males may view lack of access as a barrier to getting the vaccination.

A recent study assessed public opinion that would require middle school students to be vaccinated against HPV. Results showed that approximately 25% of the sample favored vaccination for *both* boys and girls, 35.5% were opposed in general, and the remainder were "unsure" (Crosby et al., 2008). Having a higher educational status and being white prompted people to be less inclined to have children vaccinated for HPV. These findings may indicate denial or fear of stigma among middle-class society about a problem that is generally associated with people of lower socioeconomic status.

Dr. Jonathan L. Temte, associate professor in the Department of Family Medicine at the University of Wisconsin School of Medicine and Public Health, summed up the issue in the eyes of public health: "There is probably no reason to think it would not be effective in boys, and because HPV is passed back and forth, immunizing a large part of the population would limit transmission" (Thompson, 2008).

Questions such as who should bear the costs of vaccination and whether there should be sanctions for those who choose not to get it need to be considered in current and future perspectives on males and public health. Ultimately, the best prevention against HPV is abstinence; however, realism concerning male sexual health needs to be put forth on the table and discussed.

Genital Herpes   Genital herpes (GH) is an STI caused by the herpes simplex virus-1 (HSV-1) or herpes simplex virus-2 (HSV-2) (USDHHS, 2009). HSV-2 is the most common cause of genital herpes, and according to the CDC, approximately 1 out 5 Americans has had genital herpes as an adolescent or adult. Rates are higher in females than males (1 in 4 versus 1 in 8), likely because of how the virus is transmitted (CDC, NCHHSTP, 2009; Xu et al., 2006). The virus is transmitted by open sores, usually on the genitalia, during sexual contact, but it also may be transmitted by oral-genital contact (HSV-1 type). Similar to HPV, many people with GH don't know that they are infected and therefore increase the likelihood for passing on the infection to another individual. Signs and symptoms of GH usually are obvious, as blisters and sores form in the genital area. This process may take several weeks to occur and is usually accompanied by flu-like symptoms, but it resolves within 2 to 4 weeks. Some outbreaks are very mild and may be mistaken for a rash or insect bites. People usually experience subsequent outbreaks, particularly when under stress or if they have suppressed immune systems (USDHHS, 2009). GH may predispose people to other STIs such as HIV/AIDS.

Lab tests, visual inspection, and some blood work can detect the presence of GH, and antiviral, suppressive medications can help limit outbreaks and the active infection period. There is no cure for GH at this time (Weinstock et al., 2004).

The best prevention of GH is abstaining from sexual contact. To minimize risk and exposure, people need to limit their number of sexual partners and always use protective barrier methods such as condoms. It is important to know one's infection status; therefore, health professionals should advise adolescent males who may be in risk categories to get tested on a regular basis.

Prevention of STIs

Overall, risk is high in both male and female populations, but in particular, adolescents may have a greater risk for contracting a STI. Many STIs don't have cures; therefore, a lifetime of consequences and outbreaks may ensue if proper education, advocacy, and care are not taken while a male is younger. Adolescence is a critical time to help males make good, sound sexual choices, but this is only possible with comprehensive sexuality education. The psychosocial effects of sexual pressures and cultural norms need to be understood by parents, teachers, and health educators to help adolescents make the best choices.

Safer Sexual Practices   Safer sexual practices encompass many areas. Essentially, *safer sex* is anything that reduces the risk of getting an infection, which often is confused with *safe sex* (Planned Parenthood, n.d.). The only true safe sex method is abstinence, which may not be a reality for many adolescent males due to hormonal, peer, and sociocultural influences. Safer sex indicates an awareness of the process (Planned Parenthood, n.d.). There does not need to be an exchange of body fluids for infection to occur. Skin-to-skin contact may transmit infection, so even regular use of condoms and others barrier devices are not 100% effective.

It is important for parents, educators, and health professionals to inform adolescents as to what constitutes risk. For example, many people believe that oral sex (fellatio and cunnilingus) is safer sex, but there is contact and possible exchange of bodily fluids. This will likely always be a tough health topic to impress upon teenage males because of their perceived invincibility, lack of sufficient foresight, social pressures to conform to an ideal masculine standard, sexual experimentation, surging hormones, and possible influence of drugs and alcohol. Consistent, reliable, and communicative strategies will yield better results and outcomes than simply ignoring the issue.

Not all school systems support comprehensive sexuality education; therefore, parents need to help teens process their emotions, practices, and the vast amount of sexuality information and misinformation that is out there. Quality, valid, and reliable sources of sexuality-related information as recommended by health professionals can assist in this process.

Other Male Sexual Health Topics

Contraception/Birth Control   Many adolescent males fear getting a young woman pregnant. Preventing pregnancy at an early age is important, because teens typically are not financially, emotionally, and educationally ready to support and raise a child (Planned Parenthood, n.d.). Adolescent males may not fear pregnancy as much as females do because young males often do not see themselves as the primary caretakers and supporters of the child. Teenage fathers do in fact have a responsibility to their children and need to be present in the children's life so as to break the cycle of fatherless children, especially boys.

Contraception and birth control are key prevention strategies to minimize the chances of unwanted pregnancies. Contraception does not mean protection from STIs; this should be stressed by health professionals, in educational programs, as well as in frank sexuality discussions with parents and caregivers. The main forms of contraception and birth control in teenage males are likely to be abstinence and condoms (Oberne & McDermott, 2010). Abstinence is an option, and if it is viewed as a method, it has a failure rate like other methods.

When used correctly, latex condoms are 99% effective at preventing pregnancy (Planned Parenthood, n.d.); the operative term here is *correctly*. Many males don't know how to appropriately store, apply, and dispose of condoms. Checking expiration dates and proper storage are important factors to consider so that condoms do not rip or otherwise fail to protect. Many males store condoms in their wallets, which causes friction and heat that can break down the latex. Applying a condom can present a challenge if a teen has never practiced before his first sexual encounter (Oberne & McDermott, 2010). Additionally, the intensity of the moment may cloud judgment and lead to improper application of the condom on the penis. Practice on models (dildos), fruit (cucumbers or bananas), or even on oneself can be useful, even though the boy may be embarrassed. Consider demonstrations, books, and media clips; otherwise, a young male may not feel confident or competent in using them on a regular basis and thus becomes at risk for infections and pregnancy (Oberne & McDermott, 2010). Removal of the condom is very important and often overlooked. Improperly removing a used condom can spill its contents, thereby increasing the chance of pregnancy and STI exposure (Oberne & McDermott, 2010). Contraception needs to be openly discussed with teen boys, but more important, teens need to be directed in actions they can take to reduce their risk of pregnancy and STIs.

Buying condoms can be a challenging experience for adult males, let alone adolescents. Frank discussions about contraceptive options are a good start. Health professionals should advise parents to reinforce the potential embarrassment of having to see a doctor about a STI or going to a friend's parents to discuss the fact she is pregnant in their discussions with teens. Shopping for condoms may be unnerving, but helping a teen realize it is part of responsible sexual health decisions is the ultimate goal.

Peyronie's Disease   Many younger males experience anxiety due to the fact they are not yet in control of their bodies and emotions. Males tend to compare and express concern for their genitalia, namely the penis. Other than normal physical variances in males in penis size and shape, some males experience a condition known as Peyronie's disease, which usually becomes more apparent as a male ages and his genitals grow. While it is normal for some curvature of the penis to the right or left when **flaccid** and to the right, left, up, or down when erect, the angle of curvature determines Peyronie's disease (Levine, Estrada, Storm, & Matkov, 2003).

The condition involves fibrotic changes in the connective tissues of the penis for various reasons, such as genetics, damage, and practices, such as how a male places the penis in his underwear and pants (Levine et al., 2003). Some believe that circumcision causes excessive forces to be placed on certain sides of the penis, thereby causing fibrotic changes and thus angulation (Jordan, 2006). The condition also is known as chronic inflammation of the ***tunica albuginea*** or CITA. Damage or other congenital issues can cause plaques to build up in the segments of the penis that influence how a penis will angle. The resulting scar tissue, from whatever the **etiology,** causes angulation in the penis that may affect sexual performance and even urination. The disease also is more common in males with other types of connective tissue disorders, such as when tissues tend to stick together (*contractures*) (Jordan, 2006). Diagnosis of the disease is done by a urologist. Treatment depends on the relative severity of the condition. Some males respond over time to no treatment, whereas greater than 50% tend to get worse. Nonsurgical treatments, such as vitamin E supplementation, have been met with limited success. Other medications, such as sildenfil (Viagra), have shown promise in correcting the disorder, but long-term studies need to be undertaken. Injections may help as well as surgery. The "Nesbit procedure" may surgically straighten and eliminate or reduce scar tissue in the penis. Additionally, some manual therapy (noninvasive) procedures have been met with moderate success. Some devices attempt to gradually straighten or reduce the curvature over time, but results mainly are anecdotal. If a male has concern for his genitals, he may be reluctant to talk about the issue with anyone (Jordan, 2006; Levine et al., 2003). Peyronie's disease typically will not get better on its own; therefore, open communication needs to be stressed. This type of condition may be noticed during routine physical exams or sports. Health care personnel need to pay more attention to this issue that affects 1%–4% of the population. Peyronie's disease should be accounted for in comprehensive physical and sexual health.

Erections Hormones strongly influence physical and emotional responses related to sexuality. Stimulation in adolescent males most often leads to excitement and erections. Erections are very normal and frequently occur as a boy enters and proceeds through puberty. Early on in puberty, when hormone levels may be at their highest, erections often occur without cause or stimulation. This can be the cause of embarrassment for boys as well as frustration because they may feel as if they cannot control their bodies. Many males express anxiety over random erections, particularly in social situations (Harris, 1994). While there is little to nothing that can be done from a physical perspective concerning erections, helping a teen understand how and why it happens is a good starting point. Health professionals, parents, and caregivers can help him to understand that it is normal and should be expected. Discuss the details concerning testosterone and other hormones in his system as the cause for random erections. Of course, sexual excitement also may elicit an erection, but teens are likely to know this as obvious. Most males grow to understand their bodies and how to control certain situations, erections are no different. Some males try to figure out ways in which to hide their erections. Sound advice can be found on credible websites such as "Go Ask Alice" (www.goaskalice.columbia.edu), and may allay many of a teen's fears and concerns.

The only other health-related issue of concern regarding erections is a condition called *priapism*. There are several causes of priapism, which is an extended period of an erection that can last upward of several hours. This can cause serious damage to the sensitive tissues and structures of the penis and is therefore considered a medical emergency. Some causes of priapism include drug use, black widow spider bites, trauma to the spinal cord or genitalia, carbon monoxide poisoning, and even sickle cell anemia. Occasionally, chronic compression of the *perineum* (the area between the anus and scrotum) as with cyclists, horseback riders, and motorcycle riders can cause priapism to occur (Jordan, 2006). If a teenager has a chronic erection lasting more than a few hours, he needs immediate attention for treatment. In most cases, this will not occur, but if it does, it is important to be sensitive to the issue and immediately seek help.

Nocturnal Emissions The term *wet dream* refers to a common occurrence, particularly in adolescent males, called *nocturnal emissions*. The involuntary expulsion of semen (ejaculate) occurs during one's sleep and mainly occurs due to heighten sexual responses because of hormones (Planned Parenthood, n.d.). These spontaneous orgasms may be a cause of great embarrassment or even concern for an adolescent, but it is quite normal and signifies pubertal maturation, growth, and development. An exact cause is not known, but hormones, release of sexual tension or excess semen, and sexual response to memories or dreams are some postulated causes. Some males experience many nocturnal emissions, whereas others have reported never having this happen, with much variation in between. For example, as many as 83% of males have reported at least one experience of a wet dream (Planned Parenthood, n.d.). It also is possible to have wet dreams throughout a lifetime and not just in adolescence.

Famed sexuality researcher Dr. Alfred Kinsey noted a strong correlation between masturbation and nocturnal emissions. That is, males who masturbated less often where more likely to report having more wet dreams. This finding corroborates with the hypothesis that wet dreams are related to sexual tension and its release (Kinsey, Pomeroy, & Martin, 1948). Another study found that males who received testosterone therapy later in life also experienced nocturnal emissions, further supporting the hypothesis that they are related to circulating hormone levels in the body (Mooradina & Korenman, 2006).

In antiquity, nocturnal emissions were viewed as abnormal and even a dysfunction of the male's system called *spermatorrhoea*. Some males were subjected to radical treatments such as herbal remedies, circumcision, and even **castration** (removal of the gonads). Some religious views also frown upon the issue, but more and more, culture has come to understand this as a normal part of male growth and development (Brakke, 1995).

Some common signs that a male may be experiencing nocturnal emissions include being secretive about entry into his room, insistence on doing his own laundry, particularly his bedding and sheets, uneasiness discussing sexuality or things about the body, and possible difficulty sleeping. It is important to help an adolescent understand his body so as to reduce anxiety and negative emotions concerning sexuality and sexual development. This awkward time may be a great opportunity to connect with a teen regarding sexuality, which can segue into other discussions on responsible sexual attitudes, behaviors, and practices. Parents can be advised to help the adolescent male embrace his body and the fascinating changes that accompany becoming a man. Once the initial awkwardness is breached, communication will help ensure a healthier perspective concerning his sexuality and development.

Premature Ejaculation   Similar to nocturnal emissions, some males experience premature ejaculation during sexual stimulation and arousal. There is a lack of control over sexual function to a certain extent, which decreases the time to orgasm and emission of semen (Master & Turek, 2001). While this condition is not pathological in nature, it can create anxiety and pose a problem for some males. Additionally, premature ejaculation is not necessarily an occurrence in adolescence and may continue well into adulthood, but it is more common during puberty and adolescence. It is very common, with 25%–40% of the U.S. male population reporting issues with premature ejaculation (Waldinger et al., 2005). There are several potential causes, such as emotional issues, fear, anxiety, physical damage to the reproductive system, and overactive nerves, among others (Master & Turek, 2001). Classic research by sexuality pioneers William Masters and Virginia Johnson and Alfred Kinsey demonstrated that most males ejaculate within 2–4 minutes of activity, and upward of 75% of males self-reported ejaculating within 10 minutes (Waldinger, Quinn, Dilleen, Mundayat, Schweitzer, & Boolell, 2005). The main concern is whether it interferes with sexual performance and pleasure with another person. Most males will not be overly concerned about the rate of their ejaculation until sexual experiences are shared with partners.

Younger males will exhibit less control over ejaculation and orgasm because the experience is relatively new to them. As a male gets to know how his body reacts to various sexual stimuli, he likely will increase his confidence in controlling his sexual climax and orgasm. Typically, anxiety plays a major role in why adolescent males may prematurely ejaculate; however, this is relative to the context in which it occurs. Diagnosis can be difficult. If there appears to be a real issue with this, consultation with an appropriate medical professional, such as a primary care physician, urologist, or psychiatrist, is important. Treatments can range from sexual therapies and counseling to behavioral control and antidepressant medications. Parents are advised to approach this and like issues during open communication and discussion with their adolescent teen.

Masturbation   Once thought of as a "social ill," masturbation has been misunderstood by nearly every culture on Earth. In previous centuries and other cultures, the practice was offensive and even punishable by extreme means. Religions always have had a strong presence and say in terms of masturbation. It was viewed as an offense to God and carried severe penalties, such as castration and even death.

Formally defined, masturbation and many of its euphemisms is any act of sexual self-stimulation through various means that often leads to orgasm (Stengers & van Neck, 2001). Male masturbation often involves rhythmically stroking one's penis or rubbing one's genitals in other forms. The use of other objects and materials, such as sexual toys and lubrication, may be used to enhance one's pleasure. Adolescence is a very common time for a male to seriously begin exploring his sexuality; that is, what he enjoys and what he does not. Hormones, particularly testosterone, enhance his sex drive, which may lead to frequent erections and masturbation (Harris, 1994). Also, males may masturbate at younger ages, which is normal as long as there is no suspicion of sexual or emotional abuse (Mallants & Casteels, 2008).

Every person has his or her own likes and dislikes and "style." Sexuality researchers have self-reported statistics that anywhere from 92% to 98% of males masturbate frequently (three or more times per week), with many reporting five to seven times per week or more (Gerressu, Mercer, Graham, Wellings, & Johnson., 2007). The benefits of masturbation include better self-esteem, lower blood pressure, mood enhancement (combats the effects of depression), enhanced fertility, anxiety reduction, normalized congestion within the reproductive tract, enhanced prostate health, and reduction in promiscuous sexual activity (*Badger Herald* staff, 2007). In fact, several nations in Europe have a public policy that encourages teens to masturbate on a daily basis because it releases sexual tension that otherwise may evolve into premature sexual intercourse, unprotected sex and STIs, and unwanted pregnancies (Mallants & Casteels, 2008; Treptow, 2009).

Today, most people view the practice of masturbation as acceptable and healthy. It is normal and expected behavior. It is a very personal issue that should be handled as such. Appropriateness should be stressed throughout a young male's development; chastisement and ridicule may lead to lower self-esteem and possibly abnormal views concerning sexuality and sexual health. Abnormal behaviors also can develop. Sexual compulsions and **addictions** can develop. As testosterone levels equalize during adolescence and early adulthood, masturbation may become less frequent or desired.

Stigma associated with masturbation may stem from a simple functionality perspective. If ejaculation occurs for the purpose of creating life, it has value in many cultures and societies; if it has been used simply for pleasure, it can be been met with disdain. However, if society views pleasure as health additive, masturbation certainly serves a valid purpose. In fact, in some cultures, public displays of masturbation and proof of ejaculate is a symbol of manhood and virility. Some cultures save the ejaculate in animal skin and wear it while trying to conceive a child as a sign of fertility (DeMartino, 1979). If we culturally embrace masturbation as a normal and healthy part of overall holistic health, ridicule and stigma may diminish, which may enhance overall sexual health in adolescents.

Expectations of Masculinity and Sexual Prowess

Every culture expects different things from males. Demonstrating one's masculine traits and values communicates sexual maturity and virility to others (Stibbe, 2004). Evolutionary anthropologists point out that masculine and even hypermasculine males often receive more positive attention as with better jobs and more sexual success (Leit, Gray, & Pope, 2001; Schwartz & Tylka, 2008). The strongest and most representative of the masculine ideal gets preference in jobs and mate (Schwartz & Tylka, 2008). Males may use masculinity to compete with society in general versus only other males for sexual prowess and fertility. Take, for example, the growing market for male cosmetics, cosmetic procedures, and even clothing.

A male is defined by his sex, that is his XY chromosomes, whereas culture and society help assign his gender (that is, masculine). A male's sexual prowess is commonly defined by his culture and the society in which he grows and develops (Schwartz & Tylka, 2008). Adolescence is a period of rapid **assimilation,** particularly in terms of a young male's view of his sexuality (Erwin, 2006). Some males are hypermasculine whereas others are less masculine according to societal standards. In some cultures, males care for the children rather than dominating and protecting, and still others plan events and ceremonies within their traditions and norms. Society tends to govern what is considered masculine and what is not.

Many boys learn from male role models what is acceptable and what is not. If a male experiences role models who encourage promiscuous sexual activity, or if in order to "prove" he is man, he must demonstrate certain behavior, such as dominance and aggression, the young male typically will comply. To be within the social norm means fewer challenges to a male. Many males may overexemplify and overexaggerate their perceived masculinity and sexual prowess simply to stay under the radar of potential challengers or even bullies (Schwartz & Tylka, 2008). For example, using a hypermasculine front that promotes aggression, dominance, and lack of sensitivity may create a "bad boy" image.

In some settings, people will respect a man more or leave him alone because he has "proven himself." Some women find this attractive in a male; therefore, they are drawn to potentially dysfunctional relationships. Anything considered unmasculine may be viewed as posing a threat to a male's social status (Rando, Rogers, & Brittan-Powell, 1998).

Adolescent males often tease each other with respect to their sexuality, often referring to things or one another as "gay" and "feminine." "That's so gay" is a commonly uttered phrase in the vernacular of an adolescent male. Moreover, homophobic bullying has continued to be a stain on the fabric of school health. These insecurities concerning sexuality play out in several venues. A recent online survey measuring sexual intent and respect and conducted with 1,200 teen males and young men in the United States reported results titled, "Truth About Sex: 60 Percent of Young Men, Teen Boys Lie About It." Findings showed that 45% were virgins, 60% reported lying about something related to sex: 30% lied about how far they have gone, 24% about their number of sexual partners, and 23% about their virginity status. Moreover, 78% agreed that there was "way too much pressure" from society to have sex. These results seem to reinforce that males use sex to communicate their masculinity through exemplifying their sexual prowess. This furthers the age-old double standard between males and females; among males, 53% said having a lot of casual sexual partners makes them popular, but 71% agreed that the same activities make girls less popular. On a positive note, 53% of the sample said they had talked with a parent about preventing pregnancy, but 51% reported that having sex before marriage was acceptable in their families (Jayson, 2010).

What we teach adolescent males will guide them in different directions, some positive and some negative. Males who believe masculinity is defined by dominance, aggression, and sexual conquests are less likely to be successful and healthy in the long term than are males who are encouraged to develop emotional intelligence.

Homosexuality

The topic of homosexuality is complex and never easy to navigate. Adolescent males have several unspoken and spoken pressures from family and society in general concerning sexuality and sexual matters. A boy may view his plunge into puberty as a quest to define who he is and what he feels is normal. Many boys will emerge with a strong sense of who they are and what sexuality means to them. Others may not. Some males grow up feeling one way biologically but express their sexuality otherwise. For a male growing up in a society where dominance, aggression, stoicism, and heterosexuality have been prized, valued, encouraged, and even expected, being anything but can and does present an emotional challenge (Maurer-Starks, Clemons, & Whalen, 2008). Research suggests that up to 10% of the population is gay, lesbian, bisexual, transgendered, or otherwise "non-straight" (Fay, Turner, Klassen, & Gagnon, 1989). An adolescent may struggle with expressing his sexuality because it goes against the social norm. Although gains have been made in this area over the past few decades, there still exist various forms of intolerance and even bigotry associated with "non-straight" ideals (Maurer-Starks et al., 2008).

Many younger men try to figure out their sexual orientation on their own, which can be a daunting task. Not knowing where to turn, whom to confide in, or whom they can trust can lead to risky behaviors and other physical and emotional health risks. Gender expectations play a key role in how males identify with their worlds (Schwartz & Tylka, 2008). For example, research suggests that eighteen- to twenty-four-month-old toddlers have high discrimination when recognizing gender-consistent and inconsistent roles (Hill & Flom, 2007). Teenage boys often are very protective of their masculinity and sexuality. The internal conflict of feeling one way (homosexual or gay) and acting another (heterosexual or straight) can make life a challenge in resolving one's inner feelings.

Author C. J. Pascoe notes this conflict in an ethnography written from high school interviews and experiences with many boys in her book, *Dude, You're a Fag* (Pascoe, 2007). In her eighteen months of field research in a racially diverse, working-class high school, Pascoe noted that masculinity coincided with various values and practices of male sexuality. The "specter of the fag" is discussed as a form of discipline for males, helping to assert heterosexual norms and mores while holding homosexuality at bay. Culture seems to view homosexuality as an individual issue or even a choice, but the issue of the individual is very likely to affect more than just him.

Researcher David Aveline conducted a retrospective study that interviewed parents of gay males about of their earlier development and behaviors. Nearly eighty parents were interviewed for recurrent themes concerning their sons' behaviors. Most parents recalled atypical gender roles and behaviors, such as interests in traditional female pursuits and lack of interests in sports. Aveline calls into question the notion of whether or not "atypical" gender behavior equates to homosexuality (Aveline, 2006). Behaviors or not, they are merely representations of *what* and *who* a person is. Parents, generally speaking, automatically assume a boy is heterosexual from birth, which characterizes the hetero-normative and homo-negative perspective, especially in the Western world (Maurer-Starks et al., 2008). Recent research has challenged the way we as a society view sexuality and, in particular, homosexuality. Many males who are born homosexual, because of the effects and fear of social stigma, represent their sexuality as heterosexual (Crooks & Baur, 2005).

In reparative therapy, also called *conversion therapy*, a person of same-sex orientation goes through a series of psychological batteries of tests and treatments, such as group therapy, psychoanalysis, aversive conditioning, sex therapy, and religious teaching, which is aimed at correcting his or her sexuality or sexual preference. This is a very controversial practice because it is "based upon the assumption that homosexuality *per se* is a mental disorder or based upon the *a priori* assumption that a patient should change his/her sexual [homosexual] orientation," according to the American Psychological Association (Haldeman, 1994). Many religious groups support and even sponsor such programs to correct "moral insufficiencies." However, many people view reparative or conversion therapy as flawed and based on the notion that sexual orientation is a choice.

Many self-identified homosexuals strongly refute that they made a choice to be as they are. "Why would I choose a life where I would be discriminated against, have fewer civil liberties and rights, be constantly judged by others, and constantly feel compelled to justify who I am or who I am with!?" quipped one younger male concerning being gay. On the opposite end of the spectrum, many people feel that it is less the "nature" of homosexuality and more the "nurture" of it (MacGillivray, 2000). Society influences what we perceive to be true, helps shape values and morals, reinforces norms, and guides what we do and don't do. Some people argue that openness and **acceptance** of homosexuality encourages impressionable youth to explore and experiment. Research suggests that behavior is a combination of inherited genes from both a mother and father. Sometimes genes are misplaced and cause variance. Other research has shown interesting but inconclusive findings pertaining to homosexuality (Crooks & Baur, 2005). For example, the hypothalamus (or master gland) in cadavers was found to be smaller in homosexuals. Hormonal imbalances in the body were shown to be stronger factors in another research study. Researcher Dean Hamer noted that a "gay gene" was likely and was found on the X chromosome, therefore, it was sex linked to the mother of a homosexual male (Queer Foundation, 2006).

Homosexuality in incarcerated populations often is viewed as expected, but many males claim to remain straight beyond the walls of prison. Sexuality often is viewed as being more of a fluid process than a set definition that occurs at the time of conception and birth. So, is sexual orientation a choice, defined in genetics, both, or none?

To help answer the question as to whether homosexuality is a choice or not, one needs to look at the entire scope of variance in the human population. The influence for variety in humans is their genes, which are "turned on" by certain social conditions. Genes can be suppressed, but they are still there. Viewing the spectrum of sexuality and sexual orientation as a binary condition is simply shortsighted. Society tends to employ an "either/or" mentality. But there are several variations along the spectrum of possibilities.

What do you think: Is homosexuality a choice, is it nature, nurture?

©iStockphoto.com/Chris Schmidt

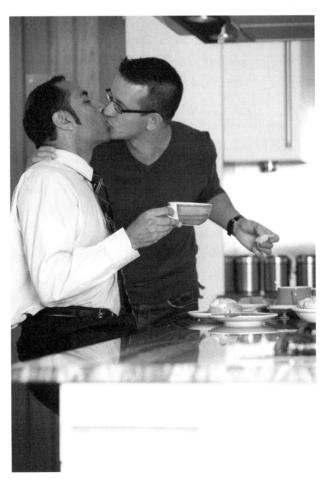

Sexual orientation carries with it health consequences and implications, particularly for homosexual, bisexual, and transgendered males. For example, gay males are more likely to be at risk for STIs, use tobacco products, use and abuse alcohol, use and abuse recreational and some hard drugs such as methamphetamine, be victims of gay bashing and domestic violence, and suffer from mental health issues such as depression (Johnson, Wadsworth, Wellings, Bradshaw, & Fields, 1992). Gonorrhea rates are on the rise in gay males because of the nature of sexual experiences (anal sex, lesions, and bacteria from feces). Additionally, gay males have higher rates of genital warts and HIV because of open lesions caused by STIs and the nature of sexual intercourse (anal sex). Infections such as hepatitis A are common even though a vaccination is available, mainly because of lack of awareness. Hepatitis A is usually transmitted through the oral-fecal route, which may be the result of anilingus, also known as "rimming." Unprotected intercourse among males (usually referred to as "barebacking") also increases the chances of hepatitis B infection, which is mainly a blood-borne pathogen.

Although awareness and knowledge of HIV/AIDS has become widely known over the past twenty-five-plus years, new HIV infections in gay males continue to increase in the United States and abroad. Cancers due to certain types of infection, such as HIV, also are more common in gay males. For example, Kaposi's sarcoma and other lymphomas have much higher rates in gay communities than others. HPV has been shown to increase the risk of anal cancers in gay males, whereas hepatitis A/B infections increase the risk for developing certain liver cancers. Lung cancer and heart disease as well as emphysema are more likely.

Males are not commonly thought of as victims of domestic violence, but many teens who identify as being gay face ridicule and physical violence from peers and even family members (Fineran, 2001). Many gay males live in a world in which being gay is thought of as being abnormal, which can affect one's self-esteem and overall mental health. Low self-esteem can lead to depression and risky behaviors. Teens who "don't care" because of self-esteem problems will take more risks than those who have self-efficacy and positive experiences.

Homophobia and homophobic bullying are a continual concern for gay youth (Fineran, 2001). Take, for example, the case of Matthew Shepard, a twenty-one-year-old University of Wyoming college student who was the victim of a hate crime pertaining to his sexuality. Matthew was beaten, tortured, and left for dead by two acquaintances he'd met earlier in the evening on October 7, 1998. He was likely targeted because he admitted that he was gay to the two individuals, who violated his trust, civil liberties, and human rights. Matthew died a day later of massive head trauma. Matthew Shepard's death prompted public outcries for better human rights for people of various sexual orientations and a stricter policy on **hate crimes.** In October 2009, President Barack Obama signed the Matthew Shepard and James Byrd, Jr. Hate Crimes Prevention Act,, which expands the definition and broadens the penalties for hate crimes, particularly for those of the homosexual and transgendered communities.

According to data from a national database that tracks calls to a child help/crisis line, males represent only 25% of all the total calls but represent nearly 60% of all calls concerning homophobia and homophobic bullying. Homophobic bullying and fear of telling their parents were the top concerns expressed by these youth. The concept of "triple isolation," from schools, friends, and their own families, concerning their sexuality was detailed in the report. These teenagers felt as if there was nowhere and no one to turn to for assistance. Many teens feel unsupported by those they expect to be there for them during times of challenges and crises (Adams, Cox, & Dunstan, 2004). To further feelings of isolation and loneliness, many boys felt that if they approached their friends or family about homophobia or bullying, they would be **outing** themselves, which may further isolate them. Keeping these feelings to themselves furthers the emotional stress and strain on a developing adolescent. In turn, these feelings of isolation and loneliness may translate or transform to hopelessness and even lead to suicidal ideation (Fineran, 2001).

Gay teen males are more than six times more likely than heterosexual males to complete suicide. The increase in these rates demonstrates the increased pressure and stress during adolescence. For a gay male, these stresses may be too much to process and therefore may prompt a suicide attempt. Clearly, health concerns in gay teenage males pose a public health issue.

- 1 in 5 HIV-positive men were apparently infected during their adolescent years (Johnson et al., 1992).

- 68% of adolescent gay males use alcohol (26% or more at least once a week); 44% use other drugs (CDC, Youth Risk Behavior Surveillance System [YRBS], 2008).

- 31% of homosexual students have used cocaine, as opposed to 7% of nonhomosexual students (CDC, YRBS, 2007).

- 62% of homosexual students smoke, as opposed to 35% of nonhomosexual students (CDC, YRBS, 2007).

- 30% of gay and bisexual adolescent males attempt suicide at least once (Remafedi et al., 1991). Gay and lesbian youth represent 30% of all completed teen suicides: extrapolation shows this means a successful suicide attempt by a gay teen every 5 hours and 48 minutes (Remafedi et al., 1991).

- Homosexual students are 4 times more likely to attempt suicide than nonhomosexual students (CDC, YRBS, 2008).

It is critical that health professionals, parents, and caregivers understand the challenges of adolescents in general. Open communication and understanding are particularly important in the life of a gay teen. Parents who support their child, regardless of his or her sexual orientation, are more likely to combat the ills previously detailed. Fostering an atmosphere of **tolerance** and love are critical in reducing health risks and their lifelong consequences. Beyond tolerance is acceptance. Parents who accept their son for who he *is* and not what he *does* will encourage positive relationships and behaviors. There is no substitute for compassion, empathy, and love.

SEXUAL DEVIANCE

Sexual deviance involves a broad range of sexual behaviors that deviate from a social or cultural norm or more and are classified as atypical. For example, a foot fetish, cross-dressing, sadism, or masochism all are types of sexual deviance (Laws & O'Donohue, 2008). The definition is influenced by the perspective and timing of the culture it is in. Twenty-first-century Western culture supports many forms of deviance and sexual acceptance. This has not always been the case. For example, Victorian era values were quite different than what we see today. Moreover, certain religious backgrounds view sexuality differently. There are minor deviations and extremes if we view human sexuality as a spectrum. What we call "normal" may be viewed as abnormal or even unacceptable by other cultures. Therefore, sexual deviance is in the eye of the beholder and is strongly influenced by the context of the culture and society in which we live. Our perspectives are defined by the summation of our previous experiences; not everyone will have the same experiences and therefore, not everyone will conform to sexual expectations.

Adolescent males begin to fully explore and experience their own sexualities at this stage. Sexual offenders tend to be male (Bureau of Justice Statistics, 2010); therefore, it is important to understand what may predispose a younger male to developing these types of feelings and resultant behaviors. As a male develops and experiences the world of sexuality, he begins to know what he likes and dislikes. When internal conflict with one's emotions combines with social forces, such as media messages, adolescents may use sex to suit their perceived needs, which may result in what society refers to as *deviance*. Sometimes he likes things that we as a society dislike or disapprove. In some cases what the young man likes may be illegal, such as pedophiles with children.

Sexuality is very closely tied in with emotions. Sexual experiences help teach and define who we are (Laws & O'Donohue, 2008). However, when emotions are connected to the physical nature of an experience, coupled with the social influences of expectations and media, emotions may become clouded or even lost in the process. This may leave the male questioning and confused as to what he feels and whether it is okay or not.

Sexual Addiction

This term has become popular in the twenty-first century. Golf professional Tiger Woods and late-night television host David Letterman are two of many high-profile males who have admitted to problems with sex intruding on their lives. But, does sex qualify as an *addiction*? Medical professionals have questioned whether gambling, overeating, and sex are truly addictions or simply vices. Some argue they are vices that become addictions, but this is not the case for everyone. Some psychiatrists are lobbying for their inclusion in the newest edition of the *Diagnostic and Statistical Manual*, 5th edition (*DSM-V*), a reference manual that helps health professionals diagnose psychiatric disorders (Laws & O'Donohue, 2008). Critics mention that these terms are being overly classified and we are running the risk of wrongly pathologizing many peoples' unique differences, whereas others claim that sexual addictions are forms of behavioral addictions that have to be studied more extensively (Wetzstein, 2010).

In a recent report, males with higher levels of testosterone were more likely to have multiple marriages and divorces, experience greater instances of cheating and infidelity, pay less attention to children, and focus more on themselves. However, once a male settles into a family pattern and has children, he begins to produce lower levels of the hormone. This may be a biological adaptation to assure better family structure, the report notes (Slatcher et al., 2011)

Several classical studies have somewhat confirmed, through the use of chemical castration of sex offenders, that testosterone does in fact lead to greater instances of sexual deviance and possibly addiction. In these studies, sex offenders volunteered to have a chemical introduced into their systems that would limit testosterone production and therefore diminish most or all of their sexual energy and desire (Grubin & Beech, 2010). The answers are not clear, but there does appear to be a connection worth exploring in the future.

Adolescent males have higher testosterone levels than at any other point in their life spans. An adolescent male needs to learn to navigate his emotions and feelings about to his sexuality and be able to process them accordingly. When adolescents don't know how to express themselves, they are more likely to substitute other behaviors, such as sexual practices. Adolescents are very pleasure seeking and use sex for different reasons than do younger and older adults. Sex addictions, whether real or over-represented, can begin to manifest at this age due to these factors.

Promoting expression of an adolescent male's emotions and furthering the development of emotional intelligence and competence is a strategy that parents and educators can consider. Good, reliable, and valid sexual information will help an adolescent learn what is accurate versus myth and inaccuracies. Parents and educators need to have an open-door policy about sex. If odd behaviors, such as secrecy, excessive requests for private use of the computer, or anxiety concerning sex, are apparent, parents and educators are advised to be ready to intervene.

Pornography

Every second, in the United States, $3,075.31 is being spent on pornography, 28,258 internet users are viewing pornography, and 372 internet users are entering adult content search items into search engines, and every 39 minutes, a new pornographic video is being created. The word *sex* is the most common search term on the internet; there are approximately 4.2 million pornographic websites, $4.9 billion is made in internet pornography sales annually, eleven years old is the average age of first internet porn exposure, 80% of fifteen- to seventeen-year-olds have viewed multiple hard-core sexual exposures online, and the United States, Brazil, and the Netherlands are the top three producers of pornography (Ropelato, n.d.). Whether it is on the internet, on television, depicted in movies or in magazines, sex is omnipresent and omnipotent in our culture. In the United States, there are differing values concerning human sexuality. Perhaps adolescent boys are simply reacting to the overwhelming number of mixed messages sent to them concerning sex.

The bottom line for adolescent males and pornography is how well it is all processed. Sexual health is very important as a boy develops. It will govern his sexual health practices, such as abstinence or safer sex precautions; help develop his sense of self; allow him to see meaning and value in his intimate relationships; and build a trust within himself and with others. Sexual health is necessary for a well-adjusted individual (Laws & O'Donohue, 2008).

Boys will be curious about sexuality as they progress into puberty and enter adolescence. The rush of sex hormones creates strong psycho-emotional-biological urges within the adolescent; therefore, he may seek various ways to express his sexuality and feed his desires. Adolescent males should be expected to venture out and peruse sexual content. If a parent or educator suspects inappropriate use of pornography in a young male's life or if it seems to interfere with his normal daily function, professional assistance and help from a counselor or other qualified medical professional should be pursued.

Pedophilia

Sexual attraction to children, particularly prepubescent ones, through physical contact, pictures, movies or any other media, is known as *pedophilia.* Pedophilia also is known as a *paraphilia,* which puts it on the spectrum of deviant sexual practices and behaviors (Laws & O'Donohue, 2008). Pedophiles seem to lack insight into the nature and severity of their actions. Statistics tell us that the overwhelming majority (approximately 97%) of pedophiles in the United States and abroad are white males who commit acts ranging from viewing pornography to sexual molestation of children (boys, girls, or both) (Holmes & Holmes, 2002). The cause of pedophilia is not well known, but some theories suggest it is caused by previous sexual abuse or violence that continues as a cycle as one ages. Not knowing how to process his own emotions about sexuality may lead a pedophile to commit acts of sexual abuse and violence against children because they are easier targets. Low self-esteem and poor social skills also have been implicated in cases of pedophilia. Treatments, such as **cognitive behavioral therapy (CBT),** behavioral therapies and modification, and chemical interventions have been met with limited success (Laws & O'Donohue, 2008). Parents need to be aware of sexual abuse in their own children as this is likely to create issues later in the boy's life. Be alert for odd behaviors and associations with children much younger than them. If pedophilia or related behaviors are suspected in adolescence, help is needed to avoid a lifetime of trouble and subsequent abuse of others.

Sexual Abuse and Rape

Boys *do* in fact suffer from sexual abuse and rape, with roughly 1 in 4 experiencing some form of abuse. One of the main issues at hand for boys and sexual abuse is the lack of cultural awareness of the expansiveness of the problem (Chandy, Blum, & Resnick, 1996; Laws & O'Donohue, 2008).

Society seems to deny that a boy can be sexually abused or conveys that it is not as serious as sexual abuse of a female.

Boys who are sexually abused follow an all-too-often, all-too-common algorithm of perpetrating abuse themselves. Lacking self-confidence, having low self-esteem, and searching for a semblance of order and control in one's life may lead an adolescent or young adult male to commit sexual crimes, such as abuse or even rape. With the overwhelming majority of sexual offenses committed by males, it is time we as a society spend more time learning how to interrupt the cycle of "silent" abuse boys may experience (Chandy et al., 1996; Laws & O'Donohue, 2008). We need to break down stigma and cultural barriers that surround the double standard of abuse in males and females. The better we promote awareness and advocacy, the better inroads can be made to curtail sexual abuse and lead to better sexual outcomes for all.

VIOLENCE, AGGRESSION, AND BULLYING

Adolescent males have a lot on their plates as they try to fit in and find out more about themselves. They may find themselves in conflict and competition not just with parents, siblings, peers, and others, but also with themselves. They may become more aggressive or withdrawn. A closer look at adolescent male behaviors often will reveal insecurities that may be masked by expressions of power and control. Higher levels of testosterone may cause a male to be more aggressive, which in turn can lead to fights and other forms of violence, such as bullying.

The plight of the male in Western society is a complex series of tests and proving oneself to others (Fineran, 2001). The competitive nature of males also seems to drive the formation of hierarchies and power struggles. More often than not, these power struggles and competitive aspects of males are handled in appropriate venues, such as sports and other structured activities. For some males; however, sports may not help them to avoid violence and acts of aggression directed at them or by them to others (Kindlon & Thompson, 2000). For example, in the educational video *Tough Guise*, director Sut Jhally and narrator Jackson Katz recount the numerous factors and examples of males perpetrating violence and aggression in society as a function of society. Many impressionable boys, adolescents, and eventually young men fail to receive and adequately process positive messages concerning their roles in society. This latter statement also carries heavy negative implications for one's health status.

In *Tough Guise*, the introduction depicts common, harsh words and video examples of male aggression in sports such as football and concludes with pictures of female domestic abuse victims. The opening scene comes from the 1939 classic movie, *The Wizard of Oz,* when the protagonist (Dorothy) and her counterparts are attempting to *see* the Wizard of Oz. The Wizard is found to be behind a curtain, controlling the image he wishes to portray to Dorothy and others. This opening is used to correlate how many young males also operate behind a "curtain" of their emotions. The portrayal of being tough, stoic, aggressive, apathetic, and otherwise dominant is likened to a "guise" to protect and maintain one's self-esteem, control, and position of hierarchy. That is, males who can "prove" themselves will be less likely to be harassed or victimized by others. This educational video exposes how and why young males feel the need to represent themselves in this light and, perhaps more important, how we as society can model better attitudes so as to enhance overall health and quality of life.

Males are more likely to be aggressive in their pursuit of exercising dominance, power, and control, particularly among other males (Kindlon & Thompson, 2000). Unfortunately, women often become victims of aggressive acts. According to national statistics on crime and other acts of violence, males commit approximately 85% of murders nationally, 95% of domestic and intimate partner violence, and 99% of rapes and other forms of sexual assault. Overall, males are the perpetrators in roughly 90% of *all* violent crimes in society (Bureau of Justice Statistics, 2010). Many popular theorists point their fingers at the all-powerful influence of media as the reason for these statistics. Certainly Jackson Katz in *Tough Guise* supports this notion.

Genetic research at Florida State University in 2009 and a few other centers has possibly isolated a gene that has been dubbed the "warrior gene." The theory works something like this: variants of a specific monoamine oxidase A (MAOA) gene, known as a "low-activity 3-repeat allele," play a significant role in the formation of aggressive behaviors. These gene sequences have been isolated to aggressive primal emotions that are part of human nature and are well supported by certain evolutionary models (Gibbons, 2004). Craig Kennedy, a researcher and professor of special education and pediatrics at Vanderbilt University in Tennessee goes further, stating, "Humans crave violence just like they do sex, food, or drugs" (Beaver, DeLisi, Vaughn, & Barnes, 2010).

Of course, these studies and implications are controversial and are widely contested by many other researchers in the field. Male behavior is affected by many influences, including genetic history and genetic code. Low-activity MAOA variants certainly are connected to some males who pursue violent activities such as membership in gangs and who display other forms of anti-social behaviors, but confirmatory research still is lacking. The MAOA gene variants affect a person's brain chemistry, specifically neurotransmitters serotonin and dopamine. These neurotransmitters affect certain aspects of mood and resultant behaviors (Beaver et al., 2010; Gibbons, 2004). These studies must be viewed with a discerning eye. As with other genetic factors, a person may possess certain sequences and express various traits yet never develop other ones. This is where Katz's discussion of social influences such as media comes into play. Future research will give us a better understanding of why people, especially males, tend to be more aggressive and violent. Until confirmatory research is performed, we believe that a confluence of psychosociobiological factors influences one's behaviors and tendencies.

An issue that has plagued society is domestic violence. Social modeling certainly plays a strong central role in causing males to batter and bully others, including their partners. Boys who grow up seeing instances of direct physical abuse perpetrated by other males, such as fathers, are more likely to model these same negative behaviors as they become adults themselves (Kim & Leventhal, 2008; Simmons et al., 2008). For example, those who bully tend to have been bullied in the past. Those who join gangs are likely in search of some form of validation, greater purpose, or even protection (Beaver et al., 2010; Gibbons, 2004). Those who are aggressive in domestic scenarios are likely acting out what they believe to be acceptable (Simmons et al., 2008).

Direct influences may not be required for learned behaviors pertaining to domestic violence. Some research suggests that media, such as popular music, videos, movies, television, and other forms, teach young boys what is the norm (Simmons et al., 2008). That is, if boys see instances of violence and aggression towards others, namely women, they are more likely to view these instances as normal. If parental figures are not there to monitor and offset these influences, coupled with biological factors, boys may not be able to figure out what is right versus what is wrong.

Many of us view these behaviors as unacceptable and simply wrong. Yet many young males may have been left up to their own devices to define acceptable norms and morality. There is certainly no excuse for domestic violence or bullying, but there is room for more understanding as to why it develops and how it can be prevented.

DRUG USE

The nature of drug use in adolescence is a complex phenomenon, because it has many roots and serves several sociocultural purposes in an adolescent's worldview. Drug use ranges from socially acceptable drugs, such as alcohol and tobacco, to harder drugs or "street" drugs, such as methamphetamine and cocaine. Drug trends among adolescents also tend to cycle; that is, drugs go through popularity stages, as does fashion and other cultural media (Reynolds et al., 2007). According to organizations and research investigations such as the Partnership for Drug Free America and the Monitoring the Future Survey, the main factors surrounding teen drug use are perceived risk, perceived social approval, and perceived availability. Drugs that carry high risk for side effects or consequences will be less likely to be used; whereas, drugs that are more available and garner social approval will be more likely to be used and abused. Drug use may be viewed as a social rite of passage for some males and an enabler for others as with sexual confidence and diminished social inhibitions. Drug use in adolescent males presents a social purpose as well as a physical purpose.

Alcohol

Perhaps one of the most commonly used and abused drugs in all adolescent populations is ethyl alcohol. Many teens begin experimenting with alcohol in their homes. Parents may not be aware that their children may be dipping into their supply of alcohol. For example, teens may consume alcohol when parents are away or at work and then cut the alcohol with water or other fluids to make it look less suspicious. Others may ask an older friend or sibling to purchase alcohol for them. Even still, some parents buy alcohol and host alcohol parties at their homes with hopes that if it is done in front of them, their children will be safer overall. Exposure to alcohol, whether in a controlled environment or not, carries risks, including tolerance and habituation, **dependence,** addiction, and several other psycho-emotional changes. One in 4 males drinks heavily in high school and college, as compared to 1 in 10 females. Alcohol dependence, which peaks at age 21, was nearly 5% among twelve- to seventeen-year-olds,. Lifelong patterns can develop from initial alcohol exposures. Additionally, heavy drinkers (those who consistently consume alcohol, for example, daily, also were more likely to use illicit drugs, such as marijuana, ecstasy, and methamphetamine than binge drinkers (those who consumed higher quantities of alcohol during one occasion versus consistently) (44% compared to 26%, respectively) (YRBS, 2008). Many males pride themselves on how much they can drink and how well they can "hold their liquor." Alcohol consumption represents a badge of masculinity to many males (Dishion, Capaldi, Spracklen, & Li, 1995).

A dialogue with an adolescent male may be richer and more effective than trying to snuff out his alcohol practices. Parents, educators, and health professionals should focus on education and discussing consequences rather than trying to instill fear in him. Parents are advised to offer their own experiences and discuss their collective morals and values concerning alcohol. Set limits, but always follow up with reasons.

If a young male does drink, parents, caregivers, educators, and health professionals should be aware of signs of abuse, such as depression, withdrawal from family and friends, problems in school, fighting, and other negative behaviors. Parents and educators should seek help from qualified counselors or medical professionals if they suspect alcohol addiction or dependence. Teens likely will experiment with alcohol; adults' primary role is helping him understand why he drinks and what it can mean for him. Keep him safe and reinforce that behaviors such as drinking and driving or buzzed driving are *never* an option. Parents, educators, and health professionals need to help him develop the management and resiliency skills that will last him a lifetime.

Tobacco

Societal attitudes toward tobacco use in males have dramatically changed over the past few decades. For example, in the 1950s and 1960s, it was commonplace to see strong males smoking cigarettes and other tobacco products on television and in the movies. Tobacco commercials permeated the airwaves. Some of the most convincing studies conducted on tobacco and different forms of cancers (namely of the lung) were conducted in the 1970s. In response to these studies, policies changed about commercials depicting tobacco use and how tobacco was marketed (Hackshaw, Law, & Wald, 1997). Attitudes toward tobacco continue to evolve, with smoke-free workplaces and statewide bans on indoor smoking. Many young males begin experimenting with tobacco in their early teens. The addictive properties of **nicotine** become evident when many males who begin as teens smoke well into adulthood.

According to the American Heart Association and the National Center for Health Statistics, 23.1% of males in the United States smoke, as compared to 18.3% for women. Moreover, the racial disparity of smoking and tobacco use is apparent with 23.5% of white males, 25.6% in black males, and 20.7% of Hispanic males. Asian males and other groups were much less likely to use tobacco (American Heart Association [AHA], 2010; Garrett et al., 2011). Tobacco often is viewed as masculine and somewhat of a rite of passage.

Social acceptance is waning, but more so for cigarettes than for other dangerous tobacco-based products. Tobacco companies have aggressively marketed to youth of different demographics for years (AHA, 2010; Garrett et al., 2011). For example, cigarillos (smaller cigarettes) have been popular in black and Hispanic communities, whereas lighter tobacco cigarettes have been pushed toward females. Cigars and smokeless tobacco, such as dip and chew, have widely been used by younger males, such as athletes. One needs to only look on a high school baseball diamond to see young men chewing a wad of smokeless tobacco or taking a pinch of dip and placing it between their lips and gums. Many adult role models, such as sport coaches, teachers, and professional athletes, use forms of smokeless tobacco as well. The wrong message is being sent to adolescent males. Many adolescents consider smokeless tobacco to be less dangerous, less addictive, and not as harmful as traditional cigarettes. This is simply not the case. Gum disease and oral and lip cancers are highly prevalent and aggressive in younger male populations who use these products (AHA, 2010; Garrett et al., 2011).

Better role modeling and social advocacy are needed to help young males refuse tobacco products. Some major league baseball players and coaches, such as Boston Red Sox manager Terry Francona, have gone public in their efforts to quit using smokeless tobacco. While this is a step in the right direction, it is the everyday images boys see in their families and among their friends who smoke and use other types of tobacco products that strongly influence their perceptions and decisions to use or not use tobacco. Study after study continues to show that firsthand, secondhand, and even third-hand smoke exposures (surfaces where smoke residue has formed and settled) raise health risks ranging from asthma and chronic bronchitis to cancer and death (AHA, 2010; Garrett et al., 2011).

Perhaps one of the more disturbing trends is e-cigarettes, which have popped up all over American malls and shopping plazas. These products claim to give people the same rich and satisfying experience of smoking without the risk of tobacco smoke. The e-cigarettes use a water, nicotine, vapor system instead of smoke. While this may be a better option, these still contain the highly addictive properties of nicotine. Some research has shown spine health diminishes, especially in adolescents, due to nicotine use, which sheds new light on chronic back pain (Mikkonen, Leino-Arjas, Remes, Zitting, Taimela, & Karppinen, 2008).

Younger males may be attracted to these gimmicks, thinking that there are no risks or health consequences, which is why health educators must be aggressive in disseminating timely, relevant, and valid information. Health consequences and deaths due to tobacco use are the most preventable forms of morbidity and mortality in the United States (AHA, 2010; Garrett et al., 2011; Hackshaw et al., 1997). We must understand what motivates boys to use these products by analyzing how they are marketed to them. It is not always the product that drives consumption, but how it is presented and marketed.

Illicit Drugs

Other types of drug use are fairly common in adolescents. Teens use marijuana, inhalants, heroin, cocaine, ecstasy, MDMA, methamphetamine, and even cough syrup, among others. Some teens host "pharm parties," which involve using prescription drugs, such as opioids like Percocet and vicodin, to get high. Common products such as cough syrup contain small amounts of alcohol or codeine, which may entice a teen to try it out of curiosity. Sniffing household chemicals and products such as glue, paint thinners, and nail polish remover (also known as *huffing*) is a common practice among teens (YRBS, 2008).

Parents and educators need to be aware of abuse patterns for any type of drug. Understanding the temptations and motivation for using is perhaps equally as important as knowing the type of drug being used by a teen. The inquisitive nature of adolescent males, coupled with their incessant drive for competition and proving their masculinity may endanger more youth than we know. Parents and educators must *create* safe and supportive environments for teaching about drug abuse. We need to *connect* with teens in terms of how they feel and what they perceive about drugs, including pressure. We need to clearly *communicate* our expectations concerning drug use (Adolescent Substance Abuse Knowledge Base [ASK], 2010).

As many risks as there are for drug use in adolescence, there are an equal number, if not more, opportunities to curtail the issue. Understanding why males use drugs is the first solid step when addressing the problem. According to the Adolescent Substance Abuse Knowledge Base, we need to know how adolescents perceive and use drugs based on trends. They note:

"The challenge we face in curtailing teen drug use is that the perceived 'benefits' of using a certain drug are known sooner and spread faster than perceived risks. The 'benefits' of a drug (the euphoric high, the energy, the 'numbness') are immediately evident and electronic forms of communication like blogs, chats, and text messages allow these 'positive' experiences to be broadcasted and spread quickly. Consequently, new drugs experience sharp increases in use for months or even years. Meanwhile, gathering information about the drug's risks takes time, but when specific evidence is gathered and aggressively distributed either via the media or friends and family, the results are dramatic." (ASK, 2010)

JUVENILE OFFENDERS AND INCARCERATION

The overwhelming majority (85%–90%) of U.S. incarcerated inmates is male (Bureau of Justice Statistics, 2010). According to the U.S. Department of Justice, in 2008, there were nearly 2.5 million people incarcerated in the U.S. justice system. The United States has the highest rates of juvenile incarceration in the world. One in every 18 males in the United States is in prison or monitored with probation and nearly 70% of prisoners in the United States are non-whites. Racial disparities permeate the justice system and are complex to analyze. For instance, approximately 10.4% of all black males in the United States between ages 18–24 have been imprisoned, as compared to 2.4% of Hispanic males and 1.3% of white males (Bureau of Justice Statistics, 2010).

When a boy feels valued, experiences meaning in his life, and develops a strong sense of self, he likely will succeed in the path he chooses. However, boys who feel undervalued and disconnected from the "system" will likely choose a troubled path, or one will be chosen for them (Kindlon & Thompson, 2000). One of the primary areas of concern is educational fallout. When boys feel disconnected with the learning process and experiences in the classroom, they are more likely to seek alternative experiences outside of the classroom and beyond (Parkin, 2007). Additionally, adolescents lack the life experience, wisdom, and brain development to make solid decisions. Development of the prefrontal cortex of the brain, which guides rational decision making, often is not fully developed until the mid-twenties.

Many boys simply cannot see the value or meaning in certain educational environments. Curricula that emphasize self-restraint, empathy, and cooperative experiences versus competition may not work well for a boy

(Parkin, 2007). A 2006 article by Gerry Garibaldi asked how a feminized curriculum "hurts" boys. Garibaldi discusses his own observations in his twenty-five-plus years of teaching that advances in making the classroom better for girls has had the opposite effect on boys, thereby promoting their disengagement, which is captured in lower graduation rates and college attendance. He also notes, "Girls now so outnumber boys on most university campuses across the country that some schools, like Kenyon College, have even begun to practice affirmative action for boys in admissions. And as in high school, girls are getting better grades and graduating at a higher rate" (Garibaldi, 2006). Parkin (2007) notes that 23,000 more university seats are offered to females than males in the United Kingdom, which shows this might not just be an American phenomenon.

This is a hotly contested assertion; many educators hold firm to the notion that sex is less of factor and educational methodologies are the center of concern. There does seem to be strong evidence that the way boys learn is very different than how girls learn. It also is true that many boys mainly are taught by female teachers in their first experiences in school (Parkin, 2007). Certainly some boys are simply disruptive and disinclined to education, but the whole sex . . . not likely. The challenge is not in pinning blame but in taking a good, long, and hard look at curriculum and how we promote learning in boys.

We must appreciate *how* boys learn versus simply focusing on *what* they are charged to learn. If a boy is not able to transfer meaning from the class-room to his own practice of life, then other social factors will step in and fill that gap, leading to negative consequences and decisions.

Maybe it is not just an educational issue, but the greater context of society itself. A male who feels empowered often feels less inclined to prove himself. However, if society sends messages to a young man that he is not enough and that he must show what type of man he is, how might he react? Society is a strong player in this stage of life. Some adolescents simply are not able to parse out what society tells them to do and what they know to be the best decision. Experience, that is, trial and error, often serves many adolescents; some with positive outcomes and others with negative ones. Males who have trouble distinguishing social pressures to act a certain way from their own values and morals may in fact become juvenile offenders.

Research has suggested that younger males are more likely to disengage and commit acts against society when they have few or no strong central role models in their lives. Replacing one's feelings with actions can lead to aggression, violence, and substance abuse (Bureau of Justice Statistics, 2010). Feeling a need to belong and desiring acceptance may provoke young males to join gangs (Beaver et al., 2010). Usually males who join gangs also experience other delinquent behaviors, such as **truancy,** drug and alcohol use, promiscuous sexual behaviors, and petty crime, such as shoplifting. Statistically significant predictive factors for joining a gang as an adolescent male include multiple factors, but namely, community, family structure, school, peers, and intrapersonal factors such as negative affect, depression, and behavior conduct disorders (Hill, Howell, Hawkins, & Battin-Pearson, 1999).

Community risk factors include extreme poverty, low levels of attachment to one's neighborhood, transient communities (people frequently move in and out), higher availability of firearms and drugs, and communities that perpetuate antisocial behaviors. Family risk problems are complex and highly variable, but according to statistical models, families that have a history of violence (domestic) or behavioral problems, poor management strategies, continuous conflict among family members, family poverty, and siblings with antisocial behaviors, were more likely to predict aggression, violence, and involvement in gangs (Beaver et al., 2010; Kim & Leventhal, 2008). School risk factors include higher failure rates in school as well as truancy or low degree of commitment to school and education (Parkin, 2007). Individual and peer risk factors include lack of autonomic arousal (that is, these boys seek extreme stimulation, often through violence and aggression, to feel connected to society), early examples of antisocial behavior when younger (introversion, isolated, abusive toward others or animals), glorification of antisocial behaviors and association with others who partake in antisocial behaviors (Kim & Leventhal, 2008).

A gang may give the boy a feeling of membership and approval, but it also takes his true sense of self and replaces it with gang **ideology.** Gang members report feeling enhanced prestige and social status among their peers as well as a sense of excitement and intrigue. Protection of oneself and one's family from other gangs is another commonly cited reason why boys join gangs (Beaver et al., 2010). Yet any deviations from the gang mentality could result in harsh retaliations against a male or the family members he wants to protect. Membership in gangs often leads to violence and criminal activities and offenses (Beaver et al., 2010). As such, many males who join gangs also find themselves in court and in jail multiple times during their lives.

There are many costs associated with violence and subsequent imprisonment. The United States leads the world in highest rates of imprisonment, with rates steadily rising each year. The states with the lowest rates of **incarceration** were Maine, Minnesota, and Rhode Island, with 148, 171, and 175 per 100,000 people in prison, respectively. Conversely, Louisiana, Texas, and Mississippi had the highest rates of imprisonment, with 816, 694, and 669 per 100,000 people imprisoned in these states, respectively. States spend approximately 7% of their operating budgets on corrections systems, and the costs of medical care for these inmates are rising by about 10% each year. For example, the United States spends approximately *$70 billion* per year on corrections. That works out to $23,000–$25,000 per inmate per year or roughly $60–$70 dollars per day (Bureau of Justice Statistics, 2010). The cost of the U.S. corrections system is costing us a tremendous amount of our national, state, community, and individual resources.

The other non-monetary costs of incarceration are the social and health impacts. Rates of communicable diseases, such as HIV/AIDS, hepatitis, tuberculosis, and many others, are markedly higher in prison populations. For example, tuberculosis, an infectious lung and respiratory disease, has been on the rise since 2003, and there were 21,987 reported cases of prisoners with HIV/AIDS infection in 2008. Of these HIV/AIDS cases, 20,075 were males or roughly 91.3% of all cases. Black males had the highest rates of these infections, which further illustrates the social disparities in health and the social justice system (Maruschak & Beavers, 2009).

While it is clear that males are more likely to be involved in violence, aggression, gangs, and crime (Bureau of Justice Statistics, 2010), there also exist tremendous opportunities to chip away at this negative trend. Knowing what predisposes males to these social ills is the first step in understanding how to better develop interventions that work. Targeting adolescent and even preadolescent males is critical in preventing future trends in violence and crime. Some suggestions for parents and educators for developing stronger and more resilient males include:

- Involving strong parental role models, especially paternal influences (not necessarily the young man's biological father)

- Taking into account community and altering the factors that can be managed to help connect a boy to his world with meaning

- Helping him express his emotions, fears, and hopes in constructive and meaningful ways

- Being aware of gangs in your community and of signs that a young man is pulling away from family, school, and community

- Helping him feel a sense of acceptance in his family

- Watching for signs of substance abuse

- Being alert for antisocial behavior

- Helping him stay connected with school and his education

Studies consistently show that the higher level of education attained, the more positive health and life outcomes will follow (Winkleby, Jatulis, Frank, & Fortmann, 1992).

SUMMARY

This chapter explored physical, emotional, and social issues pertaining to the health of adolescent males. The chapter began with an overall introduction to the period of adolescence and then discussed common physical, psychological, and emotional changes within adolescent males. Sexual health, sexuality, and other sexual topics were elaborated on, such as normal psycho-emotional development of one's sexuality and orientation. Sexually transmitted infections and their disease profiles were presented and discussed from an adolescent's risk category. Safer sexual practices, vaccinations, and topics central to birth control were discussed as they pertain to a male's sexual experience. Good foundational choices and strategies were presented and discussed at length. Other sexual health topics such as wet dreams, masturbation, and expectations of masculinity were discussed in the context of overall holistic male health. Behavioral health factors, such as homosexuality, violence and aggression, incarceration, sexual deviance, and alcohol and drug use were presented. Intrapersonal, interpersonal, and social contexts and consequences were used to illustrate each of these unique topics pertaining to adolescent male health. The period of adolescence is a transitory period. With so much going on in an adolescent's body, mind, and world, parents and educators must take into account the confluence of these factors and help each teen embrace his value and meaning in life with patience and understanding.

KEY TERMS

Abstinence	Defecation	Outing
Acceptance	Dental dams	Pap test
Acne	Dependence	Paradox
Addiction	Etiology	Paternalism
Antibiotics	Flaccid	Tolerance
Assimilation	Hate crimes	Truancy
Benign	Ideology	*Tunica albuginea*
Castration	Illicit drugs	Urinalysis
Cognitive behavioral therapy (CBT)	Incarceration	Vector
	Nicotine	

DISCUSSION QUESTIONS

1. Compare and contrast how males and females emotionally experience adolescence. What are the challenges faced by each sex?

2. What is the major challenge of adolescent males concerning sexual health? Detail recent research that supports your answer.

3. Explain why adolescent males may be resistant to obtaining and/or wearing latex condoms. What are some methods and strategies to increase compliance?

4. Compare and contrast the following three types of sexually transmitted infections: chlamydia, human immunodeficiency virus, and human papilloma virus. How are they contracted? How are they diagnosed? What is the treatment for each type of STI? Other than abstinence, what is the best method to prevent infection?

5. Should boys be vaccinated for human papilloma virus? Comment on the role of paternalism.

6. Detail how the topic of masturbation has been perceived in the 1800s, 1900s, and 2000s in the United States. How have other cultures handled this topic? With what aspects of how it is handled do you agree or disagree?

7. Discuss the commentary made by Jackson Katz in the documentary *Tough Guise* pertaining to how adolescent males portray their masculinity and sexual prowess. Do you agree with Katz's assertion or do you have other ideas? How have males changed over the last two to three decades concerning this topic?

8. Do your believe homosexuality is largely based on nature or nurture? Please pick a side to defend. Prepare your answer as if you were giving a debate response.

9. Why are males more likely to experiment with alcohol and other drugs? How does this relate to masculinity? What are some of the lifelong, long-term consequences? Present current rates and statistics in your responses.

10. What steps have been taken at local, state, regional, national, and international levels to address the issue of incarcerated males? Are there any notable programs? Describe them. How do racial disparities factor into this topic?

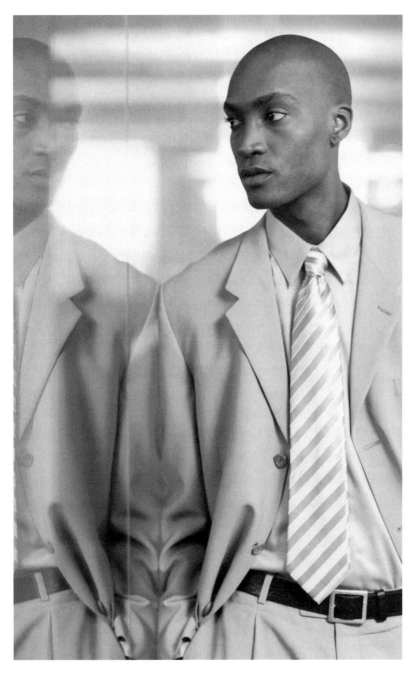

©iStockphoto.com/Grady Reese

8

Young Adulthood

LEARNING OBJECTIVES

- Identify and understand the various physical, social, and emotional variables that affect the health of young adult men
- Discuss reproductive issues facing men in young and early adulthood
- Discuss psychological and behavioral factors that contribute to adult male nutrition and body image
- Discuss the role stress plays in influencing a man's quality of life
- Identify and discuss how occupational choices affect male health

YOUNG ADULTHOOD USUALLY is considered to encompass ages from twenty to forty years. Young adulthood is an exciting yet idealized period of life for a man. A young man enters into a new phase of life that involves letting go of old ways and forging new opportunities. He might let go of his college days of parties, studying, and sleeping late in exchange for early morning alarms, hour-plus commutes to work, and late-night preparations for business presentations in his office.

Not all men will attend college or have the opportunity to do so. Underserved and marginalized men have to assume different roles in society. Men who have to immediately go to work to help provide for their families may not have the opportunity to attend college or even graduate from high school. Health is intimately related to one's level of education and resultant socioeconomic status; therefore, men who achieve less education are more likely to suffer from health **maladies** and their social consequences (Kimbro, Bzostek, Goldman, & Rodriguez, 2008). Choice may be stressful when one graduates from college, but stress also may occur for a young man who wonders whether he will be able to survive in his environment.

Data that show mortality rates for young males ages eighteen to forty-four show that injury, HIV/AIDS, and homicide are among the highest causes of death in this age range. Suicide peaks in the early to mid-twenties for men. According to the National Center for Health Statistics (NCHS) in 2008, males ages 15–34 have the highest excess mortality rates of all age groups. Many health issues during this life stage are preventable with good education and primary prevention initiatives. Injuries are inevitable, but the better the safety education (such as about seatbelt use), that can be delivered, the better the outcomes that can be expected. Infectious diseases such as HIV/AIDS are very preventable with solid education and advocacy. Safer sex education initiatives and advocating for consistent HIV testing and condom use can make a huge difference in the number of new cases of infection. Recognizing signs of depression in men and encouraging the development of emotional intelligence throughout adolescence and early adulthood also can help minimize self-harm and suicide (Parsons, 2009). Many violent crimes and homicides plague young men in the United States and abroad. For example, violent crimes such as homicide are perpetrated by younger men. Moreover, men of color appear to be at the greatest risk for violence and homicide, with the chance of being a victim of homicide at 1 in 30 for black males as compared to 1 in 179 for white males (Gremillion, personal communication, 2004).

The mission for public health professionals is clear: prevent early unhealthy behaviors, educate and advocate for men who exhibit poor health choices, and remediate how our health care system engages (or does not) men in self-determining their health outcomes. This chapter focuses on several issues pertaining to male health during early adulthood. Physical and emotional health, social health and expectations, and occupational challenges are presented and discussed in the context of developing at healthier perspective and outcome.

PHYSICAL HEALTH

The physical health of young men is usually not of major concern, mainly because most young men don't have many outward signs of physical distress or disease. Statistically, young men are more likely to die from injuries and violence than they are from heart disease or cancer (Gremillion, personal communication, 2004). However, young men may appear physically healthy while they may be harboring developing coronary artery disease, **malignant** cells that may develop into cancer, or blood pressure that can predispose them to strokes in the future. The key phrase here is "in the future." Young men's care of their physical health often functions on an as-needed basis, meaning that most young men do not routinely seek out medical care unless something is drastically wrong.

Obesity

Obesity is an epidemic in the United States and that it is likely to become a **pandemic** issue in the not-too-distant future. Of the 10 leading causes of death in the United States, 4 of them are directly related to diet (Kelishadi, 2007). Boys and young men are increasingly becoming more overweight and obese, which likely will predispose them to health issues such as diabetes, high blood pressure, heart ailments, osteoporosis, arthritis, and numerous other conditions that can cause disability (Kelishadi, 2007). Primary prevention initiatives such as good eating and nutritional practices and regular physical exercise are more effective and efficient than secondary prevention, which involves screening for diseases and related disorders. Moreover, tertiary prevention attempts to control the progression of a disease process, usually with medications and surgery. Obviously, tertiary prevention trumps secondary and primary in costs and other medical resources; Public health stresses moving toward primary prevention, the most cost-effective and efficient. The three levels of prevention are illustrated in Figure 8.1.

People in general are progressively getting fatter with each decade that passes, mainly due to cultural nutrition transitions and modifications to the food supply, such as processing and preservation practices. Growing waistlines are partially attributed to the amount and quality of food available as well as the sociocultural factors that guide how we eat it. For example, in areas (communities) of lower socioeconomic status (SES), one will find a

Figure 8.1   Levels of Prevention According to Use of Resources and Cost

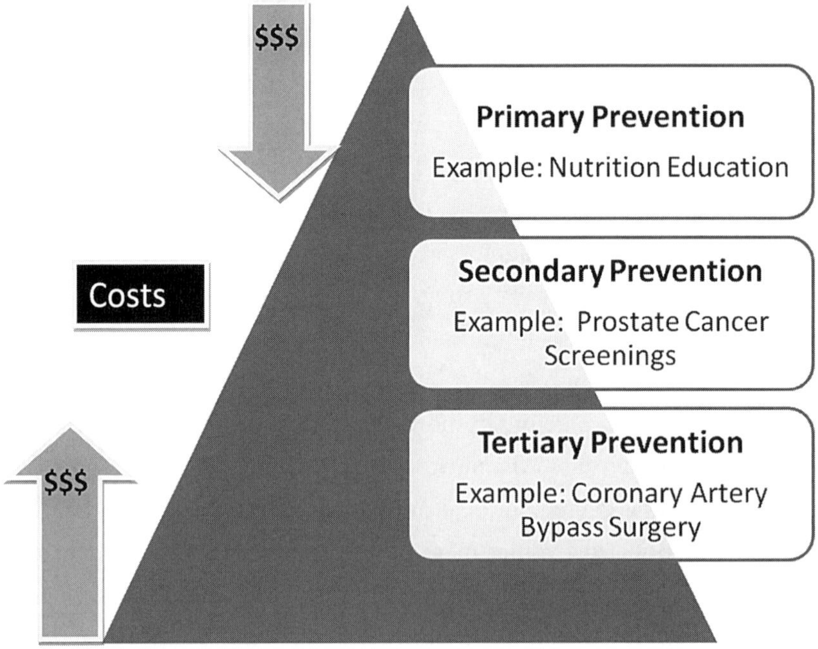

higher density of fast-food restaurant chains and options than in communities with higher standards of living. Unhealthy food options generally cost less but also serve the purpose of providing **satiety**, whereas healthier food options are usually higher in cost and less accessible to those in underserved, marginalized communities. People look for food options that cost less, feed more in their family, and stretch the dollar farther (Davis & Carpenter, 2009).

Overeating   In Western culture, men have been partially defined by how "healthy" an appetite they sport. From the earliest of ages, boys and eventually men are encouraged to consume lots of calories. Clever marketing strategies play on society's gender typing and gender bias. Manwich® and Hungry Man® dinners, among numerous others, are gender specific in that they play to men's appetites and the notion of "eating like a man." Like most aspects of society and culture, we attribute meaning and value to what people do, including the type of food we consume. A "healthy appetite" allows us to view a boy or man as robust and full of life and strength, essentially perpetuating the gender role of the man as protector. Conversely, among women, demonstrating dietary restraint likely suggests "acting like a lady."

Maintaining a Healthy Weight   Nutrition is essential to all humans. Girls and boys and eventually men and women have different dietary needs, but all people need a balance of nutrients in their lives. Food choice is one of the most critical aspects of a man's health. Knowing what healthier choices are will help men control their waistlines and improve overall quality of life. Men may think that healthy eating means sacrificing taste and quality. This is not the case; a well-balanced diet low in fat, high in fiber, rich in whole grains, vegetables, and fruit can be complemented by sweets and other higher-calorie foods.

People typically respond to all types of cues concerning food choice and eating patterns. Dr. Arthur Agatston, creator and proponent of the famous South Beach Diet, details how circulating nutrients cause hormones levels to shift and fluctuate throughout the day. With these fluctuations come signals sent to the brain that trigger hunger, cravings, and other physiological processes related to eating. Similarly, deficiencies in certain nutrients can lead to strong urges and cravings that may lead to poor food choices (Agatston, 2003). For example, a diet high in simple sugars (carbohydrates) leads to spiking of **insulin** levels in the blood, followed by a marked crash shortly thereafter. The crash leads to an increase in hunger levels and fatigue, and stresses the pancreas, which is the endocrine organ that produces insulin. Additionally, food cravings are guided by how people learn to eat from their parents and past experiences. No child is born craving a cheeseburger; it has to be introduced at some point in his or her life.

Cleansing the body of toxins from highly processed and refined foods is another step advocated by Dr. Agatston. The South Beach Diet advocates a lifestyle change. Removing simple carbohydrates (essentially sugars) and gradually replacing them with better options (complex carbohydrates) that take longer to digest is a hallmark of the diet plan. Complex carbohydrates, such as those provided in whole wheat and whole grain breads and pastas, take longer to digest (because of their fiber) and therefore help insulin levels to be gradually released, thus leading to less frequent hunger, less fatigue, and less overall stress on the body. Foods high in protein, such as meat, fish, chicken, and so on, take longer to process and digest and therefore defer hunger for longer periods of time. The type and quality of the protein source should be a primary consideration.

Fats have been a topic of concern for many people, often because of misconceptions about the role, function, and types of fat. Saturated fats come from animal sources and a few plant-based sources and should be consumed in moderation because of their propensity for negatively affecting blood cholesterol levels, which may in turn affect heart health (Agatston, 2003). Unsaturated fats, such as olive oil and other plant-based oils, should be included in men's diet more so than saturated fat sources.

Knowing how certain nutrients affect hunger and cravings also is very important. Most men know how their bodies react to food. This is their bodies' way of communicating. A continuous and sustainable number of calories through nutrients (carbohydrates, proteins, and fats) not only will eliminate hunger but also cravings. Sources of fiber include vegetables, fruits, whole grain breads, and other products that produce a sensation of fullness.

Table 8.1   A Simple Way to View Weight Management

Factor	Result
More calories out than in	Weight loss
More calories in than out	Weight gain
Equal calories in and out	Stable weight

Drinking plenty of water assures it gets into all of your cells (Agatston, 2003). Consulting the U.S. Department of Agriculture's (USDA) My Plate can help men understand what and how they eat. The site also offers great tips and suggestions as to how to improve one's diet by incorporating a diverse group of foods.

Maintaining a healthy weight is a relatively simple process. A simple formula is presented in Table 8.1.

The key variable in these formulas for weight maintenance is physical activity combined with dietary practices. Regular physical activity helps the body to effectively use calories and thereby minimize weight gain. Other key variables in maintaining a healthy weight that health professionals can recommend to male patients are four to six smaller meals per day, a variety of foods, portion size control, limited sodium intake (ideally less than 1,500 milligrams per day), limited fat and sugars from carbohydrates, increased fiber, moderate alcohol consumption, and daily breakfast. Additionally, men can be advised to take a quality multivitamin and mineral supplement; most diets are devoid of all nutrients needed to maintain optimal health (Agatston, 2003).

Other lifestyle factors related to weight include stress and alcohol use. The more stress in our lives, the more weight we tend to gain. Stress activates the sympathetic nervous system, or the "fight or flight" response. The stress hormone *cortisol* is released throughout the body, which breaks down tissues (*catabolism*) and also influences the retention of fat in the body. Therefore, managing one's stress levels is a critical factor in maintaining a healthy weight.

Bone health is directly correlated to nutritional status and physical activity levels. Although men often feel less susceptible to disease processes such as osteoporosis, men are *more likely* to develop osteoporosis-related bone fractures than prostate cancer. Osteoporosis increases with age (men over age fifty are higher risk), but the process can (and does) begin earlier in life. Factors include age, family history, race (whites and Asians are at higher risk than other populations); men with smaller body frames also are more susceptible to this disease (Perry & Schacht, 2001).

Nutritional needs continuously change throughout the life span, so health professionals should advise men to evaluate and reevaluate their diets on a regular basis for maintenance of good health.

Eating Disorders

Anorexia Nervosa and Bulimia Nervosa   Anorexia nervosa (AN) and bulimia nervosa (BN) commonly are not considered to affect men. However, of the nearly 8 million people in the United States who are diagnosed with an eating disorder, approximately 10% are men (Hudson, Hiripi, Pope, & Kessler, 2007). These rates are most likely under-reported due to the stigma of eating disorders among men. Shame and low self-esteem underpin many of the reasons why people develop eating disorders. Overweight men are more likely than normative-weight men to develop eating disorders. Moreover, eating disorders are more common in homosexual males largely due to the value placed on health, vanity, and success in the gay community (Luciano, 2001). This may worsen diagnosis and treatment in heterosexual males because of the fear of being stereotyped as gay or having a "feminine" disease. Sports such as wrestling, horse racing, and long-distance running that emphasize low body weight, eating restraint, or control of eating practices place athletes at a higher risk for developing eating disorders (Hudson et al., 2007).

Body image largely dominates how a person feels about his or her body, and when this goes awry, eating and similar disorders can result. Perfectionist traits and a need for control in one's life also contribute to the development of these disorders. The primary issue with men and eating disorders is the secrecy they commonly endure, because treatment often is tailored toward women. Men also tend to self-medicate with alcohol and other drugs rather than seek counseling and other forms of treatment. Drugs often enhance anxiety in the long term and lead to a cycle of continued use. Research has begun to investigate the link between males with eating disorders and other psychological conditions, such as attention deficit disorder (ADD) and attention deficit hyperactivity disorder (ADHD), nonsuicidal self-injury (NSSI), depression, anxiety disorders, post-traumatic stress disorder (PTSD), previous sexual abuse, obsessive compulsive disorder (OCD), borderline personality disorder, and multiple personality disorder, among others (Hudson et al., 2007). Most of the underlying causes and symptoms of eating disorders are similar in men and women; however, feeling as if one is in the minority pervades many men who are afflicted with eating disorders. Recognition and immediate management and treatment are critical for hope of a positive recovery and ultimately happiness with oneself.

DIAGNOSTIC CRITERIA FOR ANOREXIA NERVOSA

A. Refusal to maintain body weight at or above a minimally normal weight for age and height (for example, weight loss leading to maintenance of body weight less than 85% of that expected; or failure to make expected weight gain during period of growth, leading to body weight less than 85% of that expected)

B. Intense fear of gaining weight or becoming fat, even though underweight

C. Disturbance in the ways in which body weight or shape is experienced, undue influence of body weight or shape on self-evaluation, or denial of the seriousness of the current low body weight

D. Among women, amenorrhea

Source: Adapted from American Psychiatric Association (2000)

DIAGNOSTIC CRITERIA FOR BULIMIA NERVOSA

A.   Recurrent episodes of binge eating. An episode of binge eating is characterized by both of the following:

1.   Eating, in a discrete period of time (for example, within any two-hour period), an amount of food that is larger than most people would eat during a similar period of time and under similar circumstances

2.   Lack of control over eating during the episode (for example, a feeling that one cannot stop eating or control what or how much one is eating)

B.   Recurrent inappropriate compensatory behavior in order to prevent weight gain, such as self-induced vomiting; misuse of laxatives, diuretics, enemas, or other medications; fasting; or excessive exercise.

C.   The binge eating and inappropriate compensatory behaviors both occur, on average, at least twice a week for three months.

D.   Self-evaluation is unduly influenced by body shape and weight.

E.   The disturbance does not occur exclusively during episodes of anorexia nervosa.

Source: Adapted from American Psychiatric Association (2000)

Myth: It is a rare occurrence that young adult men experience eating disorders such as anorexia nervosa and bulimia nervosa.

Fact: While it is true that females experience eating disorders more than men, studies suggest that 10% of reported eating disorders are experienced by men. This accounts for nearly 3+ million men in the United States alone. Males are highly susceptible to body image disorders but may be better than women at hiding them (Cohane & Pope, 2001).

Compulsive Eating Disorder   Compulsive eating disorder, also known as *binge eating disorder,* is one of the most common forms of disordered eating and involves consuming large quantities of food in short periods of time on multiple occasions. Signs and symptoms of this disorder include eating more quickly than normal; eating until the point of discomfort; eating large quantities of food even when not hungry; eating alone due to embarrassment of food consumption patterns; and feeling guilty, disgusted, and depressed after eating episodes. The specific disorder affects more women than men, although rates are fairly comparable (3 women to every 2 men), and includes roughly 2 million Americans, with world rates not well known at this time. Obesity is more strongly correlated to this disorder as well.

DIAGNOSTIC CRITERIA FOR COMPULSIVE EATING DISORDER

A. Recurrent episodes of binge eating. An episode of binge eating is characterized by both of the following:

   1. Eating, in a discrete period of time (for example, within any two-hour period), an amount of food that is larger than most people would eat in a similar period of time under similar circumstances

   2. Lack of control over eating during the episode (for example, one cannot stop eating or control what or how much one is eating)

B. The binge-eating episodes are associated with three or more of the following:

   1. Eating more rapidly than normal

   2. Eating until feeling uncomfortably full

   3. Eating large amounts of food when not feeling physically hungry

   4. Eating alone because of being embarrassed by how much one is eating

   5. Feeling disgusted with oneself, depressed, or very guilty after overeating

(Continued)

C. Marked distress over binge eating is present.

D. The binge eating occurs, on average, at least two days a week for six months.

E. The binge eating is not associated with the regular use of inappropriate compensatory behaviors (for example, purging, fasting, excessive exercise) and does not occur exclusively during the course of anorexia nervosa or bulimia nervosa.

Source: Adapted from American Psychiatric Association (2000)

There are several theories as to why men may compulsively overeat, with the more probable reasons being lower self-esteem and diminished self-restraint. These psychoemotional factors also may be coupled with society's beliefs and values in how males consume food (Cooper & Fairburn, 2003). Western society makes it easier for males to overeat because social norms tend to guide everyday beliefs, values, and practices, particularly eating patterns. Food represents many factors beyond simple nutrition, so in order to change the struggles many men may have with consumption of food, health practitioners may need to start early in life teaching appropriate food selection and portion size control.

Infertility

A fairly common health issue and concern for many men focuses on reproductive health and viability. For millennia, men have prided themselves on their role for "creating life" through the "spreading of the seed." The importance of the male "seed" is captured in several verses in the Bible, where God scorns those who waste (spill) their "seed" without just cause. Religious overtones of fertility largely have been viewed as a function of maleness and utility in society; that is, creating life itself. This patriarchal view of the male role in procreation has lessened over past decades, particularly with the women's movement, however, if a man cannot "produce," he may develop a lesser sense of self and emotional strife.

Some men are born with **congenital** defects or develop insidious problems with the reproductive tract that can limit their fertility (Skakkebaek et al., 2001). These types of defects are relatively uncommon; however, they do affect 0.001% of the population or 125.8 births per 100,000 (Thacker, 2004). Some postulated causes of congenital reproductive defects include parental exposure to environmental toxins; individual exposures, such as in employment settings (factory work with chemicals); and abnormal genetic sequences (Lottrup et al., 2006). Some syndromes and conditions, such as Klinefelter's syndrome and fragile X syndrome (see Chapter Seven) generally result in sterility. Males who exhibit genetic traits of Klinefelter's syndrome typically are hypogonadal, meaning that the testes fail to produce viable gametes (sperm) once puberty commences.

Also, the general overall health of a man may predict his relative fertility (Thacker, 2004). Many men hold the belief that they will be able to produce viable sperm well into their seventies and eighties. While this may be somewhat true, the quality and viability of the sperm greatly depend on the relative health status of the man. Men who don't take good care of themselves will have poorer fertility status than men who do take care of their health. For instance, Mohr, O'Donnell, and McKinlay (2004) found that overweight and obesity greatly affect circulating testosterone and estrogen levels in men (that is, greater obesity led to lower testosterone) and therefore will affect sperm quality, quantity, and motility for the negative. Consumption of fatty foods, smoking, drug use (including prescription drugs), and alcohol all can affect sperm production. Toxins and other products, such as fat, affect a man's hormonal status, causing estrogen levels to rise and testosterone levels to fall. This sends feedback to the gonads to limit, or in some severe cases, shut down production of sperm. The result is limited fertility status (Mohr et al., 2004).

Injury to the testes, along with previous experiences with testicular cancer, may inhibit fertility. Damage to a testis, or to both of them, can limit sperm production or the quality of sperm, or in some cases, the testis may have to be removed (known as an *orchidectomy*). In the case of testicular cancer, radiation, chemotherapy, and removal may cause irrevocable damage to the sperm-producing cells, thereby limiting fertility (Skakkebaek et al.,

2001). Contrary to what many people believe, males who undergo the removal of a testicle due to trauma or disease don't necessarily lose all function and capabilities. Like many other body parts, the body will compensate for the loss or dysfunction of a structure. One testis often will stand in for the other in the event of damage. Additionally, supportive therapies, such as testosterone hormonal replacement, can aid the body in making sperm and thereby enhance fertility status.

Sexually transmitted infections (STIs) such as gonorrhea, syphilis, trichomoniasis, and chlamydia all can affect reproductive abilities (Weinstock, Berman, & Cates, 2004). Bacterial infections as with gonorrhea often travel into the reproductive tract, infecting vital structures such as the testes (*orchitis*) and epididymus (*epididymitis*). If left untreated, or if subsequent infections occur due to unsafe sexual practices, permanent damage and scarring may result. With 1 in 5 Americans having an infection by the age of twenty-one, STIs encompass the third most common infectious disease categories in the United States, behind the common cold and flu; therefore, reproductive health likely will be affected if an STI is not recognized, effectively managed, and prevented in the future (Weinstock et al., 2004).

Social ramifications of male infertility are many. A man may pride himself as the owner of the "seed" and his ability to help create life. When this notion is challenge by infertility, a man's self-esteem and worth may suffer. Marital or relationship strain may arise as couples struggle to conceive and comprehend their difficulties. Many euphemisms, such as "shooting blanks," also devalue the psychological stress and strain a man may experience. Embarrassment and feeling a sense of being less of a man also affects men. Many males view themselves as functional parts of society, and therefore, when they are "broken," so too is their relative position and value. The competitive nature of many men may lead to a sense of being let down. A man may experience fertility issues, whereas his best friend may "show him up" inadvertently by conceiving. Infertility is a considerable issue that should be well understood by both the man experiencing the dysfunction and the context in which he experiences it.

Possible therapies for male infertility encompass a variety of options and largely depend on the specific nature and cause of the infertility. Men who have genetic problems may not have many options. For example, men with Klinefelter's syndrome or fragile X syndrome often don't have the capacity to conceive due to primary sterility. Others may opt to seek the help of genetic counseling, which can help support couples with assisted reproductive technologies (ARTs). Men with damage to their gonads through injury or disease may respond to hormonal therapies such as testosterone replacement. For example, men who experience testicular tumors and cancer when they are younger may be best served by storing their sperm prior to treatment if they wish to later conceive. Testicular dysfunction or removal may limit future options; therefore, appropriate medical consulting and counseling may be warranted. Diseases and lifestyle issues are perhaps the most modifiable in these instances. Protecting oneself from STIs through the use of safer sex methods (condoms, limiting partners and exposures) will help avoid unnecessary exposures to diseases and infection. Taking care of one's weight through proper diet and limiting exposures to drugs (licit and illicit), alcohol, stress, and environmental toxins also can enhance one's reproductive health. Additionally, the psychosocial stress of infertility should not be taken lightly. Health professionals should encourage men to express their concern through appropriate support groups and counseling in order to understand their beliefs, attitudes, and feelings about infertility (Baraff, 1991).

Vasectomies

Controlling one's fertility status often has been a burden. Birth control pills, tubal ligations, and traditional contraceptive options, such as diaphragms and condoms, largely have been the most common options. Female options involve insertion of objects, such as intrauterine devices (IUDs), diaphragms, and cervical caps, into the vagina, which may lead to higher risk for infection. Hormonal methods such as birth control pills are very popular, but they also can be expensive and must be taken on a regular basis to be effective.

However, the popularity of male forms of birth control beyond the condom has increased over the past twenty years. Newer technologies and drug discoveries have expanded how male contraception is perceived. For example, there have been inroads made on a male form of a birth control pill (Goodman, 2008), which has added more sex-specific options for couples. Permanent methods such vasectomies also have been popularized as forms of birth control.

A vasectomy is the cutting of a section of the *vas deferens,* which is the cord that communicates sperm to the urethra during ejaculation. Alternative methods include occluding a section of the cord with sutures and even plugs to block the sperm. A relative advantage of vasectomies over other forms of contraceptive options is that it is a relatively simple outpatient procedure with minimal risks and physical consequences and faster recovery times. With the availability of such new technologies, health professionals should advise men to be more involved in exploring birth control options with their partners (Schwingl & Guess, 2000).

Penile Dysfunction

Contraception and male reproductive options are one issue, but what if the penis doesn't work correctly or at all? Penile dysfunction (including erectile dysfunction [ED]) affects as many as 1 in 10 men in the world and ranges in severity. There are many theories as to what causes ED, such as physiological (injury), hormonal, psychological (stress or depression), heart disease, obesity, diabetes, prostate disease, and a few others (Korenman, 2004). Men tend to take pride in their physical qualities, the penis notwithstanding; therefore, when something fails, a man may feel that he too fails. Failure to perform may affect a man's psyche and cause anxiety and ultimately depression. Fear of stigmatization often keeps men from expressing concerns about ED, which may limit options for diagnosis and treatment (Baraff, 1991). The recent development of ED drugs, such as Cealis and Viagra, has aided in creating an accepting and encouraging atmosphere for many men. Television and magazine advertisements and even NASCAR race cars sport logos of these and similar drugs.

One of the leading factors causing ED is completely alterable and modifiable. This factor is overweight and obesity. Being overweight or obese can cause high blood pressure (hypertension), which may limit or close off (occlude) important primary blood vessels. Since the penis is largely comprised of blood vessels, they are commonly affected by body fat. Controlling one's diet and weight can help prevent and alleviate this condition. Similarly, heart disease also has been implicated in the development of ED. Narrowing of blood vessels (*stenosis*) due to plaques that develop from cholesterol create a similar issue. Diabetes, which is highly correlated to being overweight, also may exacerbate ED. Prostate problems, such as prostate enlargement, may affect the nerves that allow for an erection to occur (Kendirci, Nowfar, & Hellstrom, 2005). Most men will experience prostatic enlargement as they age, and some undergo surgery to alleviate symptoms consistent with prostate cancer. The sensitive blood vessels and nerves can be damaged during these procedures and thus lead to ED (Korenman, 2004). Other lifestyle behaviors, such as smoking, which constricts blood vessels, also may contribute to ED (Peate, 2005).

Psychological issues also greatly affect ED. For example, men who have highly stressful lives often report higher instances of ED. Stress releases certain hormones into the blood stream that can cause the brain to become less active. When the brain becomes affected by stress, psychological health may be affected, as with depression (Baraff, 1991). Certain medications used to treat depression also may contribute to ED. Other drugs such as heart medication can affect sexual functioning in men. Popular drugs used to control blood pressure and slow heart rate are called *beta-blockers*. These drugs slow the heart, which reduces overall blood pressure throughout the body, including the penis. Men on beta-blocker therapy often experience ED as a side effect of the pharmacological treatment (Korenman, 2004).

Social and Cultural Factors   For millennia, men (and women) have viewed the penis as a symbol of fertility and thus power and status (Dillon et al., 2008). Many cultures and societies were based on a patriarchal structure, which valued what the male contributed to life, minimizing women in the process. The penis became a symbol of power and virility; therefore, the more of it, the better. Bigger is better for social status, but ironically, most men have close to the average size penis, with minor deviations (Luciano, 2001). Additionally, the true creation of life comes from the man's sperm, which is produced in his testes and not the penis. A fresco painting from ancient Pompeii depicts of the god Priapus shows him weighing his penis against a

Figure 8.2   Roman God Priapus (fresco painting)

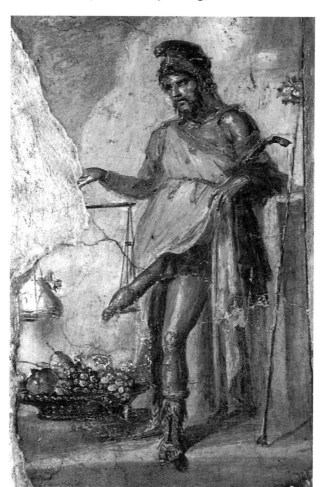

bag of gold (see Figure 8.2). The ancient Romans viewed the penis in an exaggerated state as valuable. The ancient Greeks also frequently depicted males in the nude; however, penis size was not as emphasized as with the Romans. In non-Western cultures, such as India or some tribes in Africa, the penis is depicted as large and almost always in the erect state. Illustrations from the Kama Sutra show men with abnormally large penises engaging in sexual activity.

Some common postulates for modern males' valuing of the penis include vanity, competition (alpha male mentality), sexual satisfaction, normative discontent, the symbol of power or masculinity, and others that may be less understood (Luciano, 2001). Research suggests that men appear to be more concerned with their size than are women. A 2005 internet survey of 52,031 heterosexual men and women found that only 55% of participating men were satisfied with their penis size, whereas 85% of participating women said they were "very satisfied" with the size of their partner's penis, and only 6% of women rated their partner as smaller than average (Lever, Frederick, & Peplau, 2006). In many cases this "penis panic" among men is a misperception. Men view the penis from looking down at it, thus, giving a false perception of smaller size and length. Males are naturally competitive and try to assure their dominance from the youngest of ages, so comparing penis sizes may simply be an extension of this primal male behavior. Socioculturally, myths about sexual satisfaction and a larger penis have flooded email inboxes. Again, the irony is that when polled, many partners (especially women) report that size is less of a factor than other aspects of the sexual experience, such as foreplay, intimacy, emotional connections, and how the man engages with his penis. Men tend to focus on simply the organ and how it relates to sex. In fact, most vaginas are 4–6 inches in length when aroused; therefore, length may even be less important of a factor in sexual pleasure than the girth of a penis. Men also appear to be more visual creatures and therefore value comparisons. For example, many boys and men become anxious in public settings, such as urinals or open showers, where their penises may be visible to others if they feel their penises do not "measure up."

To answer this anxiety, we explore the concept of *normative discontent.* Popularized by Rodin, Silberstein, and Striegel-Moore (1984), this concept was originally applied to women's expected unhappiness with some aspect(s) of their bodies, based on the culture in which they live. It is considered abnormal if a woman is *not* concerned about some aspect of how she looks, be it her weight, hair, shape, or other trait. The same concept can be applied to men and their body images. Men are exposed to countless media images and messages, from the earliest of ages, that suggest a "bigger is better" mentality. The norm becomes what we perceive and not necessarily what is.

According to classical research (Schonfeld, 1943) and recent studies (Chen, Gefen, Greenstein, Matzkin, & Elad, 2000; Wessells, Lue, & McAninch, 1996), most scientific evidence concludes that the average human penis is 5.1 to 5.9 inches and 4.85 inches in girth when erect, and 3.5 inches when flaccid. There are many variations; some bigger and some smaller. Some men are referred to as "showers" and others as "growers." What this means is that in the flaccid state, some men have smaller *appearing* penises, whereas some appear larger in the unerect state. These normal size variations mean little for the erect size of a penis. "Showers" typically only gain a little more size in the erect state, whereas "growers" can double (or more) relative size. Again, size doesn't necessarily relate to function.

Media such as various forms of pornography generally depict men with large genitalia, not for accuracy or realism but for fantasy and showmanship. Spam emails convey messages about not being good enough or big enough, thus playing on male insecurities to make billions of dollars annually on male enhancement products.

It is important for health professionals, partners, parents, and caregivers, and educators to be sensitive to a male's concern for penis size, whether founded or unfounded. Concerns can lead to a man's lower self-esteem, self-worth, depression, and even radical reactions, such as spending money and resources on unproven male enhancement products or even surgery. Ironically, with men knowing that so many men are concerned for their penis size, it should become more obvious that only a few males exceed well beyond the average. Health professionals are advised to have frank age-appropriate discussions with males when they are younger, and educators should not be averse to covering this topic in sexuality or even psychology and sociology classes. Educators can help dispel common myths and teach media literacy strategies and skills to help redefine the norm of penis sizes.

Options and Treatments   The medical industry has responded to males' concerns by offering many options and treatments ranging from the mild to the extreme (Korenman, 2004). Many companies offer ED products that claim to reverse ED or enhance male sexual pleasure. Unfortunately, many of the latter are little more than "snake oil." The term *enhancement* is vague. Men may perceive these claims to mean a bigger (longer or thicker) penis, while claims may refer to increased blood flow to the organ and thus more frequent and/or stronger erections. Some of the older methods of enhancing manhood include herbal remedies and physical devices such as pumps. Herbal claims include products such as yohimbe, epimedium leaf extract (horny goat weed), cuscuta seed extract, gingko biloba extract, *tribulis terrestrius*, saffron, taj, and safflower root (Gutmann, 2009). Many commercial products include these herbal products in their proprietary blends to enhance male function. Major health issues concerning these products are threefold: (1) they are largely unregulated by agencies such as the Food and Drug Administration (FDA) and therefore lack appropriate data as to their relative efficacy and safety; (2) men often are misled by the product claims and may misuse or overuse the product; and (3) men may delay treatment or medical follow-up by trying these products. Other nonhealth issues concerning these products include efficacy, financial issues, and whether they are well documented or even physiologically possible. It is not possible to "grow a larger penis," as several products claim to do, but these herbals may optimize erectile function by enhancing blood flow or encouraging systemic testosterone levels, which also has been shown to produce better, more frequent erections. Herbals have not been scientifically proven or supported to cause the penis to grow longer or thicker, but, instead they may help with what a man already has.

Nonherbal products include gadgets and devices such as pneumatic pumping devices (penis pumps), stretching (traction) apparatuses, and combinations of the two. Most of these devices provide little to no **empirical** evidence that their products do what they claim. Pneumatic penis pumps generally incorporate a suction canister connected to a pump hose that can be manually or electronically activated. Pumping causes the air to be evacuated outside of the canister, thus creating a vacuum seal around the head and shaft of the penis. This technique encourages blood flow to the penis, but does not increase size. While blood flow appears to increase the relative size of the penis, the results are temporary once the device is removed and blood flow returns to a pre-pumped state. Used over time, these devices may encourage blood to flow more freely, especially if there are blockages, scar tissue, or plaques built up in the blood vessels of the penis (Kazem, Hosseini, & Alizadeh, 2005). It should be made clear however, that there is no empirical evidence that pumping devices make the penis longer or thicker permanently.

Stretching or traction devices have recently become popular. Devices are attached to the closest part of the base of the penis as the stable end, and the far end encompasses the tip of the penis. A predetermined amount of traction force is then applied to the penis and is left on for a specified amount of time per day. The theory behind these types of products is that the erectile tissues and suspensory ligaments that stabilize the penis will yield over time and become more plastic in terms of mobility. While there may be theoretical concepts and anecdotal support for these types of enhancement devices, evidence-based empirical data are not available (Kazem et al., 2005).

Combination devices attempt to merge these two concepts. Efficacy appears to be the same. Ultimately, there is little to no strong evidence that these devices work and are little more than a novelty or fetish for some people. Alternatively, some men and their partners may enjoy the excitement and novelty of using penis enhancement products. If these are used as part of healthy sexual experience and there are no known health risks, enhancement devices can be quite enjoyable. A trained medical professional such as a primary care physician or a specialist such as a urologist can advise if a man is concerned about his penile health or related issues.

Surgical Interventions   One of the only means to increase the size and girth of the penis is through surgical intervention (Dillon, Chama, & Honig, 2008). In the vast number of cases, these are elective surgeries that are paid out of pocket by the recipient. First, a consult is required by the surgeon to determine the goals and health status of the potential surgical candidate. After the consult, the surgeon likely will go over the procedure, risks, benefits, and costs. From that point, a date is set for the procedure, which typically involves day surgery as an outpatient. Follow-up care is warranted to assure adequate healing and results. As with any surgery, there are potential risks for tissue and nerve damage, unacceptable healing or cosmetic results, need for revision of the original surgery, blood loss, infection, and even death (although rare in occurrence) (Bruno, Senderoff, Fracchia, & Armenakas, 2007).

Three of the most common surgical procedures include penile lengthening, penile widening, and glanular enhancement. Other procedures include methods to address ED and penile curvatures (Peyronie's disease). Penile lengthening generally involves cutting the suspensory ligament that secures the root of the penis to the pubic bone of the pelvis. Many men do not realize that 30% to nearly 50% of the penis is internal, as it attaches to the pubic bone. Through surgery, the penis is pulled forward, usually resulting in a gain of 1–2 inches in length. Many procedures have been attempted for girth enhancement, some with good results and others not. Recently, many surgeons prefer using dermal-matrix grafts that are placed around the shaft just under the superficial layer of skin. This matrix allows for the man's normal cells to fill in this matrix (think of scaffolding), thus creating more layers and girth. In most cases, men can expect to gain 25%–35% in girth (Bruno et al., 2007). Previous methods have included dermal fat injections usually from one's own body. Glanular enhancement attempts to increase the size (circumference) of the head of the penis, also known as the *glans penis*. Many men may choose to have this procedure in addition to length and/or girth enhancement to maintain symmetry of the overall penis. Hyaluronic acid gel is injected around the glans penis, resulting in greater circumference (up to 20% more). Results of this procedure are not permanent, however, and need to be reevaluated every 12–18 months.

Possible health complications from these procedures vary based on the skill of the surgeon, the health of the patient, and the procedure being performed. Penile lengthening can damage surrounding tissues, including the suspensory ligament, which can lead to scarring and bleeding. Ligament damage can lead to an unstable penis, which can make erections and intercourse difficult. Girth enhancement complications mainly include swelling and disproportionate distribution of fluids and tissue around the shaft of the penis. Previous methods of fat injections were more likely to cause proportion issues than recent advancements, but the risk still exists. Glanular enhancement also has similar risks as girth enhancement. Due to the need to have multiple injections to maintain the circumference of the glans penis, swelling, desensitization, and scarring can result. Risks and complications are relatively low in the United States, but procedures may be less regulated and safe in other parts of the world; therefore, caution is strongly advised (Bruno et al., 2007; Dillon et al., 2008).

There are however, actual conditions where men may suffer from penile deficiencies, such as micropenis, erectile dysfunction, and a psychological condition known as *Koro*. *Micropenis* is a condition in which the penis is less than two inches when erect. There are many possible causes of micropenis, such as genetics, endocrine system dysfunction (androgen or pituitary disorders), and environmental stress, such as pesticides and other toxins. The condition affects less than 1% of men, but it may cause significant distress in a man's life. Similarly, overweight and obesity can lead to a "buried penis," which may result in dysfunction. Excess fat may cause the penis to invaginate, which makes it appear as if it is buried within the tissue in the pubic region (Chen, Gefen, Greenstein, Matzkin, & Elad, 2000; Wessells, Lue, & McAninch, 1996). Modifying one's weight is the main way to reverse this condition, whereas micropenis may require androgen (testosterone) therapy or even surgical intervention. *Koro* is a culture-specific concern that involves the intense fear and preoccupation that one's genitals are shrinking and may eventually disappear (Chowdhury, 1998). Common in Asian countries, *Koro* is listed in the *Diagnostic and Statistical Manual of Mental Disorders* (*DSM–IV*), as a valid psychiatric condition that warrants follow-up and treatment through counseling (American Psychiatric Association, 2000). In conclusion, men value their penis and will take measures to represent it in the best possible light for a variety of psychological and sociocultural reasons. Being aware of what causes men to become preoccupied and even obsessed with penis size, in addition to schemes that prey on these insecurities, may help decrease negative health outcomes and enhance overall health-related quality of life in men.

SOCIAL HEALTH

Social health during young adulthood encompasses many areas ranging from friends and social events to relationships and communication styles. Positive social health is extremely important for men who want to lead healthy and productive lives. Challenges and imbalances of one's social health often will overflow to other aspects of one's life, such as personal health, motivation, self-esteem, self-confidence, and many other areas. The development of a positive social health perspective is a fine balance among a man's personal goals and motivations, family and social norms, and a confluence of other day-to-day events.

Younger men often value their social lives more so than at other times in their lives. Old networks from high school and college are soon challenged by that first job. Some men have families to think about, although social trends suggest people are waiting longer to begin families. Whatever scenario best fits a man's life during this stage, social health is very important in maintaining over all good health and quality of life. Strong social ties help to encourage a more positive outlook on life. They help shape what we do and how we do it. Conversely, poor social health can take its toll on a man. For example, a man who works all day and night trying to get ahead may find himself less happy overall despite his gains in status or money. People are social creatures; we need solid and frequent interactions with others to help process and modify our worldviews.

Younger men often want to keep their previous friendships and social ties strong but also develop new ones occupationally and personally. Hanging out at the bar or sports club may soon give way to working late or going on dates to find a lifetime partner. Dating and developing bonds and relationships often is a hallmark of younger adulthood. With education and occupation in check for many men, attention often turns to that next step in life. Finding a partner in order to grow intrapersonally is a key feature of social health. It is within the human condition to want to interact, be loved, love others, and feel valued as a member of society (Baraff, 1991). Some men enjoy their "freedom" and the dating "game," as many refer to it, while others aim to find the "right one" in order to settle down into family life. Every man will develop his own timeline and life goals. In the Western world, there is no standard for when a man should settle down or start a family; however, social norms often exert an unspoken pressure. In other cultures, it is not uncommon to commit earlier in life to sustain social ideals that have existed for millennia. In the United States, however, we tend to value personal choice and freedom. Either way, each individual knows what he feels is right for him, and he should let his heart and self-understanding guide his moves and goals in life during this stage.

VIGNETTE

Fresh out of college at the age of twenty-five, Ben was inspired, yet tired. He knew that he had accomplished something no one in his direct family had; he'd graduated from college! The road to a bachelor of science degree was anything but ordinary, or was it? He'd graduated from high school on time and went immediately to his college of choice. After three years of education, he grew disenfranchised from the process and dropped out to work in a professional marketing firm for the next year-plus. Ben thought this was what he was supposed to do, because he was independent now, working full-time, earning a paycheck; he'd moved out of his parents' house and was on his own. After speaking with his friends and some coworkers, Ben realized that he should finish his college education if he wanted to advance in his career. Ben applied for admission to another college, where he finished two-and-a-half years later. Ben remembers being in classes with typical eighteen- to twenty-two-year-olds, but he also noticed a greater number of older students as well. Was nontraditional now the norm? Was his path ordinary or extraordinary?

Ben now had to weigh in on his next steps. Should he attend graduate school, get a job, settle down and start a family, go on a trip around the world, or simply find himself? He thought about his life deeply. Graduate school was appealing, but he felt that he wanted to start making money and more school would delay this process; he was very excited about getting a job, but worried about what was available to him in a particularly challenging economy; he thought about settling down and starting a family only because his friends seemed to be doing that, but he realized, "I don't even have a date, let alone start a family!"; a trip around the world would be fun and exciting, but was this what he was supposed to do?; and finally, after much contemplation, he decided he did need to find himself. For now, Ben planned on reveling in his degree with his family and friends until his next life plans developed.

How men and women socially interact has been the subject of many jokes and debates. The process of being in a relationship greatly affects a man's social and personal health. Most people have heard of the book *Men Are from Mars, Women Are from Venus* by John Gray (1992), which describes how men and women seem to communicate very differently, often to the point of being at odds with one another. Men and women are biologically different, and our brains and all of the emotions and ways of communicating may be as well. (The concept is very **heteronormative** and omits men who find partners in people of the same sex.) Books such as this may help people better understand how to work on meaningful communication and better relationships. Better relationships lead to better overall quality of life, personal health, and social health. Relationships, whether traditional or not, are tricky to navigate at any age, but particularly so in early adulthood. Experience often guides people's decisions; therefore, lack of experience often leads men to making rash decisions or jumping into relationships because that is what is expected. This can lead to several negative consequences and outcomes, one of which is domestic issues and domestic violence (Bayram, Fahridin, & Britt, 2009).

Domestic violence ranges from verbal disputes all the way to murder, with everything possible in between (Robertson & Murachver, 2009). Statistics on domestic violence implicate both men and women, but younger men tend to be the perpetrators of violence more often than their female counterparts. Approximately 25% of women and just fewer than 8% of men have reportedly been sexually assaulted or physically abused by their partners. Intimate partner violence encompassed nearly seven times higher rates for women than for men. According to 2003 data, same-sex partnerships in the United States report that as high as 15% of men in same-sex relationships reported domestic abuse and violence (Tjaden, 2003). Much of the domestic violence men experience stems from past history of family violence, lack of strong male role models, substance abuse, poverty, and a confluence of other social factors (Robertson & Murachver, 2009). Men who were abused or exposed to domestic violence early in their lives are more likely to become abusers and violent later in life. It is critical that health care providers, public health professionals, and other policymakers work to break the cycle of domestic violence early on so as to foster healthy relationships and social health.

Limited communication skills plague younger men, particularly in heterosexual relationships. Poor communication often leads to frustration and disputes. Inability to positively express emotions often leads to males acting out these emotions in inappropriate and violent ways (Baraff, 1991). These frustrations may elevate to physical altercations, especially when in the presence of high-stress situations (for example, unemployment, poverty) or substance abuse. In some cases, there is a psychological issue as with **alexithymia** (the inability to appropriately express oneself), and in other cases, poor communication skills may be the result of social conditioning and norms. It is critical for health professionals, parents and caregivers, and educators to help younger boys recognize, manage, and appropriately express their emotions.

Men and Doctors

Several studies have demonstrated that men view themselves as getting sick or being unhealthy less often than do women (Barsky, Peekna, & Borus, 2001; Kroenke & Spitzer, 1998; van Wijk & Kolk, 1997). Additionally, men are more likely to postpone seeking medical care than are women, especially as problems become chronic or more severe (Eastwood & Doering, 2005). In fact, overall health care utilization by men as compared to women is strikingly different. For all age groups, men without regular physicians make up 33% of the population, as compared to 19% for women. Broken down by age, among eighteen- to twenty-nine-year-old men, 53% have no regular physician, compared to 33% of women of the same age group; and 38% of men from thirty- to forty-four years of age do not see physicians regularly, as compared to 22% of women.

Men have higher rates of not visiting a physician consistently every year than women. Overall, 24% of men don't see a doctor each year. In the eighteen- to twenty-nine age group, 33% of men did not see a doctor in the past year versus 7% in women, and 30% of men in the thirty- to forty-four-year-old age category do not see a physician each year versus 10% of women in the same age range. According to the Commonwealth Study in 2000, Louis Harris and Associates, Inc., found that only 58% of adult men who saw their doctors at least once in the past year had a complete physical examination. Of these men, 43% did not receive a blood cholesterol assessment and nearly 25% of men surveyed said that even if they were in pain or sick, they would delay seeking care as long as possible (usually one week or longer).

Social and Cultural Factors

Health care reform in the United States has become a very important and controversial issue. Partisan politics, regardless of which political side one chooses, have delayed advancements and overall improvements to delivering quality health care to all citizens. Many younger citizens do not carry health insurance because of cost, lack of access, or higher rates of unemployment. Unemployment places many young men in the conundrum of making a choice between supporting life's needs, such as food and shelter, and acquiring health insurance. Coupled with younger men's perceived lack of illness or disease risk, health insurance and doctor's visits become a very low priority for many. Of those who do have jobs and health insurance, many will adopt the lowest premium to pay, again to save money and because of their perceived lack of risk. Those who are unemployed or who are laid off have the option of Consolidated Omnibus Budget Reconciliation Act (COBRA), but this usually is not financially feasible for most young men, at the cost of upward of $700 per month (Brownlee, 2007). Fear or distrust also may underpin men's underutilization of the health care system. Many minorities avoid health care providers because of cultural expectations of quality of care. Many men of color think, "They don't care about us," which has been perpetuated by generations of family and culturally insensitive medicine (Jack, 2005; Treadwell & Ro, 2003).

Many men have been taught to use the "suck it up" mentality and to remain stoic in the face of illness. This may be due to males' fear of a social stigma of weakness. This gender role training may have set men up for a lifetime of avoiding quality health care and thus led to more negative health outcomes (Gremillion, 2004). Males often are not comfortable with health care simply because of a lack of exposure. Taking care of her body is strongly advocated for a younger woman because she may carry a child in the future. Yet men often do not see themselves as influencing the health of a baby other than what they can provide materially. However, science is showing that the relative health of a man and his sperm likely affect the genetic material conveyed to his offspring (Lottrup et al., 2006).

The functional male model seems to influence men's reluctance to access health care. When the male "machine" breaks down, he will seek care only if it is severe enough. Men don't routinely seek access to a medical specialty as do women with gynecology, which may convey men's lesser need to follow up with their health care over the course of the life span. Men may have learned to adaptively respond to health care (Parsons, 2009). They are more likely to consider the type, quantity, quality, location, and timing of pain or dysfunction in their bodies than women before making the choice to seek medical care and treatment.

Fundamentally, a cultural paradigm change is in order for newer generations of men as to how they view their bodies and their relative health. A multifaceted approach that views men's health as its own unique entity in the overall health care system may be in order. A supportive community in which everyone understands that men's health affects everyone will help shed light on this under-recognized issue (Gremillion, 2004). Health specialties that focus on male health may partially influence this positive trend in health care. If it became more of the norm for men to seek health care, more men likely would do it.

Men in general, but particularly historically underserved, marginalized minority groups, view the health care delivery system as part of an authoritarian and threatening conglomerate that sparks feelings of discord and mistrust. Attending to these attitudes and beliefs and changing them for the positive must begin at earlier ages so as to provide gender-appropriate care that reflects male values, fears, and expectations (Malcher, 2009; Treadwell & Ro, 2003). Bringing health into the workplace often encourages men to seek screenings and other forms of preventative, proactive health care more so than asking them to go to community health settings, doctor's offices, and hospitals. Sports events can be used as outlets to deliver appropriate and effective health care.

Providing vivid examples of how masculinity can successfully interact with the health care system is imperative. Fathers and other male figures acting as positive examples for younger males and generations can help correct social stigma concerning male health. There is no one formula for men's engagement in the health care process; rather a variety of social and community, as well as personal and individual, measures can be taken. Education may raise the standard of men's health. Based on research findings and national data, many men do not realize how sick they are (Barsky et al., 2001). For example, according to the Centers for Disease Control and Prevention (CDC), all 10 of the 10 leading causes of death in the United States affect more men than women; 8 of the leading 10 causes of death affect more blacks than whites; men have higher risk for life-limiting illnesses and premature death, with men of color at an extraordinarily higher risk than other categories (Kimbro et al., 2008). Making the United States "healthier in one generation" is a wonderful goal, but it must occur within the context of addressing the most underserved and marginalized groups. Strategically, through policies, and operationally, through programming, initiatives will help bridge these gaps.

EMOTIONAL HEALTH

As a man enters early adulthood, the stresses and strains of adolescence are now behind him, but they are not out of his mind and perspective. Men who experience difficulties, particularly emotional, in adolescence, may have carry-over effects into young adulthood. Society often has minimized and downplayed the emotional status of men because the social norm is for men to be strong and sturdy (Baraff, 1991). The effects can range from body image dysfunction and poor stress management strategies to physical problems such as sleep disorders. Stress and anxiety play a large role the development of psychiatric disorders such as depression. Depression and other psychiatric disorders in men change from boyhood through adolescence and well into adulthood (Treadwell & Ro, 2003). Research by Twenge and Nolen-Hoeksema (2002) found that boys of ages eight to twelve years scored slightly higher on depressive scales than did girls. In adolescence, boys' rates of depressive scores diminish; however, acting-out behaviors, school problems, and disciplinary issues seem to take center stage. As men age and enter adulthood, depression and other forms of stress lead to higher rates of diseases such as cardiovascular consequences and even death. For example, peak suicide rates for men are between the ages of twenty and forty years old, then level off until age sixty-five-plus, when they spike at abnormally high levels.

It can be **extrapolated** from these trends that at younger ages boys appear to be able to express more of their emotions and concerns; however, as society and cultural norms begin to pervade their minds and begin to take precedence, emotions are suppressed (Baraff, 1991; Kindlon & Thompson, 2000). As adulthood approaches, social standards dictate what males can and cannot do; therefore, rates of depression that most likely were under-recognized in preadolescence and adolescence reappear.

In research by Bayram et al. (2009), younger men (ages twenty-five to forty-four years old) were treated for emotional conditions at higher rates than their female equivalents. They also found higher encounter rates for psychiatric conditions in ages fifteen to twenty-four. The severity of the medical and psychiatric consults was higher in males than females; that is, females were more likely to seek consulting for psychiatric conditions, but males had more severe cases. The most common conditions in men were depression, followed by insomnia, anxiety, schizophrenia, drug abuse, tobacco abuse, acute stress reactions (panic), alcohol abuse, dementia, and post-traumatic stress disorder (Bayram et al., 2009). This research was conducted in an Australian national sample; results from Australia seem to translate to the cultural context of the United States as well. For example, in his book *Men Talk* (1991) Dr. Alvin Baraff states that a man in U.S. culture grows up feeling "innately and internally alone." He notes that because a man grows up with this sense of control and independence, "he cannot imagine ever needing to go for help and rarely considers it an option" (p. 2). Unfortunately, the average man often begins therapy at a "much more advanced stage of emotional or professional crisis; it is in most respects his last resort" (p. 3).

The under-utilization of psychological health care often skews our understanding of the emotional status of adult men. Men and women often present slightly different signs and symptoms of mental health issues. The difference in depression between men and women is how it is expressed and dealt with by the individual (Wilhelm 2009). In large-scale national studies from Canada and New Zealand, men have lower rates of anxiety and depressive disorders; however, all psychiatric conditions combined, which include substance abuse, show a different story. Men's prevalence rates equal those of women. Clearly, men handle emotional stress and strain differently. Women often report how they *feel* whereas men report what they *do* (Wilhelm, 2009). If women report how they feel, preemptive measures such as counseling and support can be provided before an issue gets out of hand; however, because men appear to be more reactionary in nature, public health often has to ask the question of why and what can be done to prevent issues in the future.

Brownhill, Wilhelm, Barclay, and Schmeid (2005) conceptualized the "big build" model to describe how younger men typically approach emotional strain and disorders such as depression. In their model, many men follow five "builds": stepping over the line, hating me and hurting you, escaping it, numbing it, and avoiding it. *Stepping over the line* includes deliberate attempts at self-harm, including suicidal ideation, highly risky behaviors, and heavy substance abuse. *Hurting me and hating you* refers to expressing feelings of aggression toward oneself and others through violence, anger, and outbursts, as well as substance use and abuse. In *escaping it* men may use drugs, violence, or sex among other behaviors to avoid their inner feelings. *Numbing it* can be explained as self-medication, using substances or activities to phase out of the current reality. *Avoiding it* involves behaviors that take a man away from the direct causes of stress and depression. A man may avoid social obligations or significant events in life. Many men are psychoemotionally predisposed to a lifetime of negative health consequences if these issues are not detected and addressed early in life or prevented altogether.

Adult Body Image

Body image may be defined as "the internal, subjective representations of physical appearance and bodily experience" (Phillips, 1998, p. 199). Body image also has been defined as "a multidimensional construct embedded in the larger, integrative construct of identity" (Graber, Paterson, & Brooks-Gunn, 1996). Body image, something all people experience, nevertheless is a complex and elusive construct (Phillips, 1998). Body image effects emotions, thoughts, and behaviors of everyday life, thereby dramatically influencing quality of life (Cash & Pruzinsky, 2004; Striegel-Moore & Franko, 2004). Many researchers have attempted to formalize a definition due to an ever-growing body of literature of both **epistemological** as well as sociologic evidence; however, capturing this human phenomenon is difficult. As people grow and develop in a physiological sense, so too does their perception of themselves. Reactions of others help to define who one is in a perceptual sense and, ultimately, allows for development of an internal portrait of the self (Phillips, 1998; Schilder, 1935). Rooted in cognitive, emotional, behavioral, and perceptual dimensions, body image is a core aspect of identity.

A strong sense of self and identity often is predictive of healthy life choices (Glanz, Rimer, & Marcus-Lewis, 2002). Conversely, a weakness in the integrity of a person's self-esteem and body image often leads to poor lifestyle choices that negatively affect health (Cash & Pruzinsky, 2004). Young adult men's mental health is a critical area to explore due to the propensity for behaviors developed during this phase of life to carry on throughout the life span.

Men in every age group may encounter body image issues. As Western culture has evolved over the past few decades, so too have our perceptions of what the ideal body should look like. Much research has focused on females. However, males also are affected by a wide range of **psychosomatic** and body image disorders, ranging from disordered eating and eating disorders to body dysmorphia and muscle dysmorphia. This social trend in males becoming more concerned and discontented with their body image can be noted in *Psychology Today*'s serial surveys. For example, in 1972, 15% of men reported they were dissatisfied with their appearance, whereas the same study found the rate had risen to 47% in 1997. Similarly, Pope, Phillips, and Olivardia (2000) found a similar trend in males reporting a frequency of 43% discontentment. When broken down by body area, 63% said they were dissatisfied with their abdomens, 45% with their muscle tone, and 38% with their chests. Additionally, 17% said they would give up three years of their life to be an ideal weight (Cash, Winstead, & Janda, 1997). Research also indicates that body image dissatisfaction occurs in countries with similar socioeconomic status as the United States (for example, Israel, Austria, Australia, and Samoa) (Lipinski & Pope, 2002; Pope, Gruber, et al., 2000; Rolland, Farnill, & Griffiths, 1997).

For centuries, men did not express much discontent with their bodies or body image because men were providers and a functional part of society. Concern for body image was never absent in males, but rather, it was not brought to the surface of the public consciousness. Today, the evolving roles of males in a **postindustrial** era have led to economic parity with females. No longer do males command industry governed by muscle and sweat; rather, today's workforce stresses ingenuity and skill of which females are aptly capable. Males may react by seizing control of the one element that remains distinct to them, the ability to overpower others through muscle (Faludi, 1999). Evolution of the "supermale," a media-endorsed conception with unattainable physical ideals, may be viewed as a contributing factor to male body image dissatisfaction (Westmoreland-Corson & Anderson, 2004).

Historically, shame and fear of public humiliation drove men with body image dissatisfaction and eating disorders underground (Anderson, Cohn, & Holbrook, 2000; Pope, Phillips, & Olivardia, 2000). Paradigm shifts in cultural standards of beauty and functionality have become paramount in contemporary society (Westmoreland-Corson & Anderson, 2004). Variations of physical attractiveness through cultures likely have origins in early childhood through adolescence with sociocultural ideals the major factors (Westmoreland-Corson & Anderson, 2004). Similar to television consumption detailed by Tiggeman (2005) and Tiggeman and Lynch (2001), Pope, Olivardia, Gruber, and Borowiecki (1999) asserted that modeling through toy action figures such as G.I. Joe may contribute to body dissatisfaction or distortion in boys and men. In this research, action figures were found to have become more muscular over time (1960s to the 1990s), far exceeding the muscularity of even the largest bodybuilders. A similar trend also was noted in *Playgirl* male centerfold models from the 1970s through the 1990s, as well as other women's magazines (Pope, Olivardia, Borowiecki, & Cohane, 2001). These factors may play a contributing role in the development of spectrum and **somatoform** disorders, such as body dysmorphia or muscle dysmorphia.

These trends contribute to a contemporary paradox of males who want to be heavier but perceive themselves as lighter, whereas females wish to be lighter but perceive themselves as almost 10–15 pounds heavier than they are. Suggested motivating factors point toward concern with physical appearance, popularity, and attractiveness to the opposite sex (Buss, 1994; Etcoff, 1999). Male body image is typically assessed through ideals such as power and dominance. The notion of the "pack leader" has been present throughout history (Etcoff, 1999). It also has been asserted that success rather than physical attractiveness defines the male ideal and his position within the male hierarchy (Buss 1994).

Men may be susceptible to a greater variety of weight concerns than females. Concern is generated due to the nature of the complexity of men's weight gain and physical appearance and strength (Westmoreland-Corson & Anderson, 2004). Men, like women, often want to change their weight but often are more preoccupied with body shape and muscularity (Pope, Phillips, & Olivardia, 2000). Appearance often is equated with success and with newer vernacular terms such as, *metrosexual*. Today's man often finds a need to react to these pressures. Reactions vary but may include obsessive exercise, dieting, use of body image drugs (Kanayama, Pope, & Hudson, 2001), and even cosmetic surgery (Westmoreland-Corson & Anderson, 2004).

Recognition and diagnosis of body image issues in males is different and more difficult than for females for a variety of reasons. Westmoreland-Corson and Anderson (2004) noted men's reluctance to admit having a "female issue" as one factor; a bias toward females in the *Diagnostic and Statistical Manual for Psychological Disorders* (DSM-TR IV; APA, 2000) as the second; and, third, male binge-eating behaviors being considered as healthy and normal guy behavior. Male concern for these behaviors is less overt than among females, making the task of predicting and intervening on behalf of male body image concerns and related consequences a clinical challenge. Follow-up studies using male samples could provide telling evidence when tracking male body image satisfaction over time. Males are more likely to respond to body image dissatisfaction preempting comorbid conditions, such as chronic depression and alcoholism (Woodside, Garfinkel, Goering, Kaplan, Goldblum, & Kennedy, 2001).

Psychosocial Disease Model   Body image dissatisfaction manifests in several ways, ranging from impaired psychological functioning to **somatic** disorders. Additionally, the term *psychosocial* implies disease characteristics, as much a social consequence as they are rooted in the individual. An individual cannot escape the reality that he or she a social creature (Schilder, 1935). As social creatures, many men are heavily influenced by the ideal that advertisers and marketers have constructed. For many years, these advertising initiatives mainly were directed toward women, but as the market grew, a whole new population was identified in that men could be marketed to as well. With these new marketing approaches came an increased perception of what being good looking meant to men (Pope, Phillips, & Olivardia, 2000).

Body Dysmorphic Disorder   Phillips (1998) defines *body dysmorphic disorder* (BDD) as having three qualities: (1) preoccupation with some real or imagined defect in appearance; for example, if a slight physical anomaly is present, the person's concern is markedly excessive; (2) preoccupation causes clinically significant distress or impairment in social, occupational, or other areas of functioning; and (3) the preoccupation is not better accounted for by another mental disorder. BDD is a subcategory of obsessive compulsive disorder (OCD) and part of the general spectrum disorders classification system (APA, 2000). Often emerging in adolescence, the defining factor of BDD is the preoccupying and obsessive nature of it. Regardless of whether there is a defect, it becomes real for the person experiencing symptoms (Phillips, 1998). It affects as many men as it does women, with men most commonly concerned with their skin, hair, nose, and genitals (Phillips & Castle, 2001).

Each person formally diagnosed with BDD must meet specific diagnostic criteria, but every individual will experience BDD differently. Severity, body areas, and behaviors are all unique to the individual, although similarities and behavioral patterns are possible. Phillips (1998) presented data on the prevalence and potential consequences of BDD in her work, *The Broken Mirror: Understanding and Treating Body Dysmorphic Disorder.* She wrote that BDD affects 1%–2% of the general U.S. population, which equates to roughly 5.8 million people; 4%–5% of people in outpatient psychiatric treatment have BDD; 8% of people with chronic depression have BDD; and up to 12% of people seeking psychiatric treatment in outpatient settings satisfy BDD criteria. Signs and symptoms of BDD include excessive checking of appearance, avoidance behaviors (such as avoiding mirrors), frequently comparing oneself to others, seeking reassurance regarding appearance, excessive time grooming, hiding parts of the body, picking at one's skin with hopes of improving appearance, use of cosmetic surgery, and many others (Phillips, 1998).

In men, BDD can lead to a series of emotional concerns, especially social physique anxiety (SPA). This condition involves anxiety experienced due to the perception that other people are evaluating one's body in a negative manner. There are many negative health consequences of SPA, including avoidance of social or public events, low self-esteem, drug use, dissatisfaction with overall body image, increased rates of disordered eating, and many others (Russell, 2002). According to Olivardia (2001), SPA in men is increasing. Lower levels of self-esteem has been postulated as a primary reason why many younger men use body image drugs, such as anabolic-androgenic steroids to meet these cultural standards and ideals (Kanayama, Pope, & Hudson, 2001). Research has established generational reasons why younger males tend to react this way as compared to retrospective feedback from males of different generations (Leone & Fetro, 2007).

Body image has been researched as a key component in social anxiety disorders and lower levels of social self-esteem (Cash & Pruzinsky, 2004). Phillips (1998) discussed BDD as a consequence of a distorted body image. Given such a long history of body image research, body image disturbance in BDD is understudied, particularly in males, and warrants further research on its impact on global self-esteem and body image in general (Phillips, 1998).

Muscle Dysmorphia and the Adonis Complex   Muscle dysmorphia (MD) was originally described by Pope, Katz, and Hudson (1993). and largely affects men in their early twenties through middle adulthood. The disorder also has been referred to as *reverse anorexia* and *bigorexia*. Pope, Phillips, and Olivardia (2000, p. 87) stated, "Muscle dysmorphia is a specific type of BDD. . . . The general category of BDD refers to all types of serious unfounded body image concerns. Muscle dysmorphia is simply the form of BDD in which muscularity, as opposed to some other aspect of the body, becomes the focus."

Causes of MD most likely include a variety of factors, ranging from sociocultural influences to genetic anomalies (Pope et al., 1993). Body esteem is a key measure and component of muscle dysmorphia (Franzoi & Chang, 2002). Unlike other disorders, such as anorexia nervosa and bulimia nervosa, identification, diagnosis, and treatment of muscle dysmorphia presents a challenge to the practitioner. This may be due to the fact that people with MD often are perceived and perceive themselves to be healthy. Behaviors and attitudes often become overt to family and friends, but the person experiencing MD remains oblivious.

Although not formally categorized as a *DSM IV–TR* disorder, several researchers have proposed diagnostic criteria for MD (Chung, 2001; Maida & Armstrong, 2005; Olivardia, 2001; Pope, Phillips, & Olivardia, 2000). Individuals experience MD differently. Muscle dysmorphia has been studied from various angles since it was proposed as a category of body dissatisfaction in 1993. For example, Leone Gray, and Sedory (2005) reviewed current trends and how the disorder can be recognized and managed in competitive athletics. Recently (2005) it was proposed that MD should be redefined as a spectrum disorder rather than a somatoform disorder based on empirical evidence over the past decade (Maida & Armstrong, 2005). This means MD may need to be reconceptualized as a psychological issue versus a body concern.

When viewed as a body image disorder rather than a collection of psychiatric and behavioral oddities, MD becomes a window through which today's evolving ideals of beauty, particularly of the male body, can be seen. Although females also are susceptible to the disorder, data suggest males are more commonly affected (Pope, Phillips, & Olivardia, 2000). From a traditional perspective, masculinity and muscle has defined the measure of a man (Dutton, 1995; Schwartz & Tylka, 2008). Muscle has come to symbolize health, dominance, power, strength, sexual virility, threat, and status (Klein, 1993; Schwartz & Tylka, 2008). When there is an actual or perceived flaw with one's muscularity, obsessive thoughts and ultimately a concern for the body may result (Dutton, 1995). Insecurity may be a cause for development of a hypermasculine persona or even insecurity with shifting gender roles (Klein, 1993).

Society likely plays a major role in the etiology of MD and similar body image disorders, particularly in males. Messages broadcast that "real men" have big muscles and that a lack thereof is unmasculine (Leone et al., 2005; Pope et al., 1993). Demasculinization often leads to a reactive approach, which may include using body-enhancing substances, such as androgenic-anabolic steroids (AAS). Many males and a few females disclosed they use AAS purely for body appearance ideals rather than for athletic ideals or goals (Buckley, Yesalis, Friedl, Anderson, Streit, & Wright, 1988; Pope & Brower, 1999; Wroblewska, 1997). A schematic of MD's relationship to other spectrum disorders is presented in Figure 8.3.

Muscle dysmorphia likely will continue to increase in prevalence due to media and societal influences (Cohane & Pope, 2001; Dawes & Mankin,

---

Figure 8.3   Obsessive Compulsive Spectrum Disorders and Their Relationships

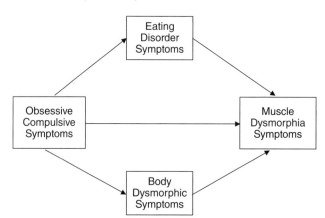

2004). Pressure to reach a muscular ideal begins at an early age and continues throughout the life span (Knoesen, 2009). Until a fundamental shift in the ideals and pressure placed upon both males and females to look a certain way diminishes, the incidence of affective body image spectrum disorders is likely to increase. It is important; however, to reinforce the fact that weight training and caring for one's body is not a bad thing; quite the contrary, exercising and weight training is excellent for optimal health and should be encouraged. Physical activity and attention to one's appearance need not be pathologized; however, exercising with the sole intent to look good and fulfill a sociocultural standard or ideal can lead to overreactions, obsessions, and possibly compulsions that negatively affect overall health-related quality of life in some men.

Cosmetic Surgery   With changing social and cultural ideals concerning youth and beauty, many men have undergone elective plastic or cosmetic surgery to improve their looks. As discussed in her book *Survival of the Prettiest: The Science of Beauty,* author Nancy Etcoff (1999) details how physical beauty has become a primary area of concern in all parts of the Western world, including among men. Most men still do not feel comfortable expressing concern for their looks, because it is deemed feminine, but the numbers of men seeking plastic surgery to enhance their looks cannot be denied nor overlooked. Women traditionally have utilized the plastic surgery sector in previous years and still do, but the rates of men seeking procedures is growing. In 1998, 9.7% of men had elective plastic surgery done to enhance their body and looks; in 2002 the rate had risen to 11.7% and to nearly 13% in 2004. Recent data suggest that as of 2010 close to 20% of men have had, plan to have, or would strongly consider having elective plastic surgery (American Society for Aesthetic Plastic Surgery [ASAPS], 2010).

   With more technology in medicine come more options for people to consider for altering their bodies and essentially their reality. Much advancement in plastic and cosmetic surgery has resulted from research done on trauma patients and soldiers returning from war. Procedures have become much safer and popularized in Western culture; many people may see it as a normal part of our society and culture. Second, the standard of living has steadily risen since the early 1900s, particularly in Western cultures such as the United States. With a higher standard of living come more money and more competition. The desire to be and look different may drive many people, including men, to seek alternatives such as plastic surgery. Third, the nature of what defines *masculine* has evolved over the past twenty years. The explosion of media detailing all types of people, expectations, cultures, and norms has chipped away at traditional gender roles. Programming such as *Queer Eye for the Straight Guy* has been implicated in changing how people view what is acceptable for men and what is not. Many men see having plastic surgery as an investment in themselves, as one would an education or even a new suit. With so many men and women achieving higher levels of education, experience, and talent, sometimes people feel that the only attribute that can set them apart from the competition is how they look.

Men are as influenced by marketing strategies as anyone else, therefore, if marketing executives in the high-rises of New York City determine men will be their next focus market, then so it will be. Men often defer cosmetic surgery until their forties, but more men are seeking consults at younger ages and having "minor" procedures, such as Botox injections to stave off wrinkles and character lines in the face, done in the meantime. Heading up the most popular procedures for men continues to be liposuction, a form of removing fat cells from various parts of the body. Liposuction is a relatively safe procedure that often is completed in an hour. Men typically target liposuction around their abdomens, chests, and lower back regions because that is where fat tends to accumulate. Injectable fat "dissolvers" (lypolysis) also have become popularized because they are less invasive. Other popular plastic surgery and cosmetic procedures for men include nose jobs, eyelid surgery, breast tissue reduction, and hair transplantation surgery (ASAPS, 2010). Many reasons are given by men who have procedures done, such as "I feel better about myself and I think it shows," "I just wanted a more professional look," and "I just wanted to look good, I didn't want to get old."

With any surgical procedures come costs and possible health risks, including permanent scarring and tissue and nerve damage if the process is not well planned. While most cosmetic and plastic surgery procedures are relatively safe, results largely vary based on the skill and experience of the surgeon, the individual health of the patient, his suitability as a surgical candidate (not everyone is a good candidate for all procedures), the complexity of the procedure, and location. Some surgeons claim to have the ability to do many types of procedures but may only have taken a cursory update course on it. Cheaper procedures or those in other countries may lack regulation from appropriate medical boards; therefore, client health may be a greater risk than at more well-established and reputable locations (ASAPS, 2010). Aside from physical risks and costs, the monetary costs associated with cosmetic and plastic surgery procedures can be substantial. Table 8.2 presents estimated costs for popular procedures sought by men.

Table 8.2   Costs Associated with Cosmetic and Plastic Surgery Procedures

Procedure	Costs	Outcomes and Comment
Liposuction	These vary, but for men approximately $3,500 including preop prep (blood work); facility costs and the procedure itself	Less fatty tissue; better self-esteem; permanent solution as it removes cells; better body weight; may cause bleeding, bruising, and scarring; costs are higher in men because of more tissue
Injection lypolysis	Costs may range from $375 to $1,500 per treatment. Up to six treatments may be needed	Less fatty tissue; better sense of self-esteem; minimally invasive; better body weight; may not be permanent solution
Hair transplantation	Most systems are $1,200, but require yearly maintenance costs that range from $75 to $650	Possible better sense of self; increase in confidence; some procedures leave scarring or poor results; often charged per graft needed

(Continued)

Table 8.2   (Continued)

Procedure	Costs	Outcomes and Comment
Rhinoplasty (nose job)	Costs vary, but on average $3,000 to $8,000 depending on need and reputation of the surgeon	Increase in self-confidence; better perceived aesthetic; permanent damage can lead to disfigurement and chronic sinus infections
Eyelid surgery	Range from $1,500 to $7,000; surgeon costs $2,500, anesthesiologist costs $700, facility fee $800	Possible increase in confidence; most people choose to have both upper and lower lids done, which increases cost; results may yield unacceptable results, leading to visual issues
Breast reduction surgery	Depends on complexity of tissue removal, but ranges from $800 to $3,000; many cases can be treated with modified liposuction procedures	Better self-esteem; improved aesthetic; reduces body weight; minimal complications

Cosmetic and plastic surgery should be a carefully thought out and planned process. Before any surgery, health professional should fully explore and discuss motivation, desired outcome, costs, and possible health issues resulting from any procedure with any man considering cosmetic surgery.

Hair Transplants

Many men lose their hair as they age as a result of genetics, environment, health status, fever or infections, thyroid dysfunction, diet, stress, and hormone levels. The primary causes of hair loss in men (also known as *male pattern baldness* or *androgenic alopecia*) are genetic factors that affect the hormones in a man's system. Male pattern baldness produces one of several familiar patterns on the scalp, such as an M-shape or "half-moon," and begins to appear in a man's twenties and thirties. The pattern is largely determined by genetics. The gene for the expression of baldness is sex linked, meaning that it is carried by a male's mother (Luciano, 2001).

At any given point of a day, approximately 85% of hairs are growing, whereas 15% are finished growing. Each hair sits within a follicle on the scalp (Rebora, 2004). The follicles shrink over time, leading to smaller, thinner hairs and eventually to none at all (Perry & Schacht, 2001). The follicle, although smaller, still remains active, which provides hope that hair can be regrown given the right environment and treatment options. One of the primary theories relates to a man's sensitivity to a hormonal byproduct of the male sex hormone testosterone called dihydrotestosterone or DHT. This byproduct affects hair follicles, causing them to thin and shrink in size, thus causing smaller hairs (Rebora, 2004).

Male pattern baldness is not necessarily a pathological condition and does not indicate poor physical health. However, in some instances, as with thyroid problems, thinning hair and balding may provoke a reason for a man to follow up with a medical consult. Other conditions warranting follow-up with a medical professional include iron deficiency, inadequate protein in your diet, cancer therapies, such as chemotherapy, as well as certain medications used to treat **gout**, arthritis, depression, heart disease, and high blood pressure. Excess amounts of vitamin A also have been implicated in hair loss. Biopsies of the skin of the scalp can help determine the health status of a man and provide better insight about treating the condition. Hair analysis can be used to determine toxins in the system, such as arsenic, lead, or other materials. Strategies to decrease exposures to such environmental toxins can be presented and discussed so as to better enhance health (Perry & Schacht, 2001; Rebora, 2004). There are options and medical treatments for men who experience hair loss regardless of the exact cause.

Most men express some concern when they begin to lose their hair. This may be because for many men, hair represents vitality and youth; the loss of their hair may signify the loss of these attributes. Losing their hair can be very psychologically distressing to some men, which can provoke symptoms of depression, anxiety, and low self-esteem (Luciano, 2001). Control also may play a role in why men may distress about their hair loss. Losing one's hair is often beyond the control that many men value; therefore, this may cause a man distress. Losing his hair at a younger age may profoundly affect a young man. As a man ages, he has older male role models with whom to compare (Luciano, 2001). However, when a man loses hair at a younger age and compares himself to others in his age or peer group, he may become distressed (Rebora, 2004).

There are options for men who experience hair loss. Hairpieces (wigs or toupees) made from a variety of materials have been used for centuries to cover hair loss or enhance the way a man looks. Hair weaving can help augment the appearance of hair by adding additional hair into a man's existing hair. Changing one's hairstyle also has been used as a popular strategy for many men. These strategies are safe and noninvasive. Cost also is less than other procedures and options.

Hair transplant surgeries vary in technique, often costing several thousands of dollars to maintain the system. Yearly maintenance fees also are commonly incurred after a procedure has been performed. Grafts are implanted at various points on the scalp based on the man's hair loss analysis. Some use "plugs," which attempt to implant stronger hairs into the existing follicles. Grafts may be from outside sources (*allografts*) or synthetic sources, or from the person himself (*autografts*), such as hair from the back and sides of the scalp. The downside of surgical procedures is the risk of infection, such as abscesses at the graft sites, or unacceptable cosmetic results.

There have been promising results from two primary drug treatments, minoxidil and finasteride. Minoxidil, otherwise known as Rogaine, is applied as a solution directly to the scalp and is used to slow hair loss by stimulating the follicles. Rogaine also may help promote a better environment for promoting hair regrowth in some men. Men have experienced mixed results with this product, but it may be a good option for some. The downside is that when you stop applying the product, the previous level of hair loss recurs. Minoxidil may be obtained without a prescription. Finasteride, also known as Propecia or Proscar, is a prescription pill that helps to limit the production of DHT. Hair loss often is slowed rather than enhanced, but this depends on each individual. Again, like minoxidil, when a person ceases taking the product, the previous level of hair loss returns (Luciano, 2001; Perry & Schacht, 2001).

Stress

Stress is ubiquitous in modern life. There are various forms of stress: physical, chemical, emotional, and occupational, among others. Stresses are the forces (both internal and external) that affect or exert an influence on an individual's system. External stress can come from a variety of sources, such as a job, personal relationships, or even the environment. Internal stress may be the result of psychological processes such as anxiety or other types of emotions when a person is presented with life experiences (Blumenthal et al., 2005).

Two forms of stress include *eustress* and *distress.* Eustress typically has been described as being positive, whereas distress is negative. The individual's perception and perspective greatly defines whether an event is eustressful or distressful (Tsigos & Chrousos, 2002). For example, being offered a new, higher paying job fresh out of college elicits a psychological and physiological stress, but most would contend that this is a eustressful event. Conversely, losing one's job would most likely elicit distress (unless the job was undesirable in the first place).

There are several psychological and physiological events that occur when a man is stressed. Increased blood pressure, muscle tension, and sweating are examples of physiological responses; increased mental alertness, anxiety, and possibly confusion typify psychological stress. One of the physiological hallmark's of stress is the release of the hormone *cortisol* into the system. Cortisol often is dubbed "catabolic," meaning that it breaks tissues down rather than strengthening them. This hormone also promotes the retention of fat cells and tissue, because the body that is chronically stressed is preparing for an adverse event in the near future (Tsigos & Chrousos, 2002). Stress is meant to alert us and make us prepared, but in today's modern world, stress often works against us, provoking several negative physical reactions.

Much of today's stress, particularly in developed nations, results from psychological factors such as anxiety and relationships. Other common stressors include money, health, school, and work. The pressures to get a good education, get a good job, start a family, provide for his family, and overall be successful can take quite a toll on a young adult male. Stresses throughout a man's life span typically change as well.

A primary goal for a person who wants to maintain good health is to recognize stress and manage it. Negative stress depletes parts of the body, such as the **adrenal gland**, because the body and mind are unable to recognize compensatory mechanisms. Signs and symptoms of chronic stress include premature aging of cells, which may produce wrinkles and gray hair, chronic fatigue, unexplained pain, inability to concentrate or focus one's attention, chronic headaches, and weight gain (Tsigos & Chrousos, 2002). These negative adaptations to stress gradually diminish the body's ability to maintain itself, and disease states such as hypertension, ulcers, anxiety, depression, and diabetes may result (Blumenthal et al., 2005).

All people experience different stresses and stressors in their lives, but how they process it varies from individual to individual. Men are more likely to hold in stress or compensate for it in unhealthy ways, such as with anger, substance use and abuse, and other forms of escapism (Baraff, 1991). Being able to appropriately and productively express feelings and emotions can help many men avert the silent pain they may feel when presented with a life stress.

Sleep Disorders

Perhaps one of the more notable and chronic manifestations of stress in life is sleeplessness. Getting a good night's rest is crucial for overall good health and well-being. Sleep helps to reset our body's systems, gives the body time to repair itself, gives the brain time to integrate its neurotransmitters and neurons, and boosts the immune system, among other benefits (Tsigos & Chrousos, 2002). The more a person invests in sleep, the greater the return in health.

Many men may not be aware that they are not getting enough sleep, chalking their tiredness up to working hard. For others, feeling tired is "doing what they are supposed to" as men by fighting through it. Most research acknowledges that people need between seven to eight hours of sleep per night for good health. Job stress is a significant cause of sleep issues in men (WebMD n.d.b). With increasing work demands and longer schedules, this may be a challenge for younger men as they strive to establish themselves in the workforce. Along with work comes stress and anxiety about events in life that make it difficult for many men to fall asleep and stay asleep throughout the night, thereby affecting quality of life. Younger men also are notorious for having full schedules that take time away from sleeping. Working late hours, going to the gym, dating, being with friends and family, traveling, and many other roles, responsibilities, and activities affect a man's ability to sleep and sleep well. Other life changes, such as getting married, moving, having a baby, losing a loved one, and having financial problems, affect sleep. Depression and other psychological issues greatly affect sleep, which often causes other life problems, such as irritability, relationship problems, and even violent outbursts. Having strong coping skills as well as seeking the help of a trained mental health professional can help avert some of these issues (Baraff, 1991). Poor health habits, such as eating later at night, consuming alcohol or stimulants such as nicotine throughout the day, or even working out too late, affect sleep. Additionally, many men believe that you can catch up on sleep, but the body and mind need consistency

Aside from stress, there are some medical disorders that affect men and their sleep (WebMD, n.d.b). Obstructive sleep apnea (OSA), narcolepsy, delayed sleep phase disorder (DSP), and jet lag and shift work disorders, as well as insomnia are a few of the more common sleep ailments in people. One of the more common sleep issues affecting men is OSA, which occurs when the tissues of the back of the throat collapse due to relaxation and gravity during sleep, resulting in limited to no air flow. This disorder causes many men to wake up suddenly multiple times throughout the night, causing them to be very fatigued throughout the next day. Men are nearly twice as likely as women to suffer from OSA (WebMD, n.d.b). Most of us snore, but loud snoring with gasps and snorts is not a normal occurrence and should be followed up. Many men don't even know that they snore until a partner makes them aware. Moreover, men may view their loud snoring as a masculine trait and something to be proud of. The opposite holds true in that men with OSA risk additional health problems aside from drowsiness, such as high blood pressure, diabetes, and even heart disease. One of the main culprits implicated with OSA is overweight and obesity. Excess body weight puts additional strain and stress on the chest cavity and sensitive throat tissues, thereby constricting and occluding tissues and structures (WebMD, n.d.b). Controlling weight is a critical and salient strategy in preventing and managing OSA in men. Other means to control OSA include continuous positive airway pressure, which is accomplished by a mask worn over the nose while you sleep that keeps a positive pressure and flow of air into the respiratory tract. Oral and nasal surgeries as well as mouthpieces (similar to mouth guards) also have shown promise in reducing symptoms of OSA.

Narcolepsy is a clinical sleep disorder characterized by extreme bouts of sleepiness and sleep "attacks" that may cause a person to inadvertently fall asleep during inopportune times, such as when working, driving, eating, or even walking. The disorder is more common in adolescence and early adulthood, with slightly higher prevalence rates in men than among women. This condition often requires medication to manage. Delayed sleep phase disorder (DSP) sounds like what it describes: people have trouble initially falling asleep, which also makes it difficult to awake in the morning. Many who experience DSP often report falling asleep two hours or more after attempting to go to bed. Natural timing of sleep can be thrown off for several reasons, but in particular stress, anxiety, and substance use or abuse (WebMD, n.d.b).

Jet lag from travel and shift work also contributes to sleep issues for men. Demanding work schedules often require men to travel for business and keep odd hours, which can affect quantity and quality of sleep. These schedules make adjusting to sleep a challenge. Also, men who work odd shifts or varying schedules can develop sleep disturbances. For example, factory workers, emergency personnel (firefighters, police officers), military personnel, and others often have to work during peak and off-peak times. The body and mind like consistency; therefore, when a man takes on responsibilities that challenge this consistency, the body may rebel by keeping him awake when he desires sleep.

Health professionals can advise men who are experiencing these conditions to regulate their sleep by avoiding excitement, food, and certain drugs a few hours prior to bedtime; avoiding bright lights; and making the sleeping environment as dark as possible. A good diet rich in nutrients, vitamins, and minerals as well as proper hydration will assure better quality sleep. **Supplements** such as **melatonin** that stimulate production of sleep hormones also can be useful additions to a regular sleep routine. For many men, finding the source of sleep dysfunction and correcting it is the solution. Normalizing the sleep experiences will pay big health dividends in the long run.

Addressing many sleep issues should suffice in restoring better sleep; however, on occasion, the use of pharmaceuticals as an adjunct therapy can be useful. Sleep aid products have become a booming business over the past decade, with as many as 45–60 million prescriptions written at the cost of multiple billions of dollars (Brownlee, 2007). Sleep aids are just that: they aid in sleep, but they should not be viewed as a solution in and of themselves. Far too many people depend on various sleep aids (prescription and over the counter) as well as herbal remedies to help them sleep when a consistent change in lifestyle and poor sleep hygiene is more in order.

NUTRITIONAL SUPPLEMENTS AND ANABOLIC-ANDROGENIC STEROIDS

Many men in younger adulthood want to feel healthy and look good. While the multitude of media messages, advertisements, and products aimed at getting men to exercise more, eat healthier, and look better seem positive (and some are), marketers and advertising executives want men to buy and consume their products. These companies dump billions of dollars into advertising per year that promote suggestive messages to men that they are not good enough and can be better than they already are. Marketing makes billions of dollars return by making men feel shamed by their health and their looks. Many young men buy superfluous exercise equipment, at-home exercise programs, dieting products, unproven, inefficacious supplements, and even illicit drugs, such as anabolic-androgenic steroids while trying to work toward this ideal.

Research suggests that most of the U.S. population has or will try a dietary supplement at some point in their lives (Juhn, 2003). One report details more than $11 billion spent on supplements in eight world countries, with Japan leading the way, followed by the United States and the United Kingdom. Sports drinks alone make up the largest segment of supplements, totaling $6.24 billion in 2001. Energy bars account for $300 million to $1 billion in sales worldwide. Rising consumer interest in health coupled with the growing awareness of the benefits of exercise has opened a portal for products designed to boost performance and accommodate busy lifestyles. Marketing ploys have targeted specific groups (for example, teens, males, females, baby boomers, and the elderly) with claims of product efficacy (Juhn, 2003; Leone, 2003). Supplements are aggressively marketed to athletes and general populations, which has generated controversy.

The term *nutritional supplements* encompasses a broad range of products, including vitamins, minerals, meal replacement powders, and the like. Certainly, there are many nutritional products that do enhance overall health and optimize performance, but for every efficacious product there is a host of others that do little. The human body needs a consistent balance of vitamins such as A, B, C, D, E, and K and minerals such as calcium, magnesium, phosphorus, zinc, and many others in trace amounts. Most people consume vitamins and minerals in their daily foods, but occasionally, they need a boost due to poor food quality, lack of variety, or not enough of it. Additionally, physical and emotional stress creates a need for more protection as found in vitamins and minerals. Several vitamins and minerals help protect the heart and other structures, such as the prostate gland. Vitamin D has been shown to reduce stress to the heart and blood vessels while also advancing bone health. Minerals such as calcium and phosphorous aid in muscle contractions, brain activity, and bone health. Many men don't realize or even think that bone loss can and will affect them, but epidemiological rates of bone disease are alarmingly high in men as they age. Zinc also has been implicated in preventing prostate cancer in older men. Prevention is key while men are younger, so that as they age, disease and infirmity are minimal.

While there is no one magic "cure all" for attaining optimal health, men can take a step in the right direction by consuming a diet rich in a balance of macronutrients, such as carbohydrates, proteins, and fats. For those lacking proper diets, a quality multivitamin and mineral supplement can help augment overall dietary health. Physicians can help to identify any deficiencies. Blood panels can help determine what is lacking and can help direct the health professional to make dietary and supplement recommendations.

Psychiatric conditions such as body dysmorphia (Phillips, 1998) and muscle dysmorphia (Pope et al., 1993) may afflict younger males more than any other population. Dietary manipulation in addition to exercise is a common way in which to craft the body to a certain look. Enter the world of nutritional and dietary supplements, a multibillion-dollar industry offering potent powders and miraculous pills and preparations that promise to give you what you want. These supplements include protein powders, amino acids, creatine monohydrate, meal replacement powders and drinks, vitamin water, and a host of other concoctions (Juhn, 2003). Younger males may be attracted to these products not for the reported added health benefits but for the performance and body image enhancement they may provide.

For example, many weight gain formulas contain fillers that promote weight but not necessarily lean muscle. Some supplements with huge amounts of protein per serving add additional stress on the kidneys, and excess is eliminated from the body versus utilized. Meal replacements may become long-term substitutes for a good, hearty meal, thus leaving out quality nutrients, such as vitamins and fiber sources. Vitamin and energy drinks often contain high levels of sugar and B vitamins and amino acids that can stress the renal system. Additionally, high levels of additives, such as guarana and caffeine can lead to jitters, anxiety, and sleep disorders in some individuals. Muscle-building supplements, such as creatine monohydrate, have some proven efficacy; however, not everyone seems to respond to them (Kanayama, Gruber et al., 2001). Overall, nothing substitutes for a well-balance diet of food and water. Supplements should be just that—supplements to a healthy diet.

For some young men, health and good diet are preceded by the desire to attain a certain physique and look, be it for vanity or athletic performance. Many younger men hit the gym hard with hopes of addressing these former areas. For some, diet and regular exercise do not yield the desired results and some opt for substances that will give them hard core results, namely anabolic-androgenic steroids (AAS).

For some young men, AAS and other "body image" drugs, such as human growth hormone (hGH) and amphetamines, provide a quick solution when trying to attain that "perfect" physique and look (Kanayama, Pope, & Hudson, 2001). Anabolic agents such as AAS are substances that promote tissue growth through nitrogen sparing and protein synthesis in the human body (Powers, 2005). The appeal and allure of these types of drugs are widespread, although prevalence rates are difficult to surmise in adult populations (Kanayama, Cohane, Weiss, & Pope, 2003). Most available prevalence data has been established with younger populations such as adolescents.

Lower levels of self-esteem and greater levels of body image dissatisfaction have been purported to influence younger men to use products such as AAS. Media pressures coupled with a drive for muscularity as part of the Western cultural norm also have been implicated in AAS use (McCreary & Sasse, 2000). The concept of AAS use in younger adults is a complex one with no clear answers. While possession of AAS remains a felony offense characterized by stiff penalties and jail time, proponents claim use should be more a matter of personal choice. U.S. law places AAS as a Schedule III controlled substance under the 1991 Controlled Substances Act. Advocates claim **harm reduction** will produce consumers who take fewer health risks, generate a new field of revenue, minimize and/or eliminate the black market for AAS, and keep people out of jail due to possession and use (Brower, 2009). Opponents cite research that implicates AAS with dependency, violence and aggression, and a variety of health consequences. Long-term, longitudinal research still has yet to establish causality between AAS use and long-term negative health effects (Kanayama, Hudson, & Pope, 2008). Anecdotal reports have surfaced over the years discussing people (mainly men) who have developed rare cancers of the brain (as in the case of former pro-football star Lyle Alzado) and liver tumors and cancers leading to death. However, there remains little empirical evidence that confirms these anecdotal reports. Short-term side effects of AAS are well documented and include (in men) acne, male patterned baldness, abscesses and infections at injection sites, infectious diseases due to needle sharing (HIV/AIDS, hepatitis), and musculoskeletal injury and damage, in addition to psychological effects such as dependence and increased aggression ("roid rage") (Brower, 2009). Unsubstantiated evidence has led many younger men to wave off the possible side effects and take the risk to gain a stronger and potentially better-looking physique. AAS, while proven to have efficacious effects in increasing lean muscle and strength, still pose potential long-term health consequences (Kanayama et al., 2008). Younger adults and all men are strongly cautioned when considering AAS use.

OCCUPATIONAL HEALTH

Many men pride themselves on their occupations. For some, what they "do" often defines how successful they are.

Conversation among men about their jobs establishes a social hierarchy, communicates relative successes and ambitions as well as his failures and inadequacies, and possibly makes or breaks him in terms of the perception of others. Men and their occupations have conveyed their role as provider, protector, and "sturdy oak." What a man does in his profession may say a lot about him as an individual. Some occupations meet our cultural expectations of a "man's man," whereas others challenge long-held beliefs.

Studies suggest men will change jobs and even professions on average of 7 to 10 times in their lifetimes (U.S. Bureau of Labor Statistics, n.d.). The type of occupation a man holds also greatly affects his relative health status. Men often occupy jobs that are higher risk, such as law enforcement, military, mining, factory and manual labor, and fire fighting. Some jobs predominated by men include surgeons, law enforcement, military, fire fighting, mining, farming, automotive jobs, and building/contractors. Of course, with jobs also come specific risks, such as factors leading to infirmity and death. According to the U.S. Bureau of Labor Statistics (n.d.), the top ten most dangerous jobs include timber cutters (loggers), fishermen, pilots and navigators, structural metal workers, drivers for sales professions, roofers, electrical power installers, farmers, construction laborers, and truck drivers. Mining is a close eleventh place with 23.5 deaths per 100,000 (U.S. Bureau of Labor Statistics, n.d.). Occupational health and safety is key for men to avoid disability and even death.

Consider, for example, lung diseases, such as cancer, chronic obstructive pulmonary disorders (COPD), emphysema, and pneumonia. Statistics show that twice as many men will die of COPD and related disorders. Smoking is more prevalent in some occupations, but exposure to various chemicals and airborne agents can cause many lung problems in men (Perry & Schacht, 2001). Lung issues are among the top causes of long-term disability in men, which affects their ability to work and provide for their families (Gremillion, personal communication, 2004). Protecting their health by reducing occupational exposures to chemicals, toxins, and hazardous situations is a solid step for men. Additionally, limiting exposure to smoking and wearing appropriate gear such as masks can help cut the risk of respiratory disorders. The Occupational Safety and Health Administration (OSHA) conducts routine evaluations for companies to comply with health standards for their employees. Men who fall out of the workforce early also limit the overall health of their families because income and other considerations become less. Moreover, a man may have lower self-worth and self-esteem if he is no longer able to work (Baraff, 1991). In a society that still views men as functional parts of the workforce, the pressure to produce may become so overwhelming that a man who is out of work may develop depression and a higher risk for suicide.

Some theorize that women's parity with males in the workplace has led to increased frustration, workplace outbursts and violence, and higher rates of substance abuse among men. Pope, Phillips, and Olivardia (2000) theorize that this gender parity has caused some men to express their masculinity by becoming overly preoccupied with their bodies, namely their muscles and hypermasculinity. Others argue that gender parity in the workforce has worked in men's favor, causing them to redefine their roles in society and become more innovative and productive (Luciano, 2001). Men still occupy some of the most hazardous professions and occupations, they have higher risks for permanent disability and death due to occupational hazards, gender parity has caused many men to reevaluate their roles in the workforce, and competition has challenged many men now more than ever to excel at what they do.

SUMMARY

This chapter explored the health challenges and opportunities of men in young adulthood. With this stage of life come many changes in physical, social, and emotional health. Men's physical health issues such as obesity, nutrition and eating concerns, and common reproductive issues were discussed. Topics such as weight management, exercise dependence, restrictive eating, and eating disorders were presented. Among social health issues covered was why men are less likely than women to seek the help of physicians. The emotional health of men is quite complex due to the dichotomous world in which we exist. Men are told not to express concern for their looks, yet many suffer in silence about various body image issues. A detailed discussion of common stresses in a younger man's life also was presented. Issues such as sleep and physical consequences of stress were detailed. Younger men's interest in nutritional supplements and body enhancing products was explored. Proper nutrition along with healthy alternatives to potentially dangerous substances was discussed. Last, issues of occupational health were considered.

KEY TERMS

Adrenal gland

Alexithymia

Congenital

Empirical

Epistemological

Extrapolated

Gout

Harm reduction

Heteronormative

Insulin

Maladies

Malignant

Melatonin

Pandemic

Postindustrial

Psychosomatic

Satiety

Somatic

Somatoform

Supplements

DISCUSSION QUESTIONS

1. Explain how cultural and ethnic practices influence how a man eats and views his nutrition. Can this be advantageous for a man's health? Explain.

2. Discuss how eating disorders such as anorexia nervosa and bulimia nervosa are similar and different in males and females. How should treatment be approached in both of the sexes? Detail particular challenges.

3. Research the rate of vasectomies in the United States. Find statistics on the relative rate of failure of this procedure. Comment on these findings. Compare and contrast the relative advantages and disadvantages of vasectomies as a form of birth control in men versus tubal ligation in women.

4. Why do you think men tend to obsess over the relative size of their genitalia, particularly the penis? Use comparisons of historical contexts and modern perspectives.

5. What factors act as barriers to seeking medical care for men? What enables access to health care?

6. What are common examples of modern media that affect and influence adult male body image? How do these forms of media affect male health overall? What are some outcomes from negative body image in men? Back up your points with relevant statistics.

7. Explain how muscle dysmorphia is likely to develop in males. What does the current research literature say about the topic?

8. Briefly describe what chronic stress does to the major organ systems of the human body.

9. What is considered to be good sleep hygiene? How does not getting enough sleep affect the health of a man?

10. Highlight three occupations that are predominantly male. Discuss how each occupation is both health positive and health negative. What are common long-term health outcomes for men who enter such occupations? Use the most recent statistics to illustrate your points.

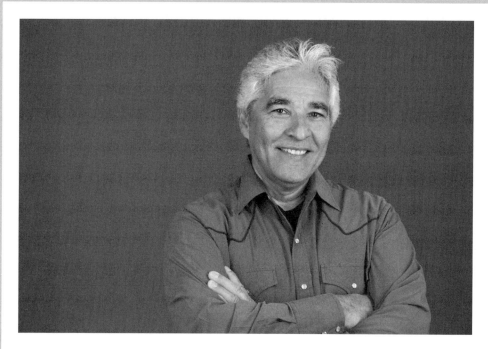

©iStockphoto.com/Alina Solovyova-Vincent

9

Middle Adulthood

LEARNING OBJECTIVES

- Identify the physical and emotion health challenges men face in middle adulthood and strategies to prevent and address challenges to their physical and emotional health

- Describe preemptive and preventative strategies, such as dietary modifications and stress reduction methods, that men can use to avoid disease and disability

- Discuss factors relating to prostate cancer, midlife crisis, and infidelity, as well as preventative strategies

- Describe issues pertaining to paternal rights and fathers' movements

IDDLE ADULTHOOD IS a relative time period in a man's life. Considering that the average life span of men in the United States is between seventy-two and seventy-seven years (Centers for Disease Control and Prevention [CDC], 2008), middle adulthood would lie roughly between the ages of thirty-six to forty years old. However, many of us would not consider thirty-six to be middle aged. This nicely illustrates that the concept of "middle age" is just that: a *concept*. The age of a man is only as meaningful as the life experiences that go along with it. For example, the average life span for the entire world is approximately 66 years, with Swaziland at 32 years at the low end and Macau at the higher end at 84.5 years of life (Central Intelligence Agency [CIA], 2010). In this chapter, middle adulthood is considered to encompass the ages of forty to sixty-five years.

No matter what age you are, it is human nature to periodically evaluate one's relative position in life. Middle age, middle adulthood, or the midlife "crisis" all come down to one common theme: *evaluation*. How a man responds to his evaluation of himself and his life experiences greatly predicts whether he will continue along a path of health and wellness or he will sink into desperation and despair.

With progressing age come physical and emotional changes. What is different during this stage of life is that how well (or not so well) a man has treated his body previously becomes readily apparent. The body breaks down with progressing age, and with that breakdown come physical challenges such as illness, injury, and disease. In this chapter we explore the physical and emotional changes, challenges, and opportunities for men of this age.

PHYSICAL HEALTH

How a man treats his body earlier in life often predicts how it will hold up later in life. Some physical events are related to a man's genes, whereas others evolve over the course of his life span. For example, male pattern baldness and hair loss in general is strongly determined by genetic factors, whereas the development of atherosclerosis (hardening of the arteries) is strongly influenced by diet and lifestyle factors. The breakdown of the physical body is inevitable, but the rate at which the breakdown occurs can be moderated by practicing good health measures such as exercise, good nutrition, and positive coping mechanisms.

Unfortunately, for many men, midlife may be the first time that they access quality medical care, usually not from a preventative mentality but from a **palliative** one. Men often react only when problems occur, often at the expense of months and years of care that could have enhanced and extended years of quality of life. Public health needs to be acutely aware of this fact and mentality; palliative care places an undue strain on the medical and financial resources of the United States and the world. Prevention will save billions, if not trillions of dollars on an annual basis (Brownlee, 2007).

Heart Disease

One of the most significant challenges for men as they approach midlife is heart health. According to mortality data from the Centers for Disease Control and Prevention (CDC), heart disease is still the number one cause of death in the United States. Heart disease claimed 631,636 lives in 2006, with rates of 187.7 per 100,000 for white males and 110 per 100,000 for white females. Moreover, death rates increase for men of color, with rates of 206.4 per 100,000 for black men. Rates were lower in Asian men, with 101.3 per 100,000 dying from the disease. This is likely due to genetic factors as well a diet lower in saturated fats, a major contributor to heart disease. In total, heart disease accounted for 1 in every 6 deaths in the United States in 2006 (Lloyd-Jones et al., 2010).

The human heart is fed by two major arteries (the *coronary arteries*) that carry blood rich with oxygen and life-giving nutrients to heart muscle tissues. Due in part to poor diet, lack of exercise, and cumulative effects of stress and genetics, these arteries can become damaged by plaques, which eventually clog (*occlude*) them. Blockages, also known as *atherosclerosis,* prevent the delivery of vital nutrients and oxygen from feeding and nourishing the tissues of the heart. Slowly, as these arteries harden, sections of the heart fail, causing pain and other physical features of heart dysfunction such as **angina**, chest pain, sweating, extreme fatigue, and lightheadedness, among other signs and symptoms. Pain typically occurs because lack of oxygen causes a condition known as *ischemia,* which provokes the release of pain modulators into the blood and thus increases the perception of pain in the brain (Lloyd-Jones et al., 2010; Perry & Schacht, 2001).

There are many reasons why men are at higher risk for heart disease. For some, genetic predisposition is evident and needs to be closely monitored as a man ages. This can be determined by examining a man's family history and his own physical features and risk factors. Diet and exercise (or lack thereof) also strongly contributes to heart health. Diets high in fat, especially saturated ones that come from animal sources, have a propensity for increasing blood cholesterol levels, which have been implicated in artery-clogging plaques (Lloyd-Jones et al., 2010; Perry & Schacht, 2001). Some men simply have a genetic predisposition for higher cholesterol (called *hypercholesterolemia*) levels than others, which can be easily determined by simple blood panels and may be treated with dietary modifications, cholesterol-lowering medications, or a combination of the two. Exercise has been shown to decrease risk of heart attacks in men. The American College of Sports Medicine (ACSM) and the American Heart Association (AHA) set forth newer guidelines on exercise for heart health in 2007, detailing the need for moderately intense cardiovascular activity for 30 minutes five days per week or vigorous or intense cardio for 20 minutes per day three days per week and eight to ten strength-training exercises twice per week (Haskell et al., 2007). Chronic stress also has been strongly implicated in the development of heart disease in men. With stress comes the release of stress hormones such as cortisol, which elevate blood pressure and cause vasoconstriction of blood vessels, making it harder for blood to reach the heart, cause muscle tension, and cause the body to retain fat more readily. High-stress lifestyles for men, particularly in their jobs, significantly contribute to the heart disease equation. For example, a recent study concluded that people who work 3–4 hours beyond that of a "normal" 7–8 hour work day increased their relative risk for a cardiac incident by 1.6 times (Virtanen et al., 2010). Men with "type A" personalities—that is, easily stressed or high strung— have been well studied as at a higher risk for cardiovascular events. Individually, each of these risk factors can increase one's chances for developing atherosclerosis and eventually heart disease.

Myth: Older men should limit their physical activity because of an increased risk of injury.

Fact: While it is true that injury can occur with any activity, the opposite holds true for men as they age. Aging men need more physical activity to stave off the effects of aging. For example, more muscle improves balance and coordination as well as keeps metabolism active, and weight-bearing exercise increases bone mass, lessening risk of bone fractures.

Most of these factors don't exist in isolation; rather, they compound to build a profile of a heart disease patient. This type of research was pioneered in 1948 with the famed Framingham Heart Study, which was launched in the town of Framingham, Massachusetts, a town approximately 20 miles west of Boston. Prior to this study, which has included the tracking of more than three generations of participants, not much was known about the risk factors of heart disease (Dawber, Kannel, Revotskie, Stokes, Kagan, & Gordon., 1959). This type of **longitudinal research** has led to a better understanding of what predisposes people to heart disease and what can be done to prevent it.

Men in middle adulthood are at high risk for experiencing a heart attack (also known as a *myocardial infarction* or MI) (Perry & Schacht, 2001). Notice that men at this age are not at risk for *developing* heart disease, but rather are likely to *experience* it. This is because developing heart disease is a lifelong process that starts at birth and culminates in a man's first episode of a heart attack, which also may be his last. The numbers are staggering, with more than 17 million adults in the United States having been diagnosed with the disease from years 2003 to 2006. Those who do not die from heart disease often become dependent on the medical system and experience lower levels of quality of life measures (Lloyd-Jones et al., 2010). The cost alone is sobering: direct and indirect costs for coronary artery disease in 2006 were estimated at $177 billion. Comparatively, in 1987, the disease cost roughly $80 billion (American Heart Association [AHA], 2010).

Prevention is key, but this may not be feasible for all men. Therefore, we must advocate for men to be proactive in getting screened via regular physical checkups with their doctors, especially if a family history of heart disease is established. Knowing a person's blood pressure values, cholesterol levels, body mass index score, waist-to-hip ratio, and other **anthropometric** features can help determine if he is at risk. Once the risk profile is known, a health professional can recommend actions that can be taken to lower the patient's chances of experiencing a cardiovascular event. Changing diet and beginning to exercise can be great first steps toward enhancing heart health. A doctor may prescribe blood pressure or cholesterol-lowering medications; however, diet and exercise typically are the best avenues for beginning a healthier regime.

Knowing the signs of a heart ailment also can be beneficial for many men. Heart attacks are typically characterized by crushing pain in the center of the chest, diffuse sweating, abnormal fatigue, headache, pain in the extremities and jaw, pain in the middle of the shoulder blades, difficulty breathing, and a general feeling of impending doom. Other less obvious signs may include chronic fatigue, especially with exertion; diminished sexual capacity, including less frequent and less potent erections; and difficulty breathing during low-intensity activities such as walking around the neighborhood or in a store (Perry & Schacht, 2001).

The good news with middle age and heart health is that heart problems typically respond well to such a proactive, multifaceted approach.

The CDC lists cancer as the second leading cause of death (COD) in men in the United States (behind heart disease) (CDC, 2006). Deaths from cancer overall are higher in men than women, with rates of 233.3 per 100,000 people compared to 160.9 per 100,000 (CDC, 2006). Cancer is highest (26.7%) in Asian and Pacific Islanders and is the leading COD in this ethnic group. White males also experience slightly higher rates than the overall national average, at 24.6% of all CODs (CDC, 2006). Many forms of cancer, such as skin, bone, liver, pancreatic, and stomach, afflict people.

Prostate Health and Prostate Cancer

Prostate cancer is the most diagnosed non-skin cancer among all men and has the highest mortality rate of all cancers in men in the United States (Men's Health Network [MHN], 2009; Wallner et al., 2008). This form of cancer affects nearly 1 in 5 men (Wallner, et al., 2008). In the United States, approximately 150,000 new cases of prostate cancer are identified each year, with 30,000 men dying from the condition or complications. African American men also appear to be at even higher risk than other groups (that is, whites, Latinos, Asians) for developing this disease. Asian, Hispanic, and white men should begin prostate screenings after age fifty, whereas African American men with a family history should begin screening sooner, at forty to forty-five years old.

©iStockphoto.com/Linda Hides

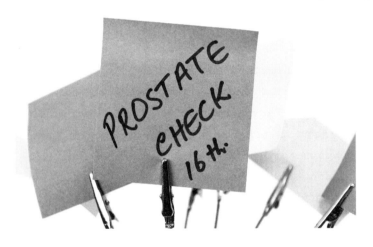

The prostate is a gland located only in the male reproductive system; it contributes fluid that comprises **semen**. The gland itself is fairly small (walnut sized), surrounds the urethra, and is in close proximity to the urinary bladder. Some anatomical studies suggest that the prostate grows as a man ages from infancy to his elder years. This growth, called *benign prostatic hyperplasia* (BPH), sometimes causes inflammation, soreness, discomfort, and urinary symptoms (Moore et al., 2009). As men age, usually into their late forties and fifties, symptoms of BPH, such as increased frequency of urination, hesitancy, weak stream of urine flow, or urinary incontinence, become more frequent. Many of these symptoms greatly affect a man's quality of life. BPH does not necessarily mean a man has or will develop prostate cancer; however, his risk increases over time.

The exact causes of prostate cancer are still largely unknown, although possible links have been identified. Testosterone and lifestyle factors play a significant role in the development of BPH and prostate cancer (Wallner et al., 2008). Obesity and diets high in fat content have been causally linked to BPH and prostate cancer. Risk of prostate cancer also appears to increase with the number of family members affected according to European research. Of more than 25,000 men with prostate cancer, 5,623 came from families with histories of the disease and were tracked in the study. Men with three affected brothers were found to be twenty-three times at greater risk than those with fewer family members affected (Kohlstädt, 2010). This is critical information for both patients and doctors; a simple screening can help improve follow-up and standard of care for this disease.

Many treatments are possible for men with BPH. Medications such as alpha-blockers and diuretics help to reduce volume and thus cause the prostate to decrease in size. Changing to a lower-fat diet, reducing body mass, eating more vegetables (especially leafy, green ones), limiting fluid intake before long trips or bedtime, avoiding caffeine and alcohol, monitoring medications (some may aggravate the condition), decreasing stress levels, and staying in contact with a primary care physician can help men manage or even prevent or eliminate BPH (Wallner et al., 2008).

Other problems can affect the prostate, causing inflammation or *prostatitis*. Bacteria, such as sexually transmitted infections (STIs) and other sources as well as nonbacterial entities, can cause the prostate to inflame. This inflammation yields pain (*prostatodynia*), urinary dysfunction, discharge from the tip of the penis, pain or itching deep within the penis, fever, pain in the groin and lower back, and sometimes blood in the urine (called *hematuria*). Some non-bacterial, non-STI-related causes of prostate inflammation include coffee, alcohol, and spicy foods as well as excessive physical activity and sitting for long periods of time (Wallner et al., 2008). For example, cyclists and men who drive long distances often report greater prostate symptoms because pressure from body weight causes stress on the gland throughout the day.

Diagnosis of Prostate Cancer   Three screenings can be performed to identify any abnormalities with the prostate. The digital rectal examination, prostate-specific antigen (PSA) blood test, and transurethral resection procedure of the prostate are the most commonly perform screenings. An annual digital rectal exam is considered to be one of the best methods to determine the health (and size) of the prostate gland. The physician inserts one to two fingers into the rectum and palpates in a superior (upward) direction to take note of the size of the prostate. The PSA is a test that notes high levels of prostate antigen markers in the blood. Levels can be monitored every three to six months or as needed to determine how active the prostate might be. Higher levels are indicative of BPH and possible prostate cancer activity. Last, the transurethral resection of the prostate (TURP) procedure can be useful in identifying abnormalities and allows the doctor to take tissue biopsies if appropriate (Pinthus, Pacik, & Ramon, 2007).

Treatment of Prostate Cancer   Diagnosis of prostate cancer is not necessarily a death sentence, but it must be understood and effectively and efficiently managed by a medical team. Along with a primary care physician, a urologist who specializes in prostate issues, in addition to a surgeon and an oncologist who specializes in cancer make up the medical team. Surgery, radiation, chemotherapy, hormonal therapy, medications, and combinations are available to treat prostate cancer (Taichman, Loberg, Mehra, & Pienta, 2007). Each therapy and option has its own benefits and side effects. Biopsy and surgical removal of parts or all of the prostate gland can rid the body of cancerous cells and tissues; however, delicate nerve structures also can be damaged, leading to erectile dysfunction. Radiation and chemotherapy can target cancer cells but may damage the gland and related neurological structures. Hormonal therapy and certain medications can be effective in shrinking prostate tissues, but not all eliminate cancer cells (Taichman et al., 2007). The type of treatment should be carefully considered by the patient and his doctor, weighing all the pros and cons of the option or procedure. Most men have concern about the sexual side effects of surgery and treatment and the possibility of urinary incontinence, bowel dysfunction, swelling in the groin, penis, and scrotum, bruising and pain, weight loss and appetite, hot flashes, osteoporosis (due to hormonal therapy), and fatigue; all should be taken into consideration by the medical team (Taichman et al., 2007; Perry & Schacht, 2001).

Current Research and Trends   The efficacy and effectiveness of screening tests are always called into question. The PSA seems to be highly efficacious because research claims that it can detect tumors on average eleven years prior to that of a digital rectal examination (Brownlee, 2007). However, not all prostate tumors develop into cancer; therefore, it is possible that many men may undergo unnecessary and invasive procedures. These procedures also may cause other problems, such as erectile dysfunction and decreased overall quality of life.

Shannon Brownlee, author of *Overtreated*, notes that "far more men die with prostate cancer than of it" (2007, p. 201). Detection and early diagnosis are good in some respects, but their limitations have to be well understood so that we are not wasting time, money, and resources when there is little evidence to support certain procedures. Brownlee notes that in ten years of epidemiologic research, more men in Seattle, Washington, than in other locations underwent PSA testing. They were five times more likely to get tested than men in Connecticut. Intuition suggests that mortality rates from prostate cancer in Seattle should be lower than those in Connecticut, but this simply was not the case. The opposite held true; men in Seattle were more likely to die from prostate cancer than were men in Connecticut, possibly due to complications from treatment and surgery.

The medical debate over PSA testing utility continues in the medical community. There is no conclusive answer to offer, but what providers can offer is communication. Discussing these pros and cons of various tests and treatment options with patients is a great first step. More medicine is not necessarily better medicine.

Recent data on radiation therapy for prostate cancer also has been called into question by the medical community. Focused radiation therapy (such as CyberKnife®), the application of a very direct dose of radiation into cancerous cells, has not been found to be superior to other forms of treatment, according to a medical panel on behalf of the Center for Medicare and Medicaid Services (CMS) aimed at controlling costs and containing extraneous medical expenditures. The panel noted, "Surgery, radiation, and simply 'watchful waiting' are all possible courses of action. But researchers are increasingly concerned that excessive screening may be leading to over-aggressive treatment when studies show many prostate cancers grow so slowly that most men will die from other causes first" (Heavey, 2010). Long-term studies are lacking, which make conclusions difficult to establish. Comparison of the evidence and long-term randomized controlled studies need to be conducted to establish reliability and validity of such treatments.

A similar study published in the *Journal of the American Medical Association* (Hu, Gu, Lipsitz, Barry, D'Amico, Weinberg, & Keating, 2009) found that minimally invasive surgery options for prostate cancer are not necessarily better than conventional methods. Robotically controlled devices, such as the da Vinci system, have pioneered these minimally invasive options, but evidence is lacking to justify this type of procedure over more conventional open surgical procedures. Patients of *less* invasive treatment were found to be *more* likely to be incontinent and have erectile dysfunction than men who underwent conventional surgery. The assumption that high-tech options are superior is simply not supported by outcome-based research studies.

New methods for the prevention and treatment of this prevalent cancer are being developed. As of 2010, the Food and Drug Administration (FDA) approved an immunotherapeutic agent called sipuleucel-T (Provenge) for the treatment of advanced forms of prostate cancer (Dubensky & Reed, 2010). The vaccine is available for men with asymptomatic or minimally **metastatic** prostate cancer who may be less receptive candidates for other therapies and treatments. The vaccine stimulates a patient's own immune system to combat the prostate cancer rather than adding an outside agent to do so. Survival rates were significantly improved in the treatment groups compared to placebo by nearly 4.1 months (Small et al., 2006). FDA panels agree that this agent is safe for use in men with this disease; however, long-term studies concerning safety and efficacy are needed (Dubensky & Reed, 2010). Regardless of treatment options, patients and health practitioners

need to be aware of risk status, consider screenings based on age recommendations, and explore all options concerning the best treatments and
highest levels of standards of care.

Men may be very hesitant or reluctant to discuss prostate issues with
their families and physicians. Because the reproductive system often is a
private matter for many men, advocacy efforts to get men to speak out
concerning their experiences with prostate cancer and recovery are limited.
There are some media advocacy initiatives in video and written forms;
however, messages may not prompt men to act (MHN, 2009). The Health
Belief Model states that people will be motivated to act if they feel a topic
is of sufficient interest, they are at risk or perceive a risk for a condition, and
the rewards outweigh the relative costs (Rosenstock, Strecher, & Becker,
1988).

Efforts to understand the psychosocial factors that encourage or discour-
age men from getting prostate cancer screenings was assessed in 2,447 men
in a large county in Minnesota from years 1990 to 1998. Men between the
ages of forty and seventy-nine completed a questionnaire concerning personal and family history of prostate cancer, attitudes pertaining to the
disease, and demographic information. Medical and laboratory records were
reviewed over a ten-year time frame. Findings showed that men who had a
family history and men who worry or have concern about prostate cancer
were more likely to be screened than those with different answers.
Additionally, the study found that married men or men living with someone
were more likely to be screened than those who lived alone (Wallner et al.,
2008). Understanding these psychosocial factors is important when devising
advocacy strategies in public health. Novel approaches bring this and similar
public health issues into male contexts. The Washington Redskins football
team promoted a prostate awareness day at one of their games, arranged
enhanced media coverage for the event, set up PSA screenings throughout
the stadium, and perhaps most important, did it in a venue where men are
likely to pay attention. This initiative was met with success in screening men
with potential prostatic issues (MHN, 2009).

Moving men past the silence and stigma that has existed for decades
concerning this disease is one of the ultimate goals of public health and

sex-specific health endeavors. Many men associate prostate cancer with uncomfortable screening procedures such as the digital rectal examination. Some men fear complications from surgery, such as loss of sexual desire and erectile dysfunction. Advocacy can make men aware that other tests can help establish their risk status. Awareness and new advances in screening and treatment options may help allay many of the fears and help men lead longer and healthier quality lives.

Prevention is the strongest message for men. Taking care of one's body is the penultimate means to reduce chances of developing prostate and other cancers.

Colorectal Cancer

One of the more common forms of cancer in men is colon and rectal (colorectal) cancer. It is the third most common form of cancer in men, trailing lung (second) and prostate (first). Many men will experience colorectal cancer; however, the good news is that cure rates are high with early detection (Jemal et al., 2008). The operative term here is "early"; left unrecognized, colorectal cancer transforms into an aggressive disease, often with deadly consequences.

The colon, or more properly defined as the large intestines (also known as the *bowel*), is part of the digestive system, which primarily functions to absorb remaining nutrients and water in the body. The large intestines have three distinct sections: the ascending, transverse, and descending colon. The rectum is part of the descending colon and primarily serves as a holding chamber for solid waste (feces). The colon and rectum are highly active structures when optimally functioning. The absorption of nutrients and water and the elimination of toxic waste products are vital to optimal health and function. Because the blood supply to the colon is extensive, it is important that waste products be removed on a consistent basis. Toxins can leach into the bloodstream and cause illness if they are not eliminated in a timely manner. Additionally, the sensitive cells of the colon and rectum can become damaged by these toxins if elimination is not consistent. Most people should have between one and two complete bowel movements per day; however, there is great variability in the population because of lifestyle choices (diet, drug use, stress, and so on) (Moore, Dalley, & Agur, 2009).

Several warning signs for colorectal cancer are generally apparent. Small tissue growths, often are referred to as *polyps,* may occur in the colon. Polyps usually are noncancerous (or benign) and present with very few symptoms; however, with age come many changes. Normally benign polyps can progress to deeper and more progressive tumors if not recognized through routine screening such as with colonoscopies (Levin et al., 2008). Lifestyle choices, such as high-fat and low-fiber diets, also play a significant role in the development of colorectal cancer. Family history plays a strong role; therefore, it is imperative that men who have family links to cancers, particularly of the colon and rectum, get routine exams. Most cancers of the colon and rectum take time to develop, with most developing by age fifty or older; however, men need to be aware of their level of risk (Jemal et al., 2008). Many warning signs are not apparent; therefore, health practitioners should advise men to be aware of changes in bowel habits (diarrhea, constipation, or consistent incomplete bowel movements); blood in the stool marked by red streaks or dark, tarry appearance; persistent abdominal pain, cramping, tenderness, or bloating; unexplained weight loss; and persistent fatigue (Perry & Schacht, 2001).

Prevention is paramount with a condition such as colorectal cancer in men. As a man ages, controlling weight through a diet high in fiber and low in fat can help offset risk of colorectal cancer. Annual **digital** rectal exams are recommended in men age forty and older but may be warranted at earlier ages if a strong history is present. After age fifty, men are recommended to have fecal occult blood tests, which attempt to spot blood in the stool. *Sigmoidoscopies* and *colonoscopies* are important (usually after age fifty) to detect polyps and other precancerous and cancerous cells in the rectum and colon. These devices use flexible tubing with cameras mounted to visually examine the colon and also can remove polyps and tissue samples for further diagnostic testing (biopsies) (Levin et al., 2008).

If colon or rectal cancer does occur, what are the next steps? The answer to this question depends on what stage the cancer is in. Some cancers affect only the intestinal lining, whereas others can proliferate (metastasize) into the blood and lymphatic system and cause many more issues. Superficial cancers often can be removed via surgery and may be treated with radiation or chemotherapy. Other cancers may require more invasive and radical procedures that remove sections of the bowel and surrounding tissues, such as lymph nodes. Radiation therapy attempts to shrink the tumor cells, whereas chemotherapy tries to destroy cells that may have traveled into the body's systems beyond the intestines. Surgery to remove sections of the colon is considered a last resort in terms of treatment (Jemal et al., 2008). A *colostomy* or *ileostomy* redirects solid waste to an internal or external pouch (referred to as a *colostomy bag*) for removal. In some cases, the procedure is permanent, and in other cases it may be temporary until the bowel heals. At a later time, surgeons may opt to reconnect the sections of the bowel if they are functional and cancer-free (Levin et al., 2008).

Colorectal cancer is a life-altering event for a man. Not only is his mortality called into question, but if he survives treatment, his health-related quality of life may be dramatically reduced. The emotional impact of this and other types of cancer needs to be addressed by physicians and family members to help a man maintain a strong sense of self. For example, many men are hesitant or reluctant to get checkups "down there" due to feelings of vulnerability and association with gay culture (this is a stereotype). Sociocultural ideals and values may preclude preemptive action on a man's part to get screened and treated. Public health has come a long way in promoting colonoscopies and screenings in men, but fear, ignorance, and social stigma still act as barriers to many men. A cultural paradigm shift is needed to reduce the incidence of new colorectal cancer in men caused simply by lack of awareness, urgency, stigma, or all three.

Breast Cancer

Although much more prevalent in women, breast cancer does occur in men. The condition is rare, 1% or less of all breast cancers. Men have underdeveloped ducts and small amounts of fatty tissue in their breasts that sometimes can develop into cancer. Lifetime prevalence in men is about 1 in 1,000 men and can occur at any age, but increases as men age (MedicineNet, n.d.). According to 2008 statistics from the American Cancer Society (ACS),

1,990 men were diagnosed in the United States, with approximately 480 deaths. These numbers pale in comparison to the nearly 40,000 deaths in women each year (American Cancer Society [ACS], 2010).

Causes of male breast cancer largely are unknown. Some common risk factors are thought to be a diet high in fat, elevated estrogen levels, stress, radiation exposure, pesticide and pollution exposure, family history, genetic diseases (such as Klinefelter's syndrome), and lesser-known factors (MedicineNet, n.d.). Common signs and symptoms of breast cancer in men include a firm nonpainful mass just below the nipple; skin changes on or directly around the nipple; retraction of the nipple; breast tenderness; blood or other discharge from the nipple; and fatigue, malaise, and weight loss (ACS, 2010; MedicineNet, n.d.).

Male breast cancer is treated similarly as other cancers, with radiation, biopsy, **lumpectomy**, **mastectomy**, chemotherapy, and hormonal treatments. Surgery is the most common treatment, and as with female breast cancer, prognosis of survival and recovery depends on how quickly the cancer is caught and at what stage (MedicineNet, n.d.). Although self examination is not routinely advocated, men (particularly older men), can check their breast and testicular tissue for consistency and to detect abnormalities.

Hypertension

Concomitant with heart disease, obesity, and diabetes is hypertension (HTN), otherwise known as *high blood pressure*. Although the CDC does not consider hypertension as a leading cause of death, the condition is arguably heavily implicated in causing mortality in men. There are several causes of HTN, including genetic predisposition, diet, hydration status, stress, and overweight and obesity (Carretero & Oparil, 2000; Perry & Schacht, 2001). As with most other conditions, there are various stages of HTN. *Primary hypertension* often refers to a higher blood pressure value for which no cause is evident and accounts for 90%–95% of cases. Secondary hypertension encompasses 5%–10% of other cases and has more severe health implications, such as heart disease, kidney dysfunction, and even death (Chobanian et al., 2003). Many people don't know their blood pressure status, which is why the disease often is called a "silent killer." In fact, up to 25% of the population (mostly men) have at-risk levels and don't know it (Chobanian et al., 2003).

Every time the heart contracts, blood is forced through the arteries, which carries nutrients and oxygen to muscles, tissues, and cells. The contraction exerts a force that can be measured through the use of blood pressure devices. Pressure against the arterial walls is very important; however, too much pressure is detrimental to a person's health. Over time, chronic HTN can lead to the heart becoming enlarged and thus less effective. Additionally, constant pressure on the arteries can cause them to weaken and possibly rupture (called an *aneurysm*) (Carretero & Oparil, 2000). Therefore, it is very important that men regularly get their blood pressure checked; it is painless, time-efficient, and may help to identify potential problems that if caught early can be corrected with minor lifestyles changes.

Blood pressure usually is measured using a stethoscope and a blood pressure cuff, which yields two numbers, *systolic pressure* and *diastolic pressure,* such as 118/82. These numbers correspond with HTN stages, which allow a patient's risk status to be more easily classified. Consistently higher values usually indicate hypertension; however, several factors, such as stress, exercise, drugs, and medications, can influence these values (Carretero & Oparil, 2000). According to the American Heart Association, people should strive for regular values below 120 systolic and below 80 diastolic to 90 systolic over 60 diastolic (AHA, 2010). Table 9.1 presents these values.

Table 9.1   Normal and Pathological Blood Pressure Values

Source: Chobanian et al. (2003).

Category	Systolic Pressure	Diastolic Pressure
Optimal	119 or less mm Hg	79 or less mm Hg
Pre-Hypertensive	120–139 mm Hg	80–89 mm Hg
Stage I	140–159 mm Hg	90–99 mm Hg
Stage II	≥160 mm Hg	≥100 mm Hg
Isolated Systolic Hypertension	>140 mm Hg	<90 mm Hg

For years, the standard of 120/80 mm Hg (millimeters of mercury to measure pressure) was considered "perfect," however, most physicians recommend that people keep values between 90/60 mm Hg and 119/79 mm Hg (Chobanian et al., 2003). Keep in mind that values should be screened occasionally, because values tend to fluctuate in certain individuals. Many drug stores offer free (or minimal cost) screenings by trained professionals as well as blood pressure machines that can give approximate values. Consistently high values should be followed up by a thorough medical consultation to identify the cause(s) of the HTN.

Men are at high risk for HTN due to several factors, but mostly lifestyle choices and lack of perceived severity of the disease affect predisposition (Carretero & Oparil, 2000; Silva et al., 2007). Younger men often perceive HTN as an "old man's" disease and are less likely to follow up with their primary care providers. According to researchers at the Medical University of South Carolina, HTN is more common in younger men than in older men and thus needs more attention at younger ages (Mainous, Everett, Liszka, King, & Egan, 2004). The cumulative damage to the heart and related structures slowly builds as a man ages until an episode occurs, such as a stroke or in some cases death. African American men are among the higher risk groups for developing HTN in the United States (Carretero & Oparil, 2000; Chobanian et al., 2003; Mainous et al., 2004; Silva et al., 2007).

A man's family history can be a good window into potential risk. Consider weight, diet, exercise patterns, life stresses, and alcohol and drug use. Overweight and obesity greatly increase blood pressure; large portions of food, especially salty foods, affect blood pressure values; lack of consistent exercise causes the heart to work harder to pump blood to its tissues and cells; stress (good or bad) elevates values; and certain drugs (including alcohol) considerably affect blood pressure, causing it to increase (possibly decrease with some drugs to dangerous values) (Carretero & Oparil, 2000).

Headaches, nausea, sweating, abnormal levels of fatigue, confusion, visual disturbances, and any other systemic changes may be clues that a man's blood pressure is off. Men who are hypertensive experience erectile dysfunction at rates of 2.5 times more than **normotensive** men (Silva et al., 2007).

Knowing the causes and individual risk factors can aid in determining appropriate, preemptive management and treatment options before the disease progresses. The ACSM and AHA both acknowledge that exercise is the best form of managing and treating HTN for most people (Haskell et al., 2007). However, at times, medications may be warranted to treat HTN. These drugs should be used in conjunction with sound exercise prescription principles versus in isolation. Specific medications include diuretics, beta-blockers, alpha-blockers, angiotensin-converting enzyme (ACE) inhibitors, angiotensin-receptor blockers, calcium channel blockers, and vasodilators (Chobanian et al., 2003). Most remove fluids from the blood and tissues, block enzymatic reactions to decrease heart rate, or keep the artery walls open (dilated).

Stroke

One of the greatest risk factors for stroke is hypertension. In the United States, stroke affects nearly 700,000 people annually. Data from the CDC lists stroke as the fourth overall leading cause of death in men in the United States, accounting for roughly 5% of all deaths. Deaths from stroke are highest in Asian and Pacific Islander men, and it is the third leading cause of death (7.6%) in these populations (CDC, 2006). A stroke, also known as a *cerebrovascular accident* (CVA), occurs when the brain is deprived of vital oxygen, thereby causing cells to die. Stroke can occur from blocked blood vessels (*ischemic stroke*) or ruptured blood vessels (*hemorrhagic stroke*) and should be considered a medical emergency. Nearly 80% of all strokes are ischemic (Donnan, Fisher, Macleod, & Davis, 2008). Attacks can occur at any age and sometimes for no apparent reason; however, the likelihood of stroke increases with age. Blocked blood vessels are more common with advancing age, and this trend appears to have accelerated over recent decades.

Arteries build up plaque over time, and occasionally these clots dislodge and block major blood vessels to the brain, causing stroke (Donnan et al., 2008). Obesity, high blood pressure, and high levels of cholesterol all affect men more so than women and African American men in particular (Treadwell & Ro, 2003). Family members who have experienced strokes are a strong risk factor. Some variables are familial in nature and need to be identified early on to prevent poor health outcomes and death. High blood pressure is one of the strongest causes of stroke in men, because elevated values exert excessive pressure on blood vessels to the brain, which can weaken them over time. Coupled with blood clots from a poor diet, trauma, and elevated stress levels, hypertension is literally a ticking time bomb for many men and their families (Chobanian, et al., 2003).

Other health conditions that exacerbate the likelihood of stroke are heart disease, diabetes, and having a prior history of strokes or TIA episodes. Plaques associated with heart disease can break off and travel in the blood stream to the brain, where blockages may occur. Often, small blockages will provoke the warning signs of stroke (Donnan et al., 2008). Diabetes and fatty deposits in the blood stream are common factors. Certain lifestyle choices also increase a man's chances for developing a stroke. Alcohol and drug use can cause blood vessels to constrict and increase pressure on delicate arteries and blood vessels (Reynolds et al., 2003). Smoking has extreme effects on blood vessels. Research has consistently demonstrated that smoking increases the buildup of fatty deposits in major blood vessels, such as the carotid artery in the neck. Moreover, smoking decreases oxygen levels in the blood; thickens the blood, increasing the chances for developing clots; and causes blood vessels to constrict, which subsequently raises blood pressure (Hankey, 1999; Wannamethee, Shaper, & Whincup, 1995).

Signs and symptoms differ among people; however, men usually report visual disturbances, diminished strength, dizziness, headache, and confusion. Blurry vision can occur in one or both eyes as the blocked blood vessel disrupts blood from the area of the brain (occipital lobe) that controls vision. A weak muscular response on one side of the body also characterizes stroke symptoms. This also may present as limp musculature, loss of tone, or drooping facial muscles on one side. Dizziness results from visual disturbances, and intense headaches can present in many areas of the head and facial regions. Disorientation and confusion typically present during a stroke as blood flow becomes limited to various areas of the brain (Donnan et al., 2008; Perry & Schacht, 2001; Goldstein & Simel, 2005).

Most people survive strokes; however, disability and long recovery periods often accompany an episode. Some people experience a *transient ischemic attack* (TIA), which is a tell-tale sign that something may be wrong and warrants a checkup immediately. For many men, a TIA often doesn't play a strong enough role to prompt a man to see a doctor. Many stroke symptoms clear up quickly, thereby lessening the emergent nature of the condition for many men. Unfortunately, at this time when the body is in a warning mode, many men ignore the signs and symptoms until they become more pronounced and frequent or they suffer a full-blown stroke.

Stroke affects the family unit in many ways. Many men who experience strokes live on. However, living on after a stroke is not a guarantee of good health or quality of life; in fact, the opposite generally holds true. Strokes rob persons of many of their physical and mental capabilities, leaving them invalids. Stroke causes brain damage and physical impairment that leaves many on a long road of rehabilitation and recovery (Mohr, Choi, Grotta, & Wolf, 2004). A man who experiences a stroke and does not die from it will put emotional, financial, and productivity strains on his family and community. Work often will not be an option, as the man must now focus on extensive rehabilitation as his primary job. Family and personal income will be greatly affected, leading to lower socioeconomic status and lower overall quality of life. A loss of self-esteem and self-worth often accompanies victims of stroke.

Stroke should be taken seriously. Knowing a man's risk factors, such as family history, overweight and obesity, diet, stress levels, and alcohol and drug use can be very helpful in recommending positive health changes that can minimize risk of stroke. It is critical that men who have diabetes keep it under control and regularly assess their blood sugar levels (Wild et al., 2004), especially if there is a family pattern. Family members are advised to encourage regular checkups, including testing for cholesterol, blood pressure, diabetes, and other predisposing factors for stroke. Additionally, family support is important in helping a man gain control of his lifestyle choices. Controlling weight, limiting alcohol consumption, avoiding drugs, decreasing stress, and quitting smoking will greatly reduce risk of stroke.

Diabetes

According to 2006 CDC data, diabetes is listed as the sixth leading cause of death in men of all ages (roughly 3%), behind stroke. It is highest in Native Americans, followed by Hispanics, African Americans, and whites (CDC, 2006). When the body is unable to properly utilize or produce the hormone insulin, a person is said to have *diabetes mellitus* (DM). Type I diabetes (also known as *juvenile diabetes*) exhibits early in life (see Chapter Six). Most men who have type I diabetes will have experienced signs and symptoms earlier in life and learned to manage it appropriately through diet, monitoring, and medication.

In type II diabetes mellitus (also called *adult onset diabetes*), cells become resistant to insulin and the metabolism is negatively altered. Type II diabetes generally results from metabolic stress brought on by overweight and obesity (Rother, 2007). Middle-aged men are at risk for the development of diabetes (especially type II) more so than other populations.

CDC data suggest that Americans are becoming more obese at alarming rates over the past decade; therefore, rates of type II diabetes will increase as well (Baskin, Ard, Franklin, & Allison, 2005). The incidence of diabetes has doubled during the past thirty years. The risk for type II diabetes increases after age forty-five, but rates are increasing at younger ages because of rising obesity. Younger children are even considered to be "prediabetic" due to poor dietary practices and lack of consistent exercise (Wild, Roglic, Green, Sicree, & King, 2004).

There are several risk factors for type II diabetes, including being overweight or obese, having a sedentary lifestyle; having a diet high in sugars, refined foods, fats, and low in fiber; and having a direct family member who has had the disease. Certain ethnicities, such as African Americans, Hispanics, Native Americans, Asian Americans, and Pacific Islanders, have increased risk factors (Rother, 2007; Wild et al., 2004). Upward of 6 million men in the United States have this disease and don't know it (Baskin et al., 2005).

Simple blood tests can be used to determine if a man's blood sugar is high and uncontrolled. Unfortunately, diabetes is a relatively silent disease process, so many men don't regularly get tested. The following signs and symptoms are consistent with diabetes: intense thirst, frequent hunger, fatigue, frequent urination (especially at night), unexplained weight loss, visual disturbances, sores that don't heal or are slower to heal, fruity smell of the breath, and dark, sticky urine (Perry & Schacht, 2001).

The good news is that type II diabetes is preventable and usually can be reversed. In a study, 3,234 overweight people with elevated blood glucose levels who followed a lifestyle change program of exercise and diet geared to losing weight lowered their diabetes risk by 58%. Further, those age sixty and over lowered their risk by 71% (Knowler et al., 2002).

Men often are less concerned for their physical health than are women, perhaps because of fear of vanity; however, as society changes, men may become more in tune with how their poor health status affects not just themselves, but their families and society in general. Public health professionals need to pay particular attention to groups of men that are at the highest risk levels for diabetes. Diabetes is not going anywhere anytime soon, but with the right awareness and advocacy efforts, men can become more proactive earlier in life to avoid conditions like diabetes that are clearly related to lifestyle choices.

Male Pattern Baldness

As men age, hair follicles atrophy (become smaller) and hair becomes thinner, eventually to the point of falling out without regeneration. This process typically occurs in one of several distinct patterns (Rebora, 2004). For most men, this is an expected part of aging, and many accept the fate of their follicles as part of that process. For some men, however, it provokes fear and uncertainty about the ever-present march toward physical decline.

Sales for hair replacement products, procedures, and drugs flood the market and media every day. Graying of the hair (loss of **pigment**) indicates physiologic changes in a man's system. A man should be aware of what may be causing these processes. Is it simply age, or does it seem to be accelerated? Abusing one's body with chemicals, poor diet, stress, and lack of sleep can greatly speed up the aging process. The cumulative effects of stress can be seen in men who possess positions of great authority and stress, such as world leaders and military personnel. Hair loss can indicate pathology in some, but for the most part, it is a natural part of many men's lives (Rebora, 2004).

EMOTIONAL HEALTH

The Midlife Crisis

Perhaps the hallmark feature of middle adulthood centers around what many have called the "midlife crisis." The perception of a midlife crisis is highly subjective and varies greatly from person to person. The midlife crisis is most commonly characterized by a period of self-doubt; however, self-reflection and self-appraisal also are common features (Jacques, 1965). The numerous and varied life changes and transitions occurring during this period of life may prompt many men to seek meaning in what they do, which can take the form of extramarital affairs, travel, changing careers, going back to school, trying to act younger, or buying the proverbial little red sports car.

VIGNETTE

Ted was sitting catty-corner from me in the waiting room of Skin Care Physicians, a private group practice in a wealthier part of greater Boston. He appeared to not fit into the setting. Ted was a man of around fifty years old and wore dark blue work pants and had thick hands with a slight hint of grit beneath his fingernails and a five o'clock shadow. What brought Ted to this establishment? Was he waiting for someone having a procedure done, like I was? Was he lost? Or was he waiting for his own appointment?

Back and forth I argued with myself on what circumstances brought him here. Finally, I asked him out of sheer curiosity or simply being nosey, "Excuse me," I said as I cleared my throat, "are you waiting for someone?" Ted looked at me with a stern expression at first, but then a warm smile came over his face. He responded, "Nope, I am waiting to see the doc. . . . How "bout you?" I informed him that I was waiting for someone. He nodded and went back to reading the sports section of the local newspaper. Again, in my nervous voice I said, "I am sorry to pry, sir, but may I ask what you are seeing the doctor for?" Expecting that he might haul off and slug me, I awaited his response. Ted said, "You know, I have always feared looking like my dad when I got older," as he grabbed the skin directly under his chin. "Chicken chin is what I call this!" I politely smiled and intently listened. "I know it is weird a guy like me is having a consultation for liposuction and a face lift, but I'll tell ya . . . when it is something that you cannot get your mind off of, it really can dampen your day." I reassured him that I would not judge him but was just curious because of a paper I was writing. He smiled and said, "Well . . . just don't let the guys at the plant know you saw me here," (he worked at a physical plant at a university in Boston). I assured him that I appreciated his perspective and that mum was the word.

Many men may experience a sense of loss in many forms: loss of youth, relationships, physical abilities, deaths of parents, and many others (Baraff, 1991). Similar to female menopause, the concept of *andropause* has been presented as a period of biopyschosocial changes within a man's life. This may be supported with evidence; as men age they tend to lose testosterone, which can lead to various hormonal changes (hot flashes, irritability, and so on) similar to those women experience (Mooradian & Korenman, 2006). A man's personality type and past psychological challenges may predispose him to experiencing a crisis during midlife (Baraff, 1991).

Some research suggests that the notion of a midlife crisis is a culture-bound phenomenon; men in cultures such as those in Asia do not have similar experiences (Kruger, 1994). Traditional Asian cultures value elders, whereas Western cultures usually praise youth and a younger status. Losing a sense youth may provoke certain people to experience the distress that has come to be called a "crisis."

In studies, 10%–15% of men expressed experiencing midlife crises, with the average age forty-six years and the stage lasting three to ten years. Age is the most commonly expressed cause of distress, but work and career changes or stress, spousal and personal relationship changes, aging or death of parents, children maturing and leaving the "nest," and physical changes appear to influence the experience of a midlife crisis as well (Lachman, 2004). Men generally experience more issues and distress related to changes in their jobs and careers than do women (Jacques, 1965; Mooradian & Korenman, 2006).

A sense of regret often accompanies a crisis. Any type of change can be met with a negative or positive approach. Those who view a crisis as a challenge are likely to rise up and learn more about themselves and life overall. Those who wallow and mire themselves in trying to figure out why are likely to be let down and may even become depressed in the process. The infinite wisdom of Buddha may have captured this period of life best, noting, "A man may conquer a million men in battle but one who conquers himself is, indeed, the greatest of conquerors."

Men may act out their emotions due to their encultured inability to express their feelings. For men, this may accompany the sense of regret, search for connections to youth, desire to be more of an individual, or search for a dream or goal they have yet to achieve (Myers, 1998). The acting out in middle adulthood may take several forms, such as substance abuse, purchasing expensive items, depression, doing things to act younger (style of dress, social excursions, plastic surgery and other cosmetic procedures), blaming themselves or others for their failures, associating with younger people, seeking sexually promiscuous experiences, or pressuring spouses or children to achieve higher goals (Kruger, 1994; Lachman, 2004; Mooradian & Korenman, 2006).

Whether real or perceived, the phenomenon of the midlife crisis brings up many psychosocial issues in middle adulthood for many men. There are periods and instances of social and personal adjustment that can challenge any man. How he responds can lead to a variety of positive and negative health issues. The stress of change should be recognized and handled like other periods of stress throughout the life span. Positive coping strategies, such as communication, deep breathing, meditation, yoga, exercise, social support, and others are important to maintaining optimal health (Baraff, 1991). Much can be learn about oneself during midlife. A man's midlife crisis, in the right context, may be revised to his midlife growth.

Divorce and Infidelity

Perhaps congruent with the midlife crisis, men may experience strain in relationships, marriage notwithstanding. Approximately half of all marriages in the United States end in divorce. Data from the CDC suggest the divorce rate is 3.5 per 1,000 people in the United States, with just over 2.1 million annually (CDC, 2006). Second and third marriages have even higher rates of divorce, at 67% and 74% respectively. Statistics show that the older a man waits to get married, the less likely his marriage will end in divorce. Roughly 50% of men who marry at age twenty-four or younger will experience divorce. Those who marry after thirty years old experience an 18.1% divorce rate.

Infidelity is a primary cause in many instances of divorce. Why people cheat on their spouses and significant others is a matter of controversy and debate. Moreover, why men tend to cheat more so than women also is a hotly contested topic. Some point to nature; that is, it is in a man's biological make-up to "spread his seed," whereas others argue it is a lack of will and weak character caused by sociocultural influences in his upbringing (Subotnik & Harris, 2005). The jury is still out on this debate and it may not be settled anytime soon. Coupled with pressures and changes during midlife, men may stray from their traditional and long-standing relationships to explore other aspects of life and their personalities (Kruger, 1994; Myers, 1998). Some men are serial cheaters, whereas others may be caught off guard by their tendencies (Subotnik & Harris, 2005). Every man is different, and it is unfair to stereotype all men as cheaters. Lack of communication and not having needs met may contribute to reasons that men get caught up in infidelity.

The stress of infidelity and possible divorce can lead to stress in a man's life, which carries severe emotional consequences (Subotnik & Harris, 2005). Divorce takes an emotional toll on people and may exhaust financial resources. Stress causes dysfunction in relationships; a man may lose contact with his children or other family members due to the breakup.

Substance abuse and depression are common reactions to divorce and relationship troubles. Moreover, some men father children outside of marriage or contract sexually transmitted infections (Subotnik & Harris, 2005). Marriage and relationships are complex no matter which stage of life; however, midlife may present additional complexities for many men (Jacques, 1965; Kruger, 1994; Myers, 1998).

FATHERS' RIGHTS

With divorce comes the separation of the family unit, which includes children. For many men, this may mean giving up certain rights and privileges that were unquestioned while married. With separation and divorce, many men lose ground and exert less influence in the lives of their children (Subotnik & Harris, 2005). This fact has given rise to various fathers' rights movements across the country that deal with family law, custody disputes, and financial considerations, such as child support. Many men desire to share equally in the lives of their children; however, the current U.S. legal system tends to side with mothers rather than fathers in many custody disputes (Bertoia & Drakich, 1993; Kenedy, 2004).

This social movement arose out of the frustration many men and some women felt in parental equality. The media has profiled mothers who have removed their child from their fathers' custody and returned to the foreign countries of their birth, leaving the fathers with little more than memories and pictures of their children. International laws and agreements make getting children back nearly impossible (Kenedy, 2004). The family court system has attempted to better calibrate the system, but there continue to be inconsistencies and deficiencies in the overall process. Shared parenting and child custody can get messy, but many parents are opting for no-fault divorce proceedings to ease the burden of this issue for their family.

Frustration and parental alienation can lead to extreme measures being taken by many men, such as domestic disputes, violence, and even kidnapping of their own children. Estranged parents may feel this is a last ditch effort to retain influence in their child's life, but the opposite results; that is, the parent likely will lose all rights and privileges because he or she has broken the law (Williams, 2002). For a man, frustration needs to be met with patience and ultimately concern for his children. Taking rash actions likely will only lead to him being further from his children rather than closer. Joining parenting groups and men's and fathers' rights groups can help advance the cause. **Social action** can bring about change, albeit slowly (Kenedy, 2004).

SUMMARY

As a man ages, his body tends to gradually break down. Knowing the risk for specific diseases based on personal and family history and through screening and diagnostic testing can help a man live a better quality of life. Prevention always is essential; however, being proactive can help alleviate many diseases, illnesses, and conditions. Some health conditions, such as balding, are simply a function of who we are; others, such as heart disease and diabetes, may be within our direct control. Knowing how to manage these life factors will alleviate much of the physical and resulting emotional stress these diseases cause in a man's life. A social phenomenon known as the "midlife crisis" sometimes crops up during this period of life. Job stress, family changes, physical aging, and many other factors can precipitate this. Adding to these stressors are the challenges of infidelity, divorce, and child custody issues. The key for a man in this stage of life is to learn to adapt to stresses and control what is in his control.

KEY TERMS

Angina	Lumpectomy	Palliative
Anthropometric	Mastectomy	Pigment
Digital	Metastatic	Semen
Longitudinal Research	Normotensive	Social action

DISCUSSION QUESTIONS

1. Why do men have a higher risk for coronary artery disease and heart attacks than women? What can be done to reduce a man's risk of developing heart disease?

2. Why do you think men tend to avoid getting regular checkups and screenings for colorectal health and prostate health?

3. Take a position on whether you think it is valuable for a man to know his prostate status or if it inflicts more harm than good. Justify your answer with facts and statistics.

4. Briefly explain the correlative relationship between hypertension and risk of stroke. How can controlling his blood pressure reduce a man's risk of stroke?

5. Briefly describe the factors associated with hair loss in men. What can be done to slow or reverse this process?

6. Do you think the midlife crisis actually exists? Justify your opinion.

7. Briefly explain the concept of andropause in men. What physical and emotional changes can result from this experience? What might moderate the effects of andropause?

8. Do you think men are "wired" to cheat? Justify your answer based on both your opinion *and* what the current research has to say about the topic.

9. Many fathers do not retain custody of their children when a separation and divorce ensue. Why is this usually the case in family law? Do you think fathers should be given more rights and access to their children?

10. Do you think the current family legal system encourages fathers to become more distant and disconnected with their children or do you think the system works? Be sure to justify your answers with specific examples.

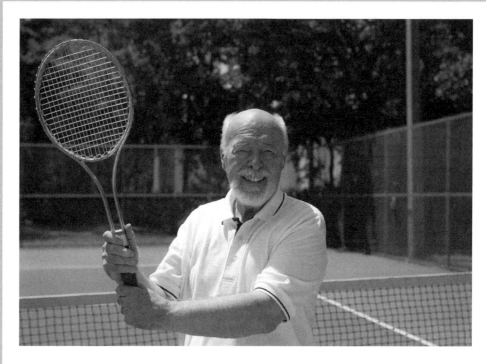

©iStockphoto.com/Lisa F. Young

10

Older Adulthood

LEARNING OBJECTIVES

- Identify the physical changes men experience as they age, such as androgen deficiency syndrome and erectile dysfunction

- Discuss strategies, such as hormone replacement therapy, exercise and nutrition, and medications, to lessen the cumulative effects of aging

- Analyze higher risk factors in men as they age, such as bone health, depression, and suicide

- Examine the changing trends in older adulthood pertaining to sexual health matters

- Appraise the emotional adjustments in older men, such as losing a spouse or a job

EARLY HEALTH ADVOCACY and nutrition pioneer Adelle Davis once equipped, "As I see it, every day you do one of two things: build health or produce disease in yourself." Statistics tell us that most American men will live to and past age sixty-five, with the mean age 74.7 years (Centers for Disease Control and Prevention [CDC], 2006a). Gone are the days when a man reached his sixties and was considered "over the hill" and only a few years out from his ultimate demise. People are living longer, but longer life doesn't necessarily mean better life. In fact, as a society, we tend to get very caught up on age. When a man reaches age sixty-five, he may view himself differently simply because society tells him he is different. Senior citizen discounts, AARP memberships, retirement, pensions, senior living communities, and the like all give perspective and help to define how a person responds to this life stage.

Older adults often reflect on past decades and looks forward to their remaining time. For some, this evokes feelings of anxiety and uncertainty; however, some men may "get it." This "getting it" is what famed psychologist and behavioralist Abraham Maslow termed *self-actualization* (Gleitman, Fridlund, & Reisberg, 2004). Many men may never find this inner peace, but with advancing age comes **wisdom**. Life experience helps us determine what has and has not worked in the past. Many previous lifestyle choices and behaviors come to fruition, some good and some not so good. A man who actively exercised, ate a reasonable diet, and balanced his social experiences is likely to be rewarded with better overall health than a man who led an imbalanced younger life. This is very apparent in conditions such as cancer, heart disease, and stroke in men (CDC, 2006b). This chapter focuses on the physical and emotional challenges and opportunities men face after age sixty-five. Topics such as changing hormone profiles, bone health, and companionship later in life are presented and discussed in detail.

PHYSICAL HEALTH

Men over the age of sixty-five have unique health needs. Often, gone are the warning signs and signals that his body made available during younger and middle adulthood. Second chances are possible, but often at the expense of quality of life and stress and burden on family members and friends. Time is *not* on a man's side in this life stage. Many of the former protective factors (youth, energy, hormones, muscles, metabolism, and so on) have worn out or have become less effective. Hormones change, which affects a man's strength, muscle efficiency, risk of falling, cognitive and mental clarity, risk of cancers, and overall wellness (Fuller, Tan, & Martins, 2007; Mooradian & Korenman, 2006). Men at this stage of life need to maintain an aggressive preventative agenda for their health to optimize health and retard the aging process. Health professionals recommend the following as a health maintenance schedule for men ages sixty-five and older (Perry & Schacht, 2001):

- *General Physical Examinations.* Men should have routine physicals every year after age sixty-five. The greater likelihood of illness and disease makes staying up to date highly important.

- *Eyes.* These should be checked every year. Changes in vision are quite common as people age, and vision can affect other aspects of life. Poor vision can predispose men to falls, misreading medication labels, and automobile accidents. Also, the development of conditions such as **cataracts** and **glaucoma** are more likely during this stage of life.

- *Teeth.* Teeth should be checked at least twice per year. This includes routine cleanings and screenings for dental caries (cavities), gum disease, and bone loss. Since bone loss is more common as men age, it can adversely affect tooth structure and overall function of the jaw, possibly inhibiting chewing and other common functions. If identified early, preventative or restorative measures can be implemented to enhance quality of life.

- *Blood Pressure.* This should be checked every year. Due to atherosclerosis, increased body mass, medications, stress, and several other factors, blood pressure is likely to elevate during later years. This increases the already higher risk of vascular accidents such as stroke. The test is noninvasive, only takes a moment, and could save a life.

- *Cholesterol.* This should be checked every three years unless a man has a higher level of risk from, for example, heart disease or liver dysfunction. High cholesterol and heart disease can limit function and quality of life. Blockages can lead to excessive fatigue, cognitive impairment, and erectile dysfunction. A simple blood test can help screen for these issues.

- *Colorectal Screenings.* Men should be screened every year for rectal bleeding and fecal blood tests. Bleeding may indicate trauma caused by lesions, cancer, medications, or many other conditions. Additionally, a sigmoidoscopy or colonoscopy should be performed every three to five years to inspect the integrity of the rectum and colon.

- *Prostate Screenings.* Because this gland continues to grow and enlarge as a man ages, the likelihood of tumors and cancers dramatically increase; therefore, men ages sixty-five and over should be screened once per year. The recommended test is a digital rectal exam; however, blood tests (such as with the prostate-specific antigen [PSA] test) also can be used to identify men at risk. Health professionals should advise men to be aware of symptoms such as increased urinary frequency, weak stream of urine, erectile and ejaculatory dysfunction, and pressure.

Androgen Deficiency Syndrome

Also known as the *male climacteric*, androgen deficiency syndrome (ADS) has been called the male version of female menopause or *andropause* (Heller & Myers, 1944; Mooradian & Korenman, 2006). While there certainly are common parallels to menopause, there are some obvious sex-based differences. Changing hormonal levels cause a host of physical and emotional changes in men. Diminishing levels of the primary male sex hormone testosterone and some others cause physical changes such as increases in body fat, less muscle tissue, lower levels of strength, hot flashes, sweating, and diminished sexual drive (*libido*) (Mooradian & Korenman, 2006). Psychological effects such as lack of mental clarity, irritability, frustration, fatigue, and several other features can occur (Heller & Myers, 1944; Mooradian & Korenman, 2006). Contrary to the female climacteric, the male reproductive system does not entirely shut down; rather it slows down production of androgens and sperm (Mooradian & Korenman, 2006). A man still can produce viable sperm well into later life; however, the quality of his genetic material has recently been a topic of scrutiny in the medical sciences. "Old" sperm have been postulated to increase the chances of fathering offspring with emotional and developmental disorders such as autism, learning disabilities, and cognitive impairment (Schmid et al., 2007). Science stills needs better confirmatory evidence, but it should be considered as men and women plan to have children, and it dashes the age-old notion that men are the invincible perpetuators of life.

VIGNETTE

Paul had two months left until he retired from his longtime job at Peterson Elementary School. He was excited, but he also felt a bit sad. It hit Paul over the weekend when he thought to himself, "What will I do during my days?" Paul had two grown children and two young grandchildren. He was recently divorced after a thirty-five-year marriage and was feeling a bit "lost," as he described it. Paul knew there were many opportunities and challenges before him. Additionally, Paul also noticed that he was feeling a bit "off" even though he had regular medical checkups. He was having trouble remembering, felt weaker than usual, and experienced a lower than normal sex drive. A friend discussed the hormone replacement therapy that he was on to help slow the signs and effects of aging. Paul was intrigued.

He thought about dating and whether it was okay for him to get back on the scene. "What would my kids think?" "

Some of Paul's friends joked about going through menopause, which rang a bell in his mind. In reading the local newspaper, Paul noticed a clinical research trial being conducted at a large research hospital in his area. The advertisement read, "Are you a reasonably healthy man over age 55? Do you sometimes have weakness, irritability, and fatigue? Are you concerned about bone health? If you answered 'yes' to any of these questions, you may be eligible for a clinical research trial on a new experimental medication to control aging, prevent/slow bone loss, and treat the effects of andropause."

"Yeah!" Paul thought to himself; "Andropause," he exclaimed. Paul got online and searched for "andropause." As he read the results his eyes widened and all of his physical and emotional feelings began falling into place. Paul had always thought men simply "just got older" and hormones, emotional changes, and similar issues were reserved for their female counterparts. Paul's perspective on health was about to change.

Men who experience ADS should not be confused with men who congenitally do not produce enough testosterone, often referred to as *hypogonadism* (Mahmoud & Comhaire, 2006). Men naturally lose approximately 1% of their normal levels of testosterone after age thirty, or roughly 10% per decade (Fuller et al., 2007; Mooradian & Korenman, 2006). So, for example, a man of age seventy has lost approximately 40% of his original testosterone values. Lower testosterone levels have been associated with male osteoporosis, **Alzheimer's disease, impotence**, and depression. Low levels of testosterone cause estrogen (the primary female sex hormone) to elevate throughout a man's body, further causing physical and emotional changes (Fuller et al., 2007; Mahmoud & Comhaire, 2006; Mooradian & Korenman, 2006).

Some people advocate that ADS prompts many men to experience the midlife crisis discussed in Chapter Nine (Diamond, 1998). Much of this work is hypothetical, and one is cautioned when interpreting these findings, as some may be overly speculative in nature and not supported by evidence-based studies. In fact, many researchers believe the concept of andropause does not exist, because men often can reproduce well into later adulthood (Juul & Skakkebaek, 2002). This latter point is **binary** and compares males to females. Males and females have very different biological systems; equating one to the other is severely limited from a scientific perspective. The loss of hormones does affect physical and psychological function in men. How these physiological changes affect men in older adulthood is of more practical use than debating whether a term bests describes what is happening.

Lifestyle is likely a strong factor in how a man's system reacts to hormonal balances during life. Many men may consume excess fat or use certain drugs (for example, marijuana) that have been shown to elevate estrogen levels and limit the positive effects of testosterone (Daling et al., 2009). Testosterone also is sensitive to levels of stress a man may experience, with higher stress correlated to lower levels of testosterone (Nilsson, Moller, & Solstad, 2009). Some men also abuse androgens with anabolic-androgenic steroids (AAS) earlier in life; this can take a toll on the body's normal production of testosterone later in life (Pope & Katz, 1994).

Not every man will experience adverse effects of the inevitable drop in his body's production of testosterone and other male hormones. The complex interactional model of human physiology, the environment, and psychosocial factors all play a role in how well (or not so well) people age. The immense variety in the human population demonstrates that not everyone will experience or respond to certain stimuli, which is why monitoring trends via epidemiological methods is so important in public health. Some men of advanced age will respond well to androgen treatments, whereas others may observe no marked effects (Juul & Skakkebaek, 2002). Unfortunately, many men view treatments and therapies, such as hormone replacement therapy (HRT) as a veritable "fountain of youth," Testosterone replacement therapy and human growth hormone (hGH) have shown some clinical evidence that adverse effects of aging can be diminished or slowed, but claims that these and similar therapies can and will reverse aging are faulty and erroneous (Raynor, Carson, Pearson, & Nix, 2007).

Hormone Replacement Therapy

In hormone replacement therapy, certain hormones, such as testosterone, are *exogenously* (outside the body) introduced into the body to help compensate for minimal or no production by the body itself (Hijazi & Cunningham, 2005; Raynor et al., 2007). Recently, the term *replacement* has been dropped, because therapies are not necessarily replacing hormones but rather attempting to augment existing levels. This type of treatment for several medical issues has been studied since the 1940s, mainly in pre- and postmenopausal women. The treatment in women came under intense scrutiny in the mid-1990s due to a correlation with elevated levels of estrogen and the development of breast cancer. Recently, in the past decade, science has examined the efficacy of HRT in males using controlled levels of testosterone to combat the effects of age-related disease and illnesses (Hijazi & Cunningham, 2005; Raynor et al., 2007). Results have been mixed, with some showing positive findings, some negative findings, and some no findings at all (Juul & Skakkebaek, 2002; Raynor et al., 2007). Currently, pharmaceutical companies have dedicated much effort and many resources to studying the beneficial effects of androgens in HRT among men to help decrease loss of muscle (*sarcopenia*) and strength and other functional limitations associated with getting older (Hijazi & Cunningham, 2005).

Because results are mixed, FDA approval for use of these types of drugs and therapies are not approved for these issues.

Some of the more common uses for HRT in men are for very specific androgen deficiencies that accompany medical diagnoses. For these diagnoses, HRT has FDA approval. Men with lower levels of circulating testosterone who experience adverse effects are candidates for HRT. These men often are referred to as *hypogonadal*. Specific indications for HRT in men include underactive gonads (testes), loss of muscle mass (often due to disease or chemotherapy treatments), diminished libido, and certain mood disorders, among others (Mahmoud & Comhaire, 2006). In fact, testosterone has been used for decades (although much less frequently since the advent of selective serotonin reuptake inhibitors [SSRIs]) to combat the effects of depression (Pope, Cohane, Kanayama, Siegel, & Hudson, 2003).

Testosterone and other androgen therapies have been shown to enhance sexual functioning in men by improving frequency of spontaneous sexual thoughts; attentiveness to erotic auditory stimuli; increased frequency, duration, and magnitude of erections; sexual activity scores and ratings; and volume of ejaculate (Bhasin et al., 2006). HRT has been demonstrated to increase skeletal muscle mass and subsequent strength (Bhasin et al., 1996; Singh et al., 2008). This is an important finding for aging men because diminished muscular strength has been implicated in several adverse health issues, including loss of balance and fall-related accidents. Men with chronic diseases, such as cancer, osteoporosis, renal (kidney) disease, HIV/AIDS-related wasting syndromes, and chronic obstructive pulmonary disorder (COPD), have been treated with mixed results (Rietschel, Corcoran, Stanley, Basgoz, Klibanski, & Grinspoon, 2000). Evidence suggests that using HRT in men with HIV and related diseases is moderately effective (Bhasin et al., 2006). More relevant to older men, some evidence supports HRT use for men with muscle loss (*sarcopenia*) and other functional limitations, which have been extensively studied for more than forty years (Feldman et al., 2002; Pirke & Doerr, 1973). For example, men who lose muscle mass and strength are less likely to weight-bear, thus limiting bone strength and increasing chances for fracture and compromised health-related quality of life. Since 20% of men ages sixty and older and 50% of men ages eighty and older were found to have serum testosterone levels in the hypogonadal range in one study (Harman, Metter, Tobin, Pearson, & Blackman, 2001), HRT may be a viable treatment in these populations, but this does not include all men in these age ranges. Additionally, many of these studies have used men in "normal" ranges in the blood (that is, >325 ng dL^{-1}) for testosterone levels. Findings from Harman et al. (2001) suggest that testosterone therapy may positively affect age-related declines in memory, spatial abilities, and executive functions. Data on sexual dysfunction are inconsistent, suggesting that HRT may not be effective in all males (Araujo et al., 2007). Bone health also may be adversely affected by low testosterone levels. Men with low levels stand a 3.7 times higher risk for developing osteoporosis and bone fractures (Ensrud et al., 2006; Laurentani et al., 2006; Mellström et al., 2006).

Overall, HRT in men has been met with mixed results. Risks and benefits remain poorly understood, yet the popularization of HRT continues in the medical world and beyond (Raynor et al., 2007). Small sample sizes in many studies and relatively healthy men of varying ages make generalizability of findings very limited. The benefits of HRT need to be carefully weighed against potential risks. For example, blood can thicken due to the increase in red blood cell production, causing vascular events such as stroke, sleep disturbances can develop or worsen, breast tissue can change (*gynecomastia*) and may increase the likelihood for developing cancer, and testosterone therapy may increase prostate activity (Hoffman et al., 2009). Clinically apparent prostate activity may prompt biopsies and even surgery, which may or may not improve patient outcomes. This has prompted discussion concerning physician-caused (*iatrogenic*) adverse medical outcomes for many men. According to the Endocrine Society's Clinical Guidelines, "Until more information becomes available, testosterone administration in older men should be individualized and limited only to older men with unequivocally and consistently low testosterone levels who are experiencing significant symptoms of androgen deficiency; in these individuals, consideration of testosterone therapy should be preceded by a careful discussion of its potential risks and benefits with the patient and rigorous monitoring of potential adverse affects" (Hoffman et al., 2009, p. S28; Bhasin et al., 2006).

Sexual Health

As people live longer, their sex lives continue as well. Sexual activity is a fairly good indicator of overall relative health in men. The theory is that if you are healthy and active enough for sex, then you are most likely healthy in an overall sense. Men may have grown up expecting to lose their sex drive and have come to expect impotence to reign over their once virile bodies. For some men, the body does lose the capacity to engage in healthy sexual activity. Overweight and obesity, stress, decreasing testosterone levels, cardiovascular disease, diabetes, high blood pressure, and several other physical factors in addition to medications can limit a man's sexual capacity (Bacon et al., 2003). Some of these factors can be addressed by healthier lifestyles. Losing weight, eating a healthier diet lower in fat, managing stress more effectively, HRT, focusing on heart health, and limiting medications all can lead to a better sexual health status. Men may not realize that their high blood pressure medication also affects their erectile capacity; that an extra 50 pounds clogs arteries that feed the penis, leading to diminished erections; and that psychological stress decreases libido and causes depression. Moreover, some medications to manage depression have side effects that diminish sexual drive in many people.

Sexual health is important even as we age. Not only is it healthy for a man's physical functioning, but it also enriches his emotional status. The capacity to enjoy a healthy sexual life is only limited to how healthy people live and approach this area of health. People are living longer, with many being healthier than our ancestors. The **geriatric** population in the United States and abroad is growing. With better health also comes engaging in sexual activity more frequently (Bacon et al., 2003). Although older men feel empowered to be sexually viable, many of the same issues that plague adolescents and younger populations hold true for older men. Sexually transmitted infections do not discriminate based on any factor, including age.

With greater than 60% of people over age sixty having sex at least once per month, risk of infection is omnipresent. Many older men do not consider themselves at risk mainly because social stereotype, reinforced by media and public health messages, imply that STIs are a younger person's problem (Levy et al., 2007; Lindau, Schumm, Laumann, Levinson, O'Muircheartaigh, & Waite, 2007). This leads many to practice unsafe sex. Many men and their partners view condom use as unnecessary because most older women are beyond their reproductive years and have a low likelihood of becoming pregnant. Also, this lack of urgency precludes many men from getting tested and screened to know their status, thus increasing the likelihood that they will transmit disease to others (Lindau et al., 2007).

Many men may forgo using condoms because they think they are not at risk for an STI or that their partner will not get pregnant.

©iStockphoto.com/Don Bayley

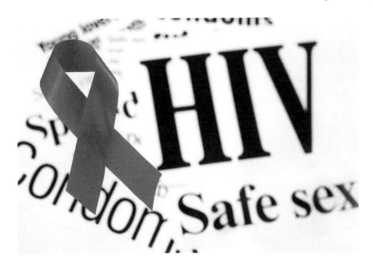

Loss of a spouse or divorce also may challenge the monogamy many men once practiced. Dating again introduces new possibilities of contracting or passing on an STI to another person. As a person ages, so too does his or her immune system, making it less likely that he or she will be able to fight off a potential infection. Some people can harbor an STI such as syphilis that can be mistaken for psychological changes associated with the aging process. HIV infection is rising in people over age fifty in comparison to people under forty, according to recent data from the CDC (Lindau et al., 2007). Men also appear to be the population most affected by HIV.

In response to this potential public health epidemic, the CDC has released new guidelines that recommend physicians consider screening people from ages thirty to sixty-four for STIs as part of their routine practices (Levy et al., 2007; Lindau et al., 2007). In addition to screenings, better educational efforts need to be undertaken to help educate older males. Bringing this education to a generation who likely grew up with principles of modesty may be a challenge for public health; some men may find the education offensive. Also, the baby boomer generation is coming of age. Many of the men in this generation grew up at a time when "free love" and the "sexual revolution" were in full swing. These cultural and generational perspectives and biases may make it a further challenge to educate men that they are at risk for infection.

Divorce rates also may have magnified this issue, with more men searching for partners in life (Levy et al., 2007; Lindau et al., 2007). Medications such as erectile dysfunction products may be contributing to the problem as men engage in more frequent sexual activity (Brownlee, 2007). Public health professionals cannot turn a blind eye to an increasing problem.

Erectile Dysfunction

Concomitant with sexual health for older men is the ability to perform sexually. As men age, the issue of erectile dysfunction (ED) often becomes magnified. The vernacular of ED changed in the late 1990s from "impotence" to "ED" with the advent of drugs such as Viagra. Changing the terminology made it much easier for men to discuss this embarrassing problem with their doctors, who were all too eager to write prescriptions for ED medications.

Myth: All men experience erectile dysfunction when they get old.

Fact: It is true that many men in fact do experience ED as they age, but it is less a fact of getting older than it is how a man takes care of his health. Clogged arteries, higher body fat, and emotional factors such as depression all enhance the likelihood of ED. These all are preventable or at least modifiable.

Pharmaceutical marketing professionals loved this shift, because it meant more men would buy their products. Impotence connoted a lack of potency or virility, whereas changing it to "dysfunction" now meant that something broke down in the otherwise normal system and it could be fixed with medication. A problem with drugs for ED is that many men began to worry that they were not performing well enough and that medication was needed to stay healthy. Medications for ED are meant to help those with actual ED and not for those who want to last longer during sex or have sex more frequently. Drugs to treat ED may send the wrong message to many older men that they need to maintain a youthful lifestyle beyond their physical, emotional, and social means. This false sense of empowerment and entitlement can lead to many physical and emotional consequences, such as diseases, empty relationships, and financial instability among older men.

Osteoporosis and Bone Health

Osteoporosis is a disease wherein the bones become less dense, more porous, and more susceptible to damage such as fracture. Overall, men suffer from osteoporosis less frequently than do women; however, the consequences of the disease are often more severe. For example, men who break a hip are two times more likely to die in six months than are women (Diamond et al., 2001).

Bone is continually changing and remodeling itself as people age, grow, and develop. Increasing stress and activity causes more bone to be added to the skeleton, whereas decreasing stress causes a loss of bone. Bone responds and adapts to what it is asked to do (United States Department of Health and Human Services [USDHHS], 2004). For example, astronauts must perform weight-bearing exercise each day while in space because weightlessness causes less stress on their bones, and their bones may become smaller and less dense. Bone loss is accelerated in men after age sixty-five because the body's ability to absorb calcium (a major constituent of bony tissue) is markedly diminished. Upward of 33% of men ages seventy-five and older have active osteoporosis, with many experiencing fractures as a result (Diamond et al., 2001; USDHHS, 2004).

There are several theories as to why some men develop osteoporosis and some do not. Bone loss occurs in most people as a natural part of the aging process, as bone tends to break down faster than it can replace itself after age thirty-five. Genetics, family history, and lifestyle and behavioral choices are thought to be the strongest influences on development of osteoporosis (Diamond et al., 2001; USDHHS, 2004). Some common risk factors include age, small frames, being white or Asian, low testosterone levels, alcohol consumption, smoking, certain medications, poor diet, lack of vitamin D, lack of physical activity, and certain systemic diseases (such as rheumatoid arthritis or celiac disease) (Perry & Schacht, 2001). While reversing osteoporosis is improbable, slowing the deleterious effects it can cause is possible. Health professionals can advise men that having regular physical checkups, being aware of bone pain or increasing fractures, and having certain urine or blood tests and bone density screenings are good ways to assess bone health as they age. Occasionally, a bone biopsy, which takes a piece of bone from the body for analysis, will be performed to confirm or refute a diagnosis of osteoporosis.

Breast Cancer

Rates of male breast cancer pale in comparison to those of women; however, risk of breast cancer and all forms of cancer increase with aging (American Cancer Society [ACS], 2010). Public health tends to focus on prostate, pancreatic, and colorectal cancers in men of advancing age; however specific groups of men need to be aware of their added risk. Men with higher levels of estrogen and/or lower levels of testosterone have an increased risk for developing this rare form of cancer (ACS, 2010). HRT possibly could offset the risk of this type of cancer as a man ages; however, results are inconclusive. Health professionals should advise about awareness and proactive screening. For example, a man can include a breast self examination (BSE) along with testicular self-examinations (TSE) as part of a daily, weekly, or monthly routine. If a man has low testosterone levels or is on HRT, risk for breast cancer may be higher. Men who develop excessive breast tissue (called *gynecomastia*) due to hormonal, genetic, environmental (pollutants or exposure to toxins), or lifestyle reasons (poor diet high in fat) also have higher risk as they age (ACS, 2010).

EMOTIONAL HEALTH

Life stresses don't necessarily attenuate as a man ages, but they do change. Concern may shift from jobs and family to health status and social networks. For example, it is inevitable that the older a person is the more likely he or she will lose friends, family members, and even children along the way. If proper coping strategies and support networks are not in place, older men can, will, and do suffer from varying degrees of depression. Left unchecked, depression can become quite profound and even result in suicide (Baraff, 1991). Cultural bias often focuses on issues related to suicide in younger populations, such as adolescents; however, suicide is a striking reality in older age as well. Men are four times more likely to commit suicide than women and account for 78.8% of all suicides, and the rates in men sixty-five and older are 38.4 per 100,000 compared to 6.0 for women in the same age group (CDC, 2005). Suicide often is preceded by substance abuse; toxicology reports from completed suicides showed that 33% tested positive for alcohol, 16.4% for opiates, 9.4% for cocaine, 7.7% for marijuana, and 3.9% for amphetamines, according to the National Violent Death Reporting System (Karch, Crosby, & Simon, 2006). This marked fact illustrates some of the drastic measures many men take when posed with stressful situations. Lack of adequate alternatives or means of expression may be a telling cause, as evidenced by the manner in which men are found to commit suicide. Firearms account for 56.8% of all deaths in men, contrasted with poisoning in 37.8% in women (CDC, 2005). Emotional health in older age for men should be no different than any other stage of life; it needs to recognized, managed and treated, and followed up by professionals and loved ones.

Social support can be a critical factor for many men as they age. Loss of a spouse due to separation, disease, divorce, or death can take an emotional toll on a man. Many men assume the role of caretaker of an elderly spouse or a spouse who becomes ill with a disease such as cancer or Alzheimer's, further adding to the emotional stress and strain. Adjusting to living single and maintaining or establishing some level of social support through companionship is a critical factor in helping older men live better-quality lives.

Companionship and Living Alone

With aging comes the possibility that relationships will fail, spouses will die, or life situations otherwise will change. For many men and women of older age, finding themselves at the precipice of a new relationship experience is a possibility. Statistically, men are less likely to live as long as their female counterparts (CDC, 2005), but some do, and this may leave a man wondering what his next step may be. To simply state that it is a well-known fact that men are more likely to die sooner than women is not enough and does little to explain and promote strategies to elucidate this paradox. Singh-Manoux et al. (2008, p. 2256) acknowledged that "a wide range of genetic, hormonal, social, and cultural factors are likely to play a role in shaping male and female patterns of morbidity and mortality."

Moreover, with divorce rates in the United States hovering around 50% or higher for the past several decades, a man is likely to find himself facing new relationships and the challenges that accompany them (Russell, 2009). Separation or divorce has been found to have a negative effect on a man's health during this life stage. A Danish study of twins revealed that depression and smoking was higher in a divorced twin compared to the other (Osler, McGue, Lund, & Christensen, 2008).

A man finding himself single from whatever cause faces issues such as increasing financial responsibility and burden, personal responsibilities, and emotional challenges (**alienation**, depression, and so on). Emotionally, men may be fearful. A younger man fresh out of relationship may move on because he knows that he has years ahead of him. But a man seventy years old or older likely will have questions.

Asthma and diabetes also were found to be increased in older men who were single because they were separated, divorced, or recently widowed (Martin, Haren, Taylor, Middleton, & Wittert, 2008). Smoking and overeating likely are the result of depression brought on by a man's loss of his relationship and companionship (Bayram, Farahdin, & Britt, 2009). Minimizing risk factors is very important during this stage of life. Men are less likely to be as physically or emotionally resilient as they once were. With aging comes the increased risk of emergent situations such as falls or heart attack and stroke.

Work provides a social support system for many men. Retiring or losing a job can strip a man of his sense of belonging, particularly if he is recently finding himself single. Single men have a higher likelihood of using drugs, alcohol, and tobacco products and adopting poor eating habits. A primary care physician and family members should monitor a man's risk of depression and suicide so as to recommend treatment (Russell, 2009).

Sexual health of single older men cannot be ignored. Age does not have to preclude sexual health and activity. With this comes responsibility of safer sexual practices. A newly single man needs to understand that responsible sexual practices will decrease the risk of disease transmission regardless (Levy et al., 2007; Lindau et al., 2007).

A man who finds himself single may react to his new life situation in several ways. Some reactions are health negative, such as substance abuse and depression, whereas others include a renewed sense of personal ability and hopefulness. Some men will enjoy their newfound freedom and sense of individuality, whereas others may become mired in fear and despair. Because responses are highly individualistic, primary care physicians, family members, and caregivers need to be sensitive and respectful of these reactions and tailor a healthy plan and approach to the situation. The stronger sense of self that a man develops, the better overall health outcomes.

SUMMARY

This chapter addressed various physical and emotional issues affecting men in older adulthood. Androgen deficiency syndrome was a primary issue. Hormone replacement therapy was discussed as a possible solution to many age-related deficits men may encounter, such as sexual health, bone health, and cancers, among others. Responsibility in sexual activity was discussed. Last, emotional health of older men was discussed. Handling the challenges of single living and seeking companionship were touched upon. Understanding the complexities of both sex (biology) and gender (social constructs) will help health professionals plan better strategies to enhance health as men age. Moreover, understanding these differences will help men and their families overcome gender barriers that preclude good health and overall quality of life.

KEY TERMS

Alienation	Cataracts	Impotence
Alzheimer's disease	Geriatric	Wisdom
Binary	Glaucoma	

DISCUSSION QUESTIONS

1. What are the hallmarks of androgen deficiency syndrome (andropause)?

2. Briefly explain how losing testosterone in men is negative in terms of their health. What are the physical and psychological effects that take place? Refer to the research concerning this issue.

3. Why do you think men who experience fractured hips because of falling often die within six months and overall have poorer outcomes than women?

4. What are some good strategies to combat and prevent osteoporosis earlier in life?

5. It was found that some women who experienced hormone replacement therapy (HRT) also increased their risk for breast cancer. Comment on HRT and any added risks associated with men undergoing this form of therapy.

6. Look up breast cancer support groups and services in your local area. Were you able to locate anything that pertains to men? Are there any recommendations for including men in these types of services if you were not able to find any in your search?

7. Briefly explain the terminology concerning sexual functioning of a man, comparing and contrasting the terms *erectile dysfunction* and *impotence*. What are the ramifications when each of these terms is used in describing the condition?

8. Do you think older men abuse erectile dysfunction drugs? Do you think so many men need these types of drugs? Briefly explain how these types of drugs work in the system.

9. What are some of the health benefits for older men who are able to maintain active sexual lives? Are there any negatives?

10. Do you think older men typically turn to multiple sexual partners when they lose a spouse due to death, divorce, separation, or any other factor? Do you think this is natural and appropriate for a man, or is it negative in terms of his health? Justify your response.

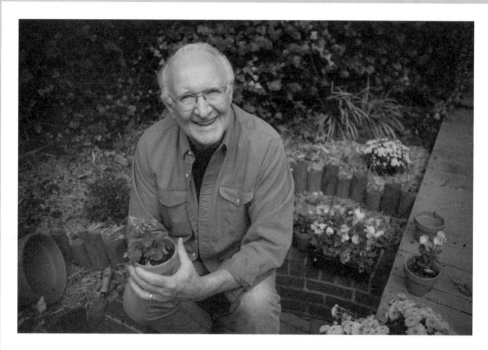

©iStockphoto.com/Steve Cole

11

Elder Years

LEARNING OBJECTIVES

- Identify the common physical and emotional challenges of elderly men
- Discuss common sociocultural biases associated with aging and determine how they can affect overall health
- Analyze misperceptions concerning Alzheimer's disease, dementia, senility, and other changes in an elderly man's psychological health profile
- Apply ways to advocate for equity in elder health matters

THERE IS NO particular age range associated with the elder years—also referred to as "old age" or "senior years." Approaching or even surpassing the average life span generally puts a person into the *elderly* category. This definition is highly subjective and varies within cultures and time periods. For example, men in cultures in which the average life expectancy is roughly eighty years, such as Iceland, would characterize elderly as closer to this number, compared to a country such as Kenya, where the average male life expectancy is just over fifty-three years (Central Intelligence Agency [CIA], 2010). Additionally, how a person perceives him- or herself can define elder status. Men who feel old, look it, or act it often are perceived as such by others in society, whereas the opposite may hold true for men who perceive themselves as vital.

Some people advocate that age is simply a state of mind. While psychological status does play into how a person feels with advancing age, some inevitable physical signs and characteristics of aging are nearly ubiquitous. As people age and enter the elder years, the body is less able to regenerate and recover from injury, illness, and disease. For some, the brain also ages, leading to bouts of forgetfulness and confusion, commonly referred to as **senility**. The study of how people age, with the intent of enhancing overall quality of life, is called *gerontology*. Physical degeneration as well as psychological impairment are concerns for men as they age. Moreover, how people perceive older men can lead to a cultural bias known as **ageism**. This chapter presents and explores some of the more common physical, psychological (emotional), and social challenges elderly men may face.

PHYSICAL HEALTH

All people can expect to experience their share of physical changes as they age. Some people more, some less, and some sooner than later; however, it is what people do to their bodies in the process that matters later in life. Putting in a little effort, such as exercising, eating right, and managing stress helps mitigate the effects of aging. Not taking care of one's health results in rapid aging, illness and disease, and even premature death. Balance is the key.

Degeneration

As people's cells age on the microscopic level, they start to see the effects at the macroscopic level, with wrinkles, graying hair, less bone mass, loss of muscle tissue and strength, and even loss of height (Panek & Hayslip, 1987; Rowe & Kahn, 1987, 1997). These changes are normal; unfortunately, Western culture in particular has pathologized aging. Physicians and other health professionals can advise men that they can slow the degeneration process through good nutrition, regular exercise, managing stress, and good sleep habits; however many men do not follow through. Not following this simple formula stresses the cells and accelerates the aging process. Drug and alcohol use also accelerates physiological aging processes (Rowe & Kahn, 1997). For example, a man who regularly smokes and drinks alcohol will typically look older than a man who does not practice these negative health behaviors.

Disease

Cumulative stress and degeneration of the body's cells can lead to diseases such as cancer, coronary artery disease, diabetes, and stroke. Many of these diseases are considered processes; that is, they occur over time rather than all at once (*acutely*). Because time is a factor with many diseases, the older a man gets, the greater the likelihood that he will experience some type of dysfunction (Panek & Hayslip, 1987). For example, a man who eats a diet high in saturated fats, doesn't exercise on a regular basis, and is chronically stressed generally experiences a heart episode or attack in his fifties, not because that is when he becomes sick, but because that is when the disease manifests.

With so many factors playing into disease models (genetics, health status, environmental and psychological stress, and social determinants), the factors that can be modified or controlled need to be a hallmark feature of public health. Research and development of innovative drugs and surgical interventions help enhance quality of life for many, but the simplest (and cheapest) method is by teaching good prevention skills to boys and men from very young ages. The financial burden of disease in the United States alone is staggering, costing an estimated $2.5 trillion in 2009 and expected to rise to $4.3 trillion by 2018 (Centers for Medicare and Medicaid Services [CMS], 2010). Consider some of these facts from the Kaiser Family Foundation 2009 report on trends in health care costs and spending:

- Health care accounted for approximately 17.6% of the **gross domestic product (GDP)** in the U.S. in 2009.

- Health care costs have grown faster than the U.S. economy since the 1960s.

- 10% of the population, many of whom are elderly, account for 63% of health care.

A small percentage of the overall U.S. population appears to be consuming the highest percentage of health care. Yet most of the elderly in the United States don't have the financial means to fund these expenditures; therefore, the costs are subsidized by insurance companies and passed on to consumers. This is very disturbing, considering that estimates suggest that by the year 2020, people over age sixty-five will comprise 17% (roughly 50 million people) of the total U.S. population. If these people are not in relatively good health, all consumers will bear the burden of increasing health care costs regardless of their individual health (Brownlee, 2007).

EMOTIONAL HEALTH

Physical health is important, but it is not the only predictor of quality of life as a man ages. How a man views himself—his body, self-esteem, self-confidence, and self-concept—can greatly affect how he conducts himself in life. A positive attitude contributes to a better sense of self in stress, image, efficacy, and several other outcome variables.

There are many factors that can aid a man in maintaining positive psychological health, such as friends, family, social networks, work, and fraternal organizations. The better connected a man feels in life, the more likely he will experience good psychological health and possibly better overall physical health as well. Augmenting psychological health often has been found to improve overall quality of life, because men who feel as if they have a purpose in life often respond with better health behaviors. Research has shown that people who feel a sense of connection to a greater cause are more likely to report higher life satisfaction and better overall social health as a result (Palmore & Luikart, 1972).

Myth: It is not possible to reverse the psychological effects of aging; once your brain is gone, it is gone.

Fact: Like other organs, the brain experiences the effects of aging; however, like bones and muscle, it can be strengthened. For example, keeping an active mind through doing puzzles, reading, socializing, and eating brain foods (Omega-3s, almonds) will stave off the unwanted effects of mental deterioration as you age (Morris, Evans, & Bienias, 2003).

Many males have been raised to repress emotions and impose a male façade to be more acceptable in society. This holds true more so in older generations of men, but as generations pass and boys develop a better sense of emotional intelligence and intellectual engagement, psychological health is likely to be improved (Baraff, 1991; Kindlon & Thompson, 2000).

Depression

One of the marked features of psychological health is the lack of it, namely depression. Depression comes in many forms and varies from person to person. Some men may be overtly depressed, whereas others effectively hide it so as to not burden others. Men also typically view depression and other psychological conditions as weakness or even unmasculine. Other men opt to self-medicate with the use of alcohol and other drugs.

Depression is common in elderly populations, with male suicide rates six times higher than those of females.

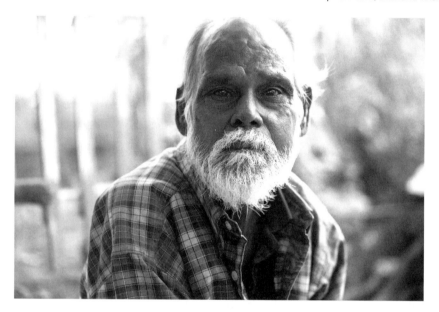

Depression is fairly common in elderly populations (Baraff, 1991); however, reactions to it greatly vary between men and women. For example, the most extreme form of handling depression (suicide) among elderly populations has been found to be nearly six times higher in males than in females (Miller, Barber, Azrael, Calle, Lawler, & Mukamal, 2009). This may be due to recent generations being taught to handle and manage their emotions or simply because people are living longer and therefore tend to experience more life events (including depression). Loss of functionality, sense of self, and loved ones all can compound to result in elderly men taking their lives (Miller et al., 2009). Fear of ridicule or not being able to appropriately express one's emotions may predispose many males to this unfortunate reaction.

Public health needs to continue advocacy efforts aimed at changing how men are managed in the health care system, particularly in psychiatric circumstances. Physicians and health care workers need to be sensitive to the unique needs of males' psychological health challenges as they age. Armed with appropriate gender-specific and gender-sensitive strategies, health care providers will be better able to help men psychologically adjust to the unique demands of their experiences as they age (Bayram, Fahridin, & Britt, 2009; Wilhelm, 2009).

Alzheimer's Disease

Alzheimer's disease (AD) is characterized by the deposition of **plaques** (hyperphosphorylated tau and aggregated β-amyloid peptides) in the brain and related nervous tissues (Hogervorst, Williams, Budge, Barnetson, Combrinck, & Smith, 2001). At present, there are no cures for AD, but researchers are working on treatments and ways to prevent the disease from occurring. Men need to be aware of this disease process not only for themselves, but for their spouses and partners who may develop it as well.

This disease process affects a person's psychological health status, but it has deeply rooted physical causes as well. The recognition and management of AD is largely based on how a man acts rather than the physical signs and symptoms that manifest. This is one area in which men seem to experience fewer effects than do women, with roughly 17% of women over age seventy diagnosed with AD, compared to 11% of men. A recent study with men and Alzheimer's disease and dementia-related Alzheimer's symptoms revealed that men with lower circulating levels of the testosterone were more likely to have AD (Hogervorst et al., 2001). This latter bit of research may lend credence to the use of hormone replacement therapy (HRT) in men.

Signs and symptoms of AD include a gradual but marked decrease in cognitive function, which can leave a person incapable of performing even simple tasks, such as caring for personal hygiene. Often referred to as **dementia**, AD affects nearly 5 million persons over age seventy in the United States alone. Plaques that develop in the brain cause tangles of neurons and interfere with nerve conduction (*synapses*). Impairment of synapses causes memory dysfunction and overall dysfunction of cognition. Many **postmortem** biopsies of brain tissue of suspected AD patients confirm the presence of plaques unique to this disease process (Hogervorst et al., 2001).

There are three stages of AD that are characterized by varying symptoms of the disease. In stage I AD, a person may become easily lost or mismanage bills and money. People in stage II AD (which can last for two to ten years) have more marked memory loss and often require assistance completing even simple daily tasks. Stage III AD lasts a couple of years and leaves a person incapacitated; unable to think, recognize people or objects, and virtually in a vegetative state. Diagnosing AD is not always a simple task (Hogervorst et al., 2001). A full medical history should be taken followed by a series of neurocognitive functioning tests. Other causes (infection, tumors, and so on) need to be ruled out before a formal diagnosis of AD is made. Some clinical tests and imaging (such as CT [computerized axial tomography] scans and brain MRIs [magnetic resonance imaging]) can be used to detect brain abnormalities. Men can take preventative measures to lessen the likelihood for developing this disease, and some treatments (Tan, 2005) have shown promising results; however, genetics and lifestyle choices factor heavily into this disease.

Elder Abuse

"I felt trapped, scared, used and frustrated," detailed famed actor Mickey Rooney. He also detailed how he and his wife Jan were made to go hungry and had medicine withheld, and that his Oscar was even sold off. "But above all, when a man feels helpless, it's terrible," said the screen legend (Silverman, 2011).

One of the social taboos that often goes unnoticed is elder abuse. While there are no formal statistics as to how many cases exist each year, it is likely that thousands of cases of abuse, neglect, and general mistreatment occur annually. There are several definitions of elder abuse, which may be why quantifying it has been such a challenge. Some privately funded organizations report that between 1 million and 2 million (2%–10%) of Americans ages sixty-five and older have been mistreated, neglected, abused, or otherwise harmed by people who were responsible for their care and treatment. These people may include family members, professionals, or a combination of the two. Abuse is not just physical but may also include emotional abuse as well as financial exploitation (Acierno et al., 2010).

Unfortunately, elder abuse often goes unreported, which further compounds the issue. Men are even less likely to report abuse than are women because of fear of being classified as invalid, weak, or simply not being a man (this fear persists well into old age for some men). Because the elderly population will only grow in the coming years (CDC, 2008), more and more instances of elder abuse are possible unless the public becomes more educated on the matter and understands how to recognize and prevent it. Physical abuse is common, and physicians and others need to be aware of the following signs: unaccounted-for instances of bruising, welts, lacerations, sprains, dislocations, broken eyeglasses, signs of being restrained or over-medicated, sudden change in behavior, or fear of being alone with a caretaker. Physical abuse is not the only form of abuse; sexual abuse occurs as well. Signs of sexual abuse include bruising, unexplained genital infections, bloody underwear, unexplained anal bleeding, or an elder's report of being sexual abused. Signs of neglect include unsanitary living conditions, dehydration, malnutrition, bed sores, and poor personal hygiene. Some elders are abandoned in living facilities or hospitals, or people simply leave an elderly person unattended for hours in public places. Financial exploitation is quite common. Some companies or individuals prey on the elderly, claiming to help them stay financially secure when in fact they are trying to bilk them of their money and resources. Because an elderly person may become confused more easily or is forgetful, people exploit this, leaving them helpless and financially vulnerable (Acierno et al., 2010).

SOCIAL HEALTH

Social Organizations

Because employment often defines men, loss of employment can take an important function and need away from a man. Substituting employment with other healthy activities as a man ages is very important. There are many social organizations and opportunities that older men can participate in and establish solid relationships. Rotary clubs, church organizations, veterans' groups, adventure clubs, and many others can provide opportunities for enhancing a man's social health. On the converse side, bars, gambling establishments, or other environments can negatively affect a man's social, psychological, and physical health if they are unmediated by other life experiences. By old age, most men have a good idea of what they like and what they do not will self-determine their likes, interests, and dislikes. Unfortunately, many men believe that they have to follow suit with what other men their age do. Health professionals can advise elderly men to branch out and eliminate one-dimensional thinking. The elderly can be advised to do things in moderation and be open to new experiences.

VIGNETTE

Manny set foot out of his car and slowly walked over to the light-brown stucco-faced building. Manny was a proud and staunch man of seventy-nine. He walked with a purpose and a slight air of hubris. As he walked into the building, he exclaimed, "Where the hell are all the cars?," in his thick Boston accent. The man behind the desk smiled and said, "Welcome, Manny. We have been waiting for you and we are glad to have you working for our company." Manny smiled and, with a boyish grin, firmly shook Ben's hand. Manny and Ben, who was in his late fifties, had known each other for years. Manny called Ben one afternoon and explained that he needed a little side work because money was tight. Ben could not understand why Manny, a man of nearly eighty years old, would want to work and where all of his money had gone. Regardless, Ben knew Manny was a good man, a solid and reliable worker, and highly personable with the clients of his company. Manny would be driving clients to and from the local airport five days per week. Pick-up times often would be very early in the morning, but Manny did not mind it since he always had trouble sleeping in. Manny's wife was lonely at home, but she knew they needed money to supplement their meager monthly Social Security stipend.

Manny and his wife had been born and lived through a time when the average life expectancy was only in the late fifties or early sixties. Social Security was enough for the few remaining years after one retired, but Manny and his wife were now well into their seventies. Where would the extra money come from? How could they make ends meet when they never planned to live this long?

One afternoon after his shift, Ben asked Manny, "Hey, old man, how are things, you enjoying this or what?!" Manny smiled and said, "Ya know, after two weeks, I forgot what it was like having a little work, money, and social time with friends, so yeah, I'm liking it." Manny realized that it was not just the money; it was that he felt a sense of purpose and he enjoyed some downtime socializing with "the gang" at the local hotel as they awaited their calls from the dispatcher. Manny would go on to work for the car pick-up service until he was eighty-five, when he reluctantly left the business because Ben had died of an apparent heart attack and the new management did not endorse having an eighty-five-year-old driver.

Manny felt he lost a sense of functionality in his life as he returned home to be with his wife. He had enjoyed the extra money, but he really missed the social health he experienced while working for the company. Soon thereafter, Manny experienced a fall one early winter morning, causing him to fracture his hip. After a four-hour surgery, Manny's chances of full recovery were not in his favor, since most men over age seventy-five who fracture a hip die six months post-fall. Manny, however, beat the odds, endured intense home-based physical therapy sessions, and was soon back on his feet, only a little slower. What does the future hold for Manny? He did not know, but he did know that life always was changing and that "when you give up, you're dead!"

It is important for men and their loved ones to realize that the life span is a continuous educational experience. From birth until death people are capable of learning and growing from their experiences. Membership in formal and informal social organizations is highly relevant and important for men's health.

Caring for Others

An elderly man sometimes is in a position of caring for an aging spouse, partner, or loved one. Anyone who has to care for another may experience a multitude of physical and emotional stresses that can negatively affect his or her health. Many men believe it to be their duty to care for their families, as it was earlier in life when they went to work and earned an income. Some men may lack the empathy skills to fully care for a loved one; others will be resistant to ask others for help. Also, some elderly men may be faced with the tough decision of when it may be appropriate or necessary to place a spouse or loved one in a long-term care facility. Some fear the financial strain as well as the physical and emotional loneliness that comes with it. In some instances, men choose to join their spouse in an elder care facility even though they may be independently functioning.

Take Roger, for example. Roger and his wife, Elly, had enjoyed nearly sixty-five years of marriage when Elly was diagnosed with Alzheimer's disease. Five years passed when Elly took a turn for the worse; she began forgetting everything, even Roger's name. After consulting with family it was decided that it would be best to place Elly in a long-term care facility for constant care and monitoring by medical staff. Roger decided to sell their home of fifty-three years and join Elly in the facility. Many men don't have this option, as finances tend to dwindle as we age. Good investment strategies exercised earlier in life can help.

Assuming the role as a caregiver is not impossible given the right social support and life experiences. The more expansive gender roles we allow boys and men to experience, the more capable they will be to assume these roles if the time should come.

Isolation and Alienation

Men often view themselves in terms of their functionality or roles in life rather than through most other life factors or experiences. Provider, protector, worker, and father figure, among others—all traditionally characterize how a man defines himself in his world. When a purpose is altered or is even taken away (such as losing a job, being forced to retire, and so on), a man may feel estranged from his emotions and purpose, possibly leading to feelings of isolation and alienation (Schwartz & Tylka, 2008). People die, family moves or loses touch, schedules are busy, and life seems to just start losing meaning. Social networks are critical in keeping a person engaged. Networks established earlier in life tend to sustain many men as they get older. Health professionals, families, spouses, friends, and others should encourage involvement in multiple activities and social venues as a man ages to keep the mind fresh and the soul fulfilled.

Most people must continually be reminded and remind themselves that nothing is permanent in life, and it is how individuals respond to change that makes them better human beings. Spencer Johnson, M.D., made it the premise of his book, *Who Moved My Cheese?* (1998). When people realize that their comfort zones always will be challenged, they can develop positive and healthy coping mechanisms to persist and live better for it. Men can be advised not to be caught off guard as they age. Life *will* change. Those who stay connected will weather most changes and fare better in their emotional and social health.

Driving and Aging

Driving is a touchy subject for many older Americans who wish to retain a sense of independence but also may realize they are not as safe as they once were on the roads. With advancing age also come slower reflexes and reaction times, diminished eyesight, less coordination, slower cognitive and decision-making skills, and other physical and cognitive impairments. Some elderly people experience medical emergencies that increase with aging, such as heart attacks and strokes, while driving. Alcohol and other drugs can severely impair a driver's ability to react, think, evaluate road scenarios, see and hear stimuli, and maintain control of a vehicle.

Reports of elderly drivers getting into serious car accidents and even causing fatalities have gotten the attention of some lawmakers. For instance, currently there are 5.6 million elderly drivers (ages eighty-five and older), a number that is expected to grow to 9.6 million by 2030. Rates for fatal and nonfatal automobile-related crashes increase after age seventy-five and notably increase after age eighty (CDC, 2005). Males had higher death rates than female drivers, with 17.5 deaths per 100,000 in 65–69 year olds, progressively increasing to 20.5 for ages 70–74, 24.0 for ages 75–79, 27.8 for ages 80–84, and 31.2 for ages 85 and older, respectively (Insurance Institute for Highway Safety [IIHS], 2008). Figure 11.1 presents these statistics as a graph.

The rates are undeniably startling and warrant public health action. What can (or should be) done to assure elderly drivers are safe and the health and safety of the general public is protected? For some groups, legislation is the answer, whereas other groups cry foul and cite ageism as the impetus for these movements. Some states, such as Massachusetts, have proposed

Figure 11.1   Senior Auto Accidents Deaths (per 100,000)
Source: Insurance Institute for Highway Safety [IIHS] (2008)

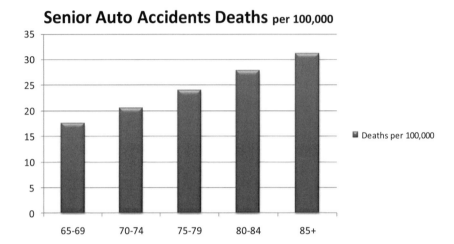

legislation aimed at testing a senior's abilities while not solely focusing on age (Schworm, 2009). Better advocacy and education for elderly drivers may help decrease mortality rates caused by auto accidents. Possessing the physical and cognitive abilities of the elderly to operate a vehicle needs to be determined without granting immunity because a person proved him- or herself capable at a younger age.

Primary care providers should discuss driving as a potential health issue during regular physical checkups with men. Elders can take steps to enhance their physical health, which may allow them to drive longer and more safely; however, when personal and public safety are at risk, driving needs to be viewed as a privilege and not a right.

Long-Term Care Facilities

With greater numbers of men and women living well past ages where they are self-sufficient, the topic of care has become highly relevant in Western society. More and more people are living into their 100s (centenarians) and even the 110s (supercentenarians), leaving many families with the decision of how to best take care of their aging loved ones. Many men and their spouses face the difficult decision of when to relinquish individual freedoms for the relative security of assisted living communities, senior living, and long-term care facilities, also known as nursing homes (Acierno et al., 2010). For some elderly people, the transition is gradual as they learn and appreciate their limitations as they age, whereas others may suddenly be forced into this option as with disease or illness, such as a stroke.

Men usually are outnumbered in nursing facilities because of higher mortality rates and lower years of life expectancy than their female counterparts. For many, entering into a nursing home or senior community creates a sense of loss for many men. Creating new roles for residents has become a primary objective for many of these communities and facilities as they strive to allow their residents to determine their needs but do so in the safety of assisted living or nursing facilities (Banaszak-Holl & Copen, 2002). Unfortunately, many public nursing facilities are state run and are strapped for funding. Poorer quality care leads to greater instances of neglect, abuse, and overall poor health (Acierno et al., 2010). Understanding how to support men as they enter into this phase of life is more complex than simply making a bed available. If we are to provide quality care to our deserving elderly community and populations, we first need to understand their reservations, fears, and unique needs.

We all deserve quality care and respect regardless of age or health status, but unfortunately many people's attitudes change as they view the elderly. The "nuisance" of the elderly is one of the vast inequities and social injustices of our age. Dismissing or ignoring the elderly plight is skewed and is ethically and morally unjust. As the population advances in age, this potential public health crisis will be revisited if we do not pay attention now.

SUMMARY

This chapter presented and discussed the physical, psychological, and social health challenges that many senior men face. Degeneration and diseases of the body become more common, which can lead to necessary lifestyle alterations. These changes in life can cause many men to become depressed and even suicidal. Some men will develop the neurocognitive disease process known as Alzheimer's disease, which robs them of their memories and life experiences. Men also face social health challenges as people move away, family structures change, and friends die. Some men become caregivers to aging spouses, partners, or even children, adding to the stress during a life stage when the body is least capable of effectively handling it. Controversial issues, such as when elders should and should not be permitted to drive, were discussed in addition to how (and where) elders should reside in their later years. The elder years are no different than others in terms of maintaining good health; how we go about doing and promoting it is a challenge.

KEY TERMS

Ageism	Plaques	Senility
Dementia	Post-mortem	
Gross Domestic Product (GDP)		

DISCUSSION QUESTIONS

1. What are some physical, social, and nutritional strategies that have been shown to improve mental health in elderly men? Cite the evidence and research.

2. Why do you think elderly men are less likely to report instances of abuse?

3. How might you help educate elderly people to protect their financial assets and interests from potential predators?

4. Why are social networks and social support systems so critical for elderly men?

5. What are three national or international organizations that are solely geared toward advocating for the rights of elderly people? Briefly describe what each organization does to accomplish its mission.

6. Do you think there should be an age limit as to how long a person can keep his driver's license? Refer to safety statistics as well as ethical arguments.

7. What strategies are being implemented at the state or national level to assure the safety of elderly drivers while also maintaining their individual liberties? Give specific examples.

8. What are current annual costs for long-term care facilities for the elderly? How might this system be improved so all people receive equitable care?

9. How can public health be more active in engaging elderly men in their own health care? Consider what is presently available to them when formulating your answer.

10. Do you believe men of the next few generations will experience better or worse overall health in their elder years than they experience currently? Justify your responses.

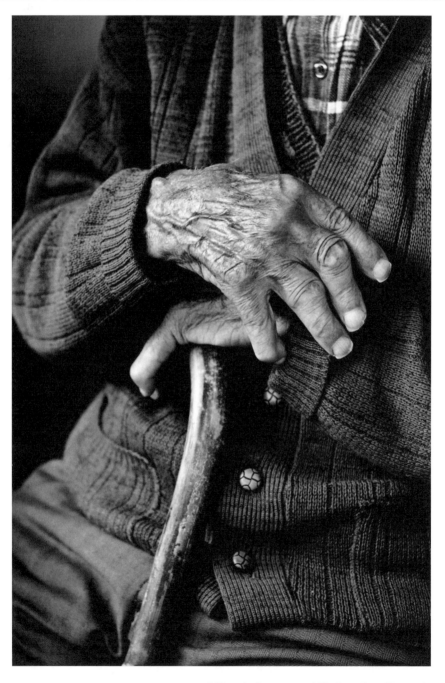

©iStockphoto.com/Christopher Farrugia

12

Death

LEARNING OBJECTIVES

- Evaluate the role death plays in life matters and decisions for men
- Identify ways in which men should plan for their deaths at various life stages
- Analyze the personal and social ramifications of death in the family structure
- Identify ways to incorporate death education into the early lives of boys and younger men

MANY PEOPLE PLACE a certain value on the *number* of years a person lives versus the *quality* of those years. Is there a *right* time to die? Statistics tell us that most males in the United States will live to approximately seventy-five years old (Centers for Disease Control and Prevention [CDC], 2008). Clearly, the quality of life one experiences greatly affects the legacy one leaves behind. Death almost always is viewed as being a sad experience; however, those who are left behind usually find good and positive aspects to reflect on concerning their loved one's lived life and experiences.

Death has been dubbed the "great equalizer" because all people will experience it. The events leading up to his death generally characterize a man's health. For men, maintaining good health needs to be a priority. Higher rates of heart disease, cancer, injuries, stroke, HIV, and suicide all afflict men more than women. For some men, death may be seen as a relief from his life struggles. This brief chapter explores the experience of impending death and the event itself. It provides strategies for embracing death, processing loss, and grieving in a healthy way.

THE SEVEN AGES OF MAN

Perhaps one of the world's most interesting (and possibly the first account) of the life span of male health comes to us from writer and poet William Shakespeare.

Shakespeare writes of the "Seven Ages of Man" in the play *As You Like It*. The poem nicely captures how he viewed a man's life.

All the world's a stage,

And all the men and women merely players,

They have their exits and entrances,

And one man in his time plays many parts,

His acts being seven ages. At first the infant,

Mewling and puking in the nurse's arms.

Then, the whining schoolboy with his satchel

And shining morning face, creeping like snail

Unwillingly to school. And then the lover,

Sighing like furnace, with a woeful ballad

Made to his mistress' eyebrow. Then a soldier,

Full of strange oaths, and bearded like the pard,

Jealous in honour, sudden, and quick in quarrel,

Seeking the bubble reputation

Even in the cannon's mouth. And then the justice

In fair round belly, with good capon lin'd,

With eyes severe, and beard of formal cut,

Full of wise saws, and modern instances,

And so he plays his part. The sixth age shifts

Into the lean and slipper'd pantaloon,

With spectacles on nose, and pouch on side,

His youthful hose well sav'd, a world too wide,

For his shrunk shank, and his big manly voice,

Turning again towards childish treble, pipes

And whistles in his sound. Last scene of all,

That ends this strange eventful history,

Is second childishness and mere oblivion,

Sans teeth, sans eyes, sans taste, sans everything. (Act II, Scene VII)

The seven ages detail the progression of the infant, the schoolboy, the lover, the soldier, the justice, the lean and slippered pantaloon, and the second child. The passage gives the reader a complete overview of how Shakespeare sees the progression of life in general. Some of the description focuses on the physical and social, whereas other lines refer to the mental and emotional challenges of life. In his younger years, a man often may tempt and even cheat death, relying solely on chance occurrences or his abilities to regenerate his body. In middle age, he becomes more tempered and his perspective matures to that of a well-seasoned man. In older age, he becomes jolly and, as Shakespeare details, "childish" in his nature. Is this the description of every man? No. However, there are clear and apparent truths in most of what Shakespeare has detailed in this passage.

VIGNETTE

Three men are chatting as they await their passage on to the "other side."

TIM: "How'd you go?"

ROGER: "My heart gave out. You?"

TIM: "Colon cancer."

PAUL: "Well, I've got you both beat! I was killed in an accident on the job!"

ROGER: "Guys, guys, why are we all comparing still now that we are dead?"

PAUL: "I guess some things never change about guys!" [*chuckle*]

What does death hold for a man? Often fearless, men are culturally groomed to defy and even mock death. Fearing this experience may be viewed by others as feminine and weak (Baraff, 1991). Risk taking may be biologically programmed into males (Erwin, 2006). Death leaves behind family members to **grieve** and other reminders of who the man was in life. People usually are not taught how to grieve loss and may turn to negative coping methods. Defining a successful life as a man is as vague, **nebulous**, and as individual as each man himself. For some men, it will be about career and financial success, whereas others view accomplishments in friends and family. Each person will have to reflect on these types of questions as they rise in life. There are no right or wrong answers, only those that have relevance for the individual. One point is certain; approaching death affords a man opportunity to reflect on his life. Most people are not taught how to grieve or die; they simply do it.

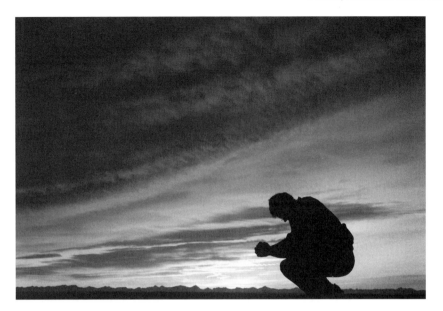

GETTING ONE'S MATTERS IN ORDER

Dying carries certain responsibilities. Health care proxies, wills, financial and family considerations, funeral arrangements, and many more topics need to be discussed and finalized before one's death. Most experts agree that planning earlier is better than waiting until one gets sick or even dies prematurely. Men hold important places in the family as role models, father figures, financial support systems, and influential decision makers. Losing a person of this capacity leaves many gaps in the fabric of the family structure (Jack, 2005).

Men are advised to establish living wills in their forties or early fifties. Some men may wish to do this sooner if they have families and dependents or if they are at risk due to family history or occupational hazards (law enforcement, military personnel, construction workers, and so on). A living will provides legal guidance as to what should be done in the event of premature disability or death. These difficult and often controversial questions need to be discussed in advance so that if misfortune does occur, loved ones know how to proceed. This gives a man social time with those who care about him.

Myth: When a man dies, so does his debt.

Fact: It is true that you cannot pay for something after you die, but your family and loved ones can. The estimated costs of a burial service in the United States are $12,000 to $15,000. Adding to this, end-of-life care (facilities, medical procedures, and so on) push the end-of-life price tag even higher. A man needs to account for this by planning early in life so as to avoid unexpected costs that add to the sadness of his demise.

Living Wills and Advance Health Care Directives

Living wills help a person to specify his wishes in the event he is unable to do so for a number of physical reasons (for example, stroke, being on life support). Some conditions leave a person in a vegetative, incapacitated state and unable to express his wishes to loved ones. An advance health care directive (that is, living will) will take much of the guessing and anguish out of the scenario for family members and other loved ones. A living will is different from a last will and testament that informs how your estate and legal matters (for example, burial arrangements, monetary issues, and so on) are to be handled upon your death. Some points of interest included in living wills include stating whether a person desires life-sustaining treatment (for example, blood transfusions, organ replacement, life support, CPR, and dialysis); whether to have life support or choose to die "naturally"; whether pain medications will be used to ease the dying process; whether a person will accept artificial means of nutrition and hydration such as feeding tubes or intravenous hydration, and whether the person's organs will be donated upon death. It also is common for people to have a Do Not Resuscitate (DNR) order in the event of a life-threatening situation (Mayo Clinic, n.d.a). There are numerous online services that can be used to assist in the planning of a living will and advance health care directive. Additionally, consulting with an attorney also can help plan for these events. Living wills stand in effect as long as the person is alive. Because a living will cannot cover all possibilities and scenarios, it is a good proactive strategy to appoint a power of attorney (PoA) to help in guiding care.

Power of Attorney

Appointing a power of attorney may help alleviate tension that can develop within a family structure during times of duress. Suggestions for selecting a PoA/health care agent include finding someone the person trusts (likely a family member, but not in all cases), someone who is level-headed even in distressful circumstances, has one's best interests at heart, and is comfortable having direct, frank conversations. Men are advised to choose a person based on qualifications rather than out of loyalty or a sense of guilt or obligation. Men should find their state's forms and fill them out; it also may be advisable to go over them with an attorney.

Once a man has approved the forms, he should share them with the person appointed PoA, family members, and his primary care physician. Occasionally people complete the process but forget to inform others as to the whereabouts of their documents. Men are advised to review and revise the PoA and advance medical directives from time to time (Mayo Clinic, n.d.a) This process helps keep everyone involved in the loop and aware of any changes a man may wish to enact.

SUMMARY

This chapter detailed some aspects of death in the context of a man's life. Shakespeare's "Seven Ages of Man" presented a perspective and overview of the life stages of people in general, but men in particular. The importance of men's coming to some conclusions about their final years and getting their personal affairs in order in advance of death was discussed. Leaving his family and friends with a sense of meaning and closure is one of a man's final acts of compassion.

How a man defines his life and how his legacy will be remembered beyond his death has been a topic for millennia. As with all life stages, as people approach death they learn more about themselves and life; when we die, it is other people's turn to learn from the tales we leave behind. A man's death can be a highly valuable experience in helping future generations of males lead healthier and more productive lives.

KEY TERMS

Grieve

Nebulous

DISCUSSION QUESTIONS

1. Do you think Shakespeare's poem, "The Seven Ages of Man," accurately depicts how men age? What (if anything) stands out in this poem?

2. Do you think males "mock" death? Give specific examples.

3. What is a living will or advance health care directive? Under what circumstances should a man have one? When should one be prepared?

4. What is meant by the term "end of life care"? Give specific examples as to how this pertains to men. What are the costs associated with this?

5. What are some strategies to advance how males view death?

6. Do you think that if men changed how they viewed death that they would increase their overall life span compared to that of women? Justify your comments.

7. In general, how does death teach us about the human condition and experience? That is, what can be learned through the inevitability of death?

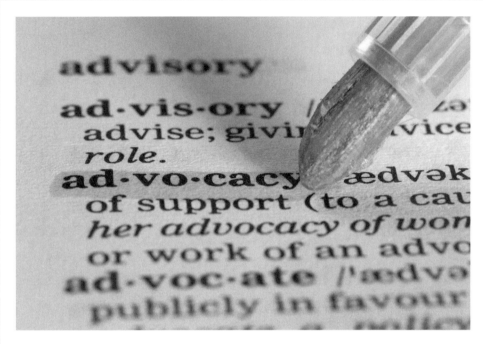

13

Promoting Male Health

LEARNING OBJECTIVES

- Identify common advocacy topics pertaining to male health, including challenges facing a male health agenda in the United States

- Identify and access advocacy groups and organizations focused on male health

- Define *misandry* and recognize other forms of social injustice directed toward males

- Apply strategies by which to close gaps in health disparities in males, particularly in racial, ethnic, and other minority groups

WITH GOOD REASON, men should be concerned for their health, but not to the point of despair or inaction. Many men may simply accept their fates because other male family members got diseases or died early in life. It is the role of the public health professional and educator to help males realize that their health future is malleable and that they can self-determine their outcomes by advocating for themselves.

Many of the health concerns that males face are alterable; however, these health consequences will not change unless there is a fundamental paradigm shift in the way we in the United States approach male health. For example, addressing the issue of men and violence that leads to incarceration is great, but approaches are usually one-dimensional. This problem is multifaceted and therefore needs multifaceted solutions. Many men, particularly those of color, may be arrested and incarcerated for drug offenses rather than for violent crimes. This in turn takes a man out of the community and his family, possibly increasing disparities based on social determinants of health (Xanthos, 2008).

The simple fact of being male often carries with it social stereotypes that lead to specific health consequences. An example is the way boys are influenced in the current public educational system. Schools attempt to control for behavior issues, such as attention deficit hyperactivity disorder (ADHD); the behavior may not be ADHD but simply a boy being a boy (Parkin, 2007). These early judgments can set the course and tone for a boy's lifetime (Xanthos, 2008). Medicine has made tremendous advances in health care, but social health care and medicine seems to be lagging behind for 50% of the **populace**.

This chapter highlights the major efforts and advances in male health during recent decades and presents future challenges and opportunities in advocacy, academic disciplines and research, social movements, health care, social justice, and racial disparities. The study of male health and the social forces that contribute to it are brought into focus for future academic and social endeavors. Future trends and opportunities to become involved at many levels are presented and discussed.

ADVOCACY AND RESEARCH

Understanding the human condition and advancing quality of life is the major goal of most forms of health research. Research provides scholars with the evidence that something is improving, getting worse, or staying the same; it generates answers to hypotheses and it also formulates new questions and areas of thought for future inquiry. When health educators and public health professionals have a full understanding of what the data say, effective solutions and proposals to eliminate health issues and disparities are made possible. Although research is performed mostly by people trained in specific disciplines (health, public health, psychology, behavioral sociology, and such), advocacy is possible by almost anyone with the passion to pursue a cause. *Advocacy* is a process aimed at changing or encouraging progress in a personal or social condition through affecting rules, laws, and public policy. Influencing the decision-making process is the ultimate goal of advocacy, which comes in many forms, such as campaigning, lobbying, media, public speaking, debate, and disseminating research to other groups to advance change (Jernigan & Wright, 1996). Research drives advocacy, as advocacy drives research in this reciprocal relationship.

Males in general tend to express reluctance to seek help when they are ill, or they feel less at risk than other groups. Men tend to delay medical care by a few days when they are ill, in pain, or are otherwise concerned about their health, according to a recent study (American Academy of Family Physicians, 2008) in *Vitality*. In this study, 92% of the more than 1,000 men surveyed confirmed that they wait a few days to seek medical advice, and more than 55% had not been to the doctor for a physical examination in the past year. Similarly, 80% rated their health as "excellent" or "good," when in fact 42% claimed they had one or more chronic illnesses (Drummond, 2008). The latter point suggests that men may overestimate their relative health and clearly delay care of potentially serious medical issues.

Many of these factors have been engrained in the psyches of males since birth, but the tide is changing. Overall health movements have encouraged males to value their health more, realizing that in doing so, not only years of life will be extended but also the quality of those years.

The Real Men Wear Gowns campaign was an effort put forth in 2008 by the Agency for Health Care Research Quality (AHRQ). This major initiative targets older men and advises them to get preventative screenings due to their lower likelihood to regularly visit a doctor each year (Agency for

Health Care Research Quality [AHRQ], 2010). The Ad Council had a major role in the development of this awareness program. Critiques concerning this approach are that it is age specific, which is not entirely a negative thing, but it may inadvertently send a message to younger men and boys that they need only to become aware and proactive in their health matters when they are older (that is, 40+).

Men's Health Network

One of the more active organizations geared toward advancing male health is based out of Washington, D.C. The Men's Health Network (MHN), formed in 1992, organizes and participates in a wide array of activities at the national level to advance male health. Some examples of their work include screenings at conferences and conventions, education through websites and public service announcements, holding community and corporate health fairs, developing informational brochures, and planning events associated with National Men's Health Week, which corresponds with Father's Day each year in June. More details and information can be found on the organization website at www.menshealthnetwork.org/.

National Men's Health Week

Much of the national concern and exposure for men's health became evident in the United States and abroad in the early 1990s. In 1987, the popular magazine *Men's Health* helped to spark interest in this academic and political area of concern. So was born National Men's Health Week (NMHW).

This event was created in 1994 by Congress with the support of then-Senators Bob Dole and Bill Richardson. The purpose of this week is to heighten awareness of health issues affecting men and boys that often are preventable with screenings and better recognition. One of the major initiatives is encouraging men and boys to seek regular medical advice, follow-up care, and early treatment for issues affecting their health (MNH, 2003). Many organizations, including the Men's Health Network, coordinate and organize activities that attempt to influence males in venues where they are likely to have interest, such as sporting events, corporate arenas, fraternal and religious organizations, and nonprofit and governmental organizations. Advances in public health policy, law, media, and roles of health care providers are focal points of this annual event. Some notable participants in NMHW include Home Depot, HBO, Boston Children's Hospital, the U.S. Naval Clinic in San Diego, and Dow Chemical. These and similar initiatives follow suit and parallel many of the advocacy efforts of the National Women's Health Week, held a month earlier in May (American Alliance for Health, Physical Education, Recreation and Dance [AAHPERD], 2010).

These are tremendous efforts to encourage health among the male population; however, many have commented on the title of this event. *Men's* versus *male* sends a message that health becomes more of a focus when one is considered a man, often at the expense of understanding and advocating for the many health-related issues that affect younger males and boys. Screenings for disease processes are a step in the right direction, but there also needs to be a stronger emphasis on primary prevention efforts if public health is to make any significant long-term headway with males.

Office of Men's Health

There are currently seven federal offices dedicated to women's health, and still there remains a paucity of organizations dedicated to male health. There is some legislative advocacy concerning male health. Bills such as the 2003 Men's Health Act (S 1028 and HR 1734) and stronger funding efforts for prostate cancer screenings (through the National Institutes of Health, National Cancer Institute, and the Centers for Disease Control and Prevention), research, the development of state men's health commissions, and welfare reform, in addition to recent health care reform in the United States, have created a more positive atmosphere for advancing male health. However, bills to create an Office of Men's Health (OMH) have lagged behind since the introduction into Congress in 2003. Advocacy continues, led by Representatives Baron Hill and Tim Murphy, who introduced HR 2115 in April 2009 during the 111th U.S. congressional session. The newest bill aims to coordinate the fragmented men's health awareness, prevention, and research efforts by centralizing them into a common office. The office would be modeled after the Office of Women's Health. For more information on the advocacy and history of this bill and the development of this office, see www.menshealthpolicy.com/OMH/index.html.

Certainly legislative and advocacy efforts are a critical linchpin for guiding the success of male health movements. Without them, funding and other critical factors would not be possible; however, **grass-roots** efforts also need to be appreciated as well.

MALE STUDIES

A call for the study of the male condition and all determinants affecting social well-being and health, similar to women's studies, has been proposed. Male studies programs have been developed but are offered only in a few settings and academic institutions. Like most academic disciplines, male studies aims to advance cultural understanding of how and why things happen as they do. Male studies attempts to bridge the gap between males and females in many areas of concern, such as sociology, medicine, biology, economics, law, health care, psychology, education, and policy, among many others (personal communication, June 11, 2010). Understanding what makes males tick is the goal of these types of studies and the academic discipline as a whole.

Myth: Men's health programs are included in gender studies curricula.

Fact: More appropriately termed "male studies" programs in the United States are grossly under- or unrepresented in most gender studies programs in the United States, which often focus on female gender issues. Several programs, such as the Male Studies program at Wagner College in New York and Akamai University's Men's Studies and Fatherhood Program in Hawai'i are offered, considered, or in the development process.

The nature of male studies is inclusive of males of all ages and stages of life, whereas *men's studies* or *men's health* imply older ages. The value of understanding the male condition has many positive outcomes that will help to advance not just males, but society and culture in general. These types of studies may focus on the learning environment, behavioral issues, violence, talents, stereotypes, behaviorism, and literacy, all of which can help alleviate many of the cultural woes experienced by men and women, such as violence and extreme risk taking. With this new knowledge and understanding, disciplines such as health can then more effectively draft, devise, and implement strategies that work to lessen the morbidity and mortality burden of men.

VIGNETTE

"The truth lies somewhere in the middle," Todd exclaimed in response to a student's question concerning whether or not men are the weaker sex. The student was referring to a course reading from a *New York Times* article that asserted that, based on morbidity and mortality statistics, men were the weaker biological sex.

A few years earlier, Todd had been approached by his associate chairperson and was asked about his interest in teaching an experimental course on men's health. Todd had done his doctoral work in the area of adolescent male health, so he thought, "Why not?" In developing the course, Todd realized that there were only a few resources and courses offered in this area in the entire country. He searched several college and university course catalogs under "gender studies," only to find a heavy emphasis on females and women's studies electives. "What is going on here?," he thought to himself.

Todd continued his search for course concepts and materials to use in this new course. A few students stopped in to ask what he planned on doing in this new elective offering. The excitement and intrigue about this course encouraged Todd.

While pulling articles from numerous research-based journals, articles from popular magazines and Web forums, resources from national health websites and databases, Todd noticed a disturbing trend: most of the literature pointed to a male health crisis, but very little in terms of resources and study was dedicated to this area. Clearly, evidence based in national statistics and registries, such as the Centers for Disease Control and Prevention, Youth Risk Behavior Surveys, and other epidemiological datasets were not faulty in reporting that males were more likely to die sooner, be the victims of

(Continued)

violent death, perpetrate crimes, be incarcerated, die at higher rates for seven out of the top ten leading causes of death, less likely to receive health care, less likely to pursue preventative health care, have higher infant mortality rates, be more likely to end their lives via suicide, and even have weaker immune systems.

Todd knew he had quite a bit of work to do in preparing this course offering, but he was both encouraged and troubled by the resources and data he had come across. The tremendous opportunities to advance health for one-half of the world's nearly 7 billion people were evident.

Three years after introducing this experimental elective class, Todd was aware of more men's health course offerings, journals seemed to be devoting more topics to these issues, conferences were introducing male health, and the study of male health (andrology) was being developed. It seemed like health education, health promotion, and public health were recognizing and getting on board with the male health movement.

Todd concluded his class in which the student had asked about men as the "weaker sex" by stating, "Advocacy and further research is critical in this area of health if we are going to help males lead better lives and increase the quality of them." As he packed up his briefcase, he thought to himself, "We really have a lot of work to do in this area. So many people take these statistics for granted or don't even know about them. Males really could lead better lives that could enhance overall quality of life for everyone in the family, community, and social unit."

Promoting male health was going to be a challenge, but in every challenge exist fantastic and exciting opportunities. As he left the classroom, Todd thought, "Indeed, the truth is somewhere in the middle."

ANDROLOGY

Some health professionals and educators have called for a stronger medical specialty for males, known as *andrology* (Jack, 2005). Similar to gynecology, andrology is a field of study that deals with male health. Unlike gynecology, andrology has been a specialty only since the 1960s and is much less known (American Society of Andrology [ASA], 2010). Typically, andrology handles male health issues such as infertility, penile and testicular problems, cancers, urological disorders, and prostate gland dysfunction.

The American Society of Andrology (ASA) fosters a multidisciplinary approach to male reproduction and promotes scientific exchanges in this area (ASA, 2010).

Some researchers have called for an expansion of this specialty to become more inclusive of male medicine or gender-specific medicine (MHN, 2009). Focusing on male reproductive issues is useful, but only a limited sector of men may be exposed to these services. If andrology were expanded to include regular male health checkups; screenings; sexual history; health promotion efforts; sex-specific, age-appropriate patient education; and many other male health topics, overall male health might drastically improve. Males need to become familiar with the medical system more than they do at present. Research suggests that men are 25% less likely than women to see a doctor on a yearly basis and are even less likely to get three- and five-year follow-ups; expanding andrology may help improve this dismal statistic (AHRQ, 2010).

Routine testing and clinical evaluation can screen for diseases in their early stages and educate a patient so as to prevent disease and illness from occurring. This process of course would take time to implement, perhaps even a generation or so. The previous statement aligns well with the recent Healthiest Nation in One Generation plan advocated by the American Public Health Association (American Public Health Association [APHA], 2010). A younger boy would be introduced into a preventative health care system that puts him at ease with the changes in his body, particularly during puberty. A yearly follow-up could educate him concerning not only his sexual health but also allow for patient education to enhance psychosocial health as well. For many younger males, knowing that someone else has an interest in their health may enhance their beliefs about health for the positive and lead to better outcomes, including a lifelong investment in their own health. It may be time for andrology to become a more prominent medical specialty and be introduced into the male **vernacular** at earlier life stages.

MISANDRY AND SOCIAL JUSTICE

Misandry is the hatred or contempt for men and boys, similar to *misogyny* for women and girls. There are various levels of misandry, ranging from insults to movements and violence against males (Ferguson & Bloch, 1989). For example, calling a male a "mama's boy" may be considered a milder form of misandry, whereas extreme groups may try to harm males in various capacities, as advocated in the *S.C.U.M. Manifesto* (Solanas, 1967). Feminism is certainly not synonymous with misandry, but people and groups that attempt to harm or impede the rights of males would be considered misadrogenistic. In fact, all forms of bias do little to advance the health of people and society. Racism, ageism, sexism, and any other type of "ism" holds back human advancement in establishing social justice principles and quality of life for all.

Men's movements are similar to other social movements, such as women's rights and liberation, gay rights, father's rights movements, and many others. Equal treatment and social fairness has given rise to many men calling for reducing biases that are levied against them (Ferguson & Bloch, 1989; Ruxton, 2009). For example, many fathers lose custody rights when they get divorced, often losing contact with their children or feeling less involved because their spouse is favored by the judicial system. Some men are singled out as perpetrators of domestic violence and may be ignored in instances of female-based domestic violence against them (Ruxton, 2009). Some men will not report instances of domestic issues because of fear of being viewed as less masculine, further exacerbating the issue.

Male therapy groups and support groups have grown in number (Baraff, 1991) during recent years because men have identified the negative emotions and consequences that follow misandry and related concepts. Many of these movements and reactions of men parallel elements consistent with social justice. *Social justice* is what it sounds like: justice principles imparted to a social context for all people. Elements include equality, **human rights**, and the application of justice in several social instances (Ruxton, 2009).

Racial and Other Disparities and Health Outcomes

Disparities come in many forms, such as lack of insurance coverage, lack of a consistent source of care, lack of financial abilities and resources, legal and structural barriers, scarcity of providers, language barriers, poor **health literacy**, lack of diversity in the health care force, age, and lack of preventative emphases for health care (Davis, Kilburn, & Schultz, 2009). Health disparities need to be viewed as the disproportionate distribution of health and disease, access to health care, and health outcomes in various populations and communities.

Racial Disparities   Health and health-related outcomes are poorer for males of color than for other groups. ADHD may be more harmful in boys of color than in other races. Nearly 40% of black men prematurely die of heart disease (including stroke and hypertension). Men of color have higher rates of prostate cancer, diabetes, homicide, and HIV/AIDS infection (five times higher) than any other group. Average life expectancy for all males in the United States is approximately 75.2 years and 75.7 years in white males; however, the number dips to 69.8 years in black males. Moreover, black males have roughly a 1 in 30 chance of being victims of homicide, as compared to 1 in 179 for white males. Men of color are less likely to receive consistent health care, are more likely not to have health insurance coverage, and are more likely to have poorer overall health outcomes, particularly in certain areas of the United States, such as California (Davis et al., 2009; MHN, 2009).

Exact causes of these disparities are complex and warrant better research such as longitudinal, prospective investigations (Jack, 2005). For instance, socioeconomic status plays a significant role in health care and some health outcomes, but so too does place of residence, type of occupation (if any), age, past medical history, family medical history, cultural factors, and issues pertaining to health accessibility (Williams, 2003). Perhaps the strongest factors accounting for racial differences in health have nothing to do with race in and of itself but lie more within the social determinants of health. Receiving treatment and the ability to access health care is one of the strongest influences in terms of the health of a man (Tudiver & Talbot, 1999).

Blacks have some of the highest cancer rates; however, they feel less at risk for it (Braithwaite, Taylor, & Treadwell, 2009; Davis et al., 2009; MHN, 2009). Perceived risk determines whether or not a man follows up with a health care provider; therefore, among black men, lower perceived risk is likely to lead to more severe health outcomes (Braithwaite et al., 2009;

Tudiver & Talbot, 1999). A recent Health Information Trends Survey (HINTS) found that blacks were far less likely to follow up with cancer screenings due to low perceived risk. The authors note, "Believing that we could develop cancer in our lifetime can motivate us to undergo tests, such as colonoscopy or mammogram to detect cancer early." Knowing what predisposes this type of thinking in minorities can help plan better education and intervention efforts (Orom, Kiviniemi, Underwood, Ross, & Shavers, 2010).

Men of color may resist seeking health care due to an inherent distrust of it. Dating back to the 1930s and through the early 1970s, the Tuskegee Syphilis Study was a clinical research study geared toward treating and eradicating the sexually transmitted infection syphilis. The subjects were African Americans living in the Tuskegee, Alabama, area (Katz et al., 2006). While the intent of the research was **beneficent**, the population and procedures used were highly unethical. The research studied the natural course of the disease; in order to understand how to cure the disease and treat its symptoms, researchers treated some people successfully whereas others received no treatment at all. For more than forty years, stories of these unethical health practices have been passed from family to family and generation to generation, possibly explaining why some men of color have distrust for the medical community.

Sexual Orientation Disparities   Youth as well as adult males in the gay, bisexual, and transgendered (GBT) community are at risk for many health consequences, such as lack of access to health care; higher rates of depression, suicide, and substance abuse; and higher rates of HIV/AIDS infections as well as other STIs (Hamilton & Mahalik, 2009). As can be seen through national and world statistics, youth and GBT males need more focused attention to help reduce these health disparities. Ignoring sexual orientation as a predictor of health is a direct threat to better standard of care for all people. Heterosexist medicine only will further cleave communication and advancement of health care for all males; therefore, patients and providers are strongly encourage to discuss this very important health topic as part of an overall holistic model of male health and wellness.

If we are to address and eventually reduce health disparities (as called for in *Healthy People 2010* and *2020*) (U.S. Department of Health and Human Services, 2010), evidence-based standards of care need to be enhanced. The delivery of this care needs to be culturally sensitive and exercise the best standard of care based on the most recent, reliable, and valid evidence to support the care provided. Culturally sensitive care does not mean that all people are treated equally; doing so probably would reduce quality of care. Adjusting sociocultural, competent care means to view each case as unique and as an opportunity to help the person and not just the illness, disability, or background from which they come. Males in general certainly need an overhaul of how they view their behaviors in relation to their health outcomes (Williams, 2003). Educating boys and men in how their unique culture and behaviors affect their health outcomes will be a major initiative and challenge for public health well into the next generation. The answers may lie in how well health educators and community practitioners engage men at the community level to help build stronger **coalitions** and develop appropriate interventions in the process (Brach & Fraser, 2000; Braithwaite et al., 2009).

THE FUTURE

There are tremendous opportunities in the area of male health and male studies. The goal is not simply to reduce death rates in men but to increase overall health-related quality of life as well. Males can take simple steps, such as exercising, to enhance their health. A recent study published in the journal *Circulation* noted that physically fit men were found to have a 70% lower death risk than men who were not physically active (Kokkinos et al., 2008).

Yet many men may simply not get the message. All too often, good data like those found in *Circulation* may simply be used only in future publications and research. Making data *real* for men is one of the primary concerns and obligations of public health. Data needs not only to inform researchers but to translate to practice and public policy.

Men now are considered an at-risk group in the United States and abroad (Jack, 2005). An active health care agenda will help to reduce disease burden, lessen the socioeconomic impact of morbidity and mortality, and assure that future generations receive the basic right of good health. The future holds the opportunity to change our way of thinking about males and male health. Realizing the complexity of the human experience and the social determinants of health are likely to be more productive than attacking diseases and disorders at the individual level (Glasgow, Litchenstein, & Marcus, 2003). In order to fully reach men and boys, public health needs to appreciate where they live, what they do, what they don't do, what they like, what they fear and why, and where they play.

Like marketing companies, health advocates need to know how to get males to buy into their health as they do any other product. Social marketing theory, which uses the systematic approach of marketing (advertising, population demographics, desires, wants, needs, and so on) to influence the adoption of positive health behaviors and goals for the overall good of society, is one way to accomplish this task (Lefebvre & Flora, 1988). Additionally, collaborative efforts within and among health care entities, such as the medical profession focusing on palliative care and health education and public health focusing on prevention, need to be accessed and strengthened.

Health care expenditures in the United States in 2009 were nearly 18% of the U.S. gross domestic product, and projections are not very encouraging for the future (Kaiser Family Foundation, 2009). With health care costs spiraling out of control, any steps that can be taken to alleviate the burden of disease in at-risk populations seems to be a salient idea and approach. Now is a good time to begin this process to embrace the multidimensional aspects of sex and gender and their influences on health (Jack, 2005).

Male health has been a topic of concern for many years. The health issues are there, but for some reason, many social institutions have ignored it, making male health "invisible" (Treadwell & Ro, 2003). One needs only to look at national and worldwide statistics to infer the disparate trends in male health. Health is not just a right of wealthy males, but of all human beings. Poor health outcomes, poverty, hazardous occupational health conditions, higher rates of incarceration, and many other social determinants make putting male health a top priority on the national health care agenda.

Figure 13.1 Male Health as a Community Priority

©iStockphoto.com/Alex Slobodkin

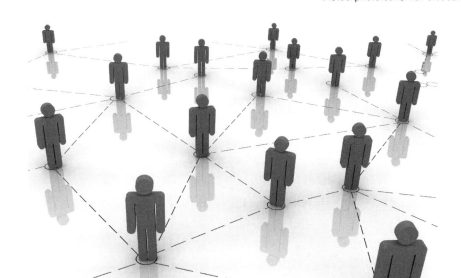

Sustaining this form of social change is highly complex, but it is possible. The future is rife with opportunity to make male health a high priority. Forming coalitions and partnerships for male health will allow stronger advocacy efforts in the future by advancing one strong voice versus several fragmented comments. Treadwell and Ro (2003) nicely attended to advocacy in their statement, "Leave no poor father, brother, uncle, nephew, or son behind, as they too have a right to the tree of life" (p. 707).

SUMMARY

This chapter presented key concepts as they relate to research and advocacy in male health. Organizations and advocacy efforts, such as the Men's Health Network and National Men's Health Week, are actively engaging at advancing the male health agenda. The development of an Office of Men's Health was discussed. Exciting new academic disciplines such male studies and a male subspecialty in medicine known as andrology were reviewed. The advancement of a social paradigm shift toward healthier alternatives is warranted. Social justice concepts and social action that will allow public health to close the gaps in racial and other male health disparities were outlined. The future is bright, but there is much to be done on all fronts. The major factor is being involved and *staying* involved!

KEY TERMS

Beneficent	Health literacy	Populace
Coalition	Human rights	Vernacular
Grass-roots		

DISCUSSION QUESTIONS

1. Several physicians have stated that males are not less likely to go to the doctor than females, but that females have more reasons to see a doctor more frequently. Take a stance on this assertion, and justify your comments with evidenced-based research.

2. What are some grass-roots efforts in your local community that advance male health? If there are none, what would you suggest?

3. Access an online listing of "men's health" or "male health" programs or courses. Describe what you find. Do you think these courses will advance male health? If so, describe in what manner.

4. Do you think male health programs in college and universities are competing with gender studies or women's studies programs? How are these types of programs likely to affect one another, if at all? Do you foresee programs working with each other versus in separate disciplines?

5. How does the concept of misandry threaten the future of male health and health initiatives?

6. How do racial and other social disparities negatively affect male health in the United States?

7. Briefly describe how ignoring or not prioritizing male health issues in the public and political agenda may affect the overall health of the nation. Identify present factual information and speculate on what the future may hold.

8. Do you think male health will be enhanced in the future, remain the same, or get worse? Justify your answer based on expected trends in this field of study. How can national public health initiatives, such as *Healthy People 2010* and *2020*, better advocate for the advancement of male health into the future?

GLOSSARY

Abstinence   The process of avoiding sexual intercourse and sexual contact; this method is advocated to prevent sexually transmitted infections (STIs) and unplanned pregnancies

Acceptance   A process of not only tolerating a person or something but also embracing him or it; by getting to know something or someone in terms of their experiences so that an empathic trust and bond can be developed

Acne   A skin disorder characterized by areas of blackheads, white heads, and reddened areas, also called *pimples* or "zits"; common in adolescence because of hormonal changes causing an increase in oil gland production and bacteria formation; acne can occur at any point in life

Addiction   A physical and psychological condition in which individuals become dependent on psychoactive substances, such as drugs, or other external sources, such as work, food, gambling, pornography; often characterized by a period of recovery or withdrawal symptoms

Adrenal Glands   A pair of endocrine system glands that sit atop each kidney and secrete hormones that moderate the stress response, particularly epinephrine (adrenaline); secretion of these hormones can cause a "rush" such as excitement or fear

Advocacy   Measures taken by individuals or groups to ensure that their rights or interests are appropriately and sufficiently represented

Ageism   A form of discrimination or bias based on age

Alexithymia   The inability to express emotions and feelings through words

Allergies   Reaction of the immune system to an external agent, such as a protein, chemical, dust, or pollen; often causes inflammation, redness, itching, and fatigue

Alienation   Feelings and emotions that one is alone, isolated, or otherwise not connected to a majority group

Alzheimer's disease   A common form of dementia that typically affects older people (the elderly); usually characterized in people over age sixty-five by cognitive impairments, difficulty remembering facts, numbers, or names and progressively worsening to the point at which a person cannot care for himself

Americans with Disabilities Act   An act of law passed in 1990 in the United States that assured equal rights to people with disabilities; the law changed the ways buildings are accessed and how policies are interpreted to advance the rights of people with various types of disabilities

Amniocentesis   A diagnostic medical procedure that attempts to identify any fetal abnormalities by removing a small sample of amniotic fluid from the amniotic sac in which a developing baby is encased; the fluid contains cells and other markers that can be used to identify genetic defects

Analgesia   The process of providing relief from pain

Anesthetics   Different type of medicinal preparations that alleviate pain or painful stimuli

Aneurysm   A rupture of a blood vessel (artery) in the body (typically in the brain or aorta of the heart) caused by a widening of the vessel; weakened areas burst, causing various negative health consequences including death

Angina   Pain or discomfort in the chest around the heart region, often confused with a heart attack; muscles of the chest become ischemic and painful due to a lack of oxygen; there are various types of angina

Anorexia nervosa   A psychiatric condition characterized by extreme restriction of food, a primary focus on low body weight, distortion of body image, dependence on exercise or other methods to reduce weight; often results in death if not treated accordingly; primarily affects females but also affects some men

Androgen   Hormones that produce masculinizing traits and characteristics such as muscle mass, strength, aggression, and body hair, among others

Anthropometric   Referring to measurement and measurable features of the body, such as height, weight, and limb circumferences

Antibiotics   A medication used to eliminate various types of bacterial infections; use is very common in modern medicine, which has led to some strains becoming resistant "super-bacteria"

Anxiety   An emotional and physiologic state marked by worry and fear as well as elevated heart rate, blood pressure, and sweating, among other symptoms

Assimilation   The act or process of becoming accustomed to or similar to another culture or group; for example, learning the language and art of a culture

Asthma   An inflammatory disorder of the airways (trachea, bronchi, and lungs) that results in difficulty breathing and ultimately can lead to death if not managed appropriately; caused by several factors including the environment, allergies, autoimmune dysfunction; often managed with anti-inflammatory medications

Autonomy   The feeling or ability to make one's own decisions; to self-direct one's experiences

Balanoposthitis   Inflammation of the glans of the penis and prepuce (foreskin) if the male is uncircumcised; the condition is more common in uncircumcised males

Bar mitzvah   A religious tradition in Judaic culture in which a preadolescent boy is called upon to "become a man" through various readings of scripture and acknowledging more responsibilities in life, usually at age thirteen

Beneficent   Characterized by performing acts of charity or kindness; having good intentions for one's actions

Benign   Harmless or not very serious

Binary   Referring to two processes

Biofeedback   A process of becoming aware of one's physical and emotion status and functions by using various different types of techniques and instruments that measure these reaction; for example, heart rate, blood pressure, and body temperature can be used to note relaxation, fear, anxiety and many other bodily functions

Birth rate   The number of births occurring per 1,000 people; most birth rates are used to track live births and can be used as an estimate of population demographics

Body language   Also known as *paralanguage;* the manner in which a person expresses himself in a nonverbal manner

Bris (B'rit) Milah   The traditional practice of circumcision on the eighth day after birth in Jewish males, performed as a religious rite or covenant; the procedure is usually performed by a Rabbi or *mohel*

Bulimia nervosa   A psychiatric condition characterized by extreme spectrums of eating, which focus on ridding the body of consumed food; people often binge, consuming as many as 10,000 calories at a time, followed by purging through vomiting, laxatives, excessive exercise, or similar methods; the disorder mainly focuses on control

Calories   A metric unit in food that indicates how much energy the food yields; especially important when considering weight gain or loss; for example, 3,500 calories equal 1 pound of body weight

Castration   The removal or destruction of one or both testes in males; often used as a punishment in criminals and offenders; however, some males, such as religious figures, were castrated to eliminate sexual desire and urges; the use of chemicals (also known as *chemical castration*) has been used in sex offenders and prison populations

Cataracts   Clouding of the crystalline lens of the eye resulting in reduced vision; progressively may result in total blindness

Chromosomes   Organized structures consisting of proteins and genetic material (DNA) that gives people particular characteristics and traits (such as hair color, height, sex)

Chronic traumatic encephalopathy (CTE)   Evidence of damage to portions of the brain from acute and chronic trauma such as concussions; in response to the trauma, the brain forms scars and abnormal tissue characterized by the presence of *Tau* proteins seen under a microscope

Circumcision   The surgical excision of the tissues covering the glans of the penis; usually performed during infancy; often linked with religious, sociocultural, and medical practices

Coalition   An alliance of groups or individuals for a common cause; groups often join together to have a stronger, more unified voice on a topic

Cognition   The ability to think and use mental functions

Cognitive behavioral therapy (CBT)   A very common form of psychotherapy that bases treatment on the assertion that thoughts create feelings and experiences, not simply the experiences themselves or external objects (such as spiders); therapy focuses on attending to the irrationality of thoughts, usually in the presence of the object or experience that provokes fear and anxiety, which gradually will lessen until it is no longer an issue

Communicable diseases   Diseases that are fairly easily transmitted person to person, such as the common cold or blood-borne diseases such as hepatitis

Concussion   A jarring or shaking force to the brain and its constituents causing damage to delicate blood vessels; characterized by confusion, headache, visual and auditory disturbances, and balance issues, among others

Confound To cause something to become confused or unclear; interfering with something else

Congenital Of or referring to a defect or anomaly that develops in a person as a fetus; occurring prior to birth; a person is born with a defect or pathological trait

Coping mechanism A psychological strategy used by people to overcome, hide, or otherwise deal with some type of physical or emotional stress; for example, using alcohol or other drugs

Cortisol A steroid hormone (glucocorticoid) that is released into the body during periods of stress by the adrenal gland of the endocrine system; the mechanisms of action include elevating blood pressure, heart rate; and serves to break down tissues and structures (catabolic action); often cortisol is not associated with optimal health

Culturalia Of or referring to popular culture in a society

Cultural competence The ability to effectively interact with people of different cultures or groups

Defecation The process of eliminating solid waste from the body

Dementia Serious loss of cognitive abilities and a progressive advancement of physical inability, mainly as people age; common in geriatric populations

Dental dam A sheath of material usually made of latex or polyurethane that is used as a barrier method during oral sex

Dependence A strong need for something (physically or psychologically), such as drugs, when a tolerance has been established; therefore, when the substance or experience is removed a person may experience withdrawal symptoms

Dermatologist A physician who specializes in care and treatment of various disorders of the skin

Digital Of or referring to the fingers; using one's fingers

Disparity   An inequity between one person or group and another

Down's syndrome   A genetic mutation on chromosome 21 (also known as *trisomy 21*) that causes varying levels of mental impairment as well as diverse physical features (wider-set eyes, prominent brow ridge, shorter stature, and so on); incidence is roughly 1 in 800–1,000 live births and usually occurs in children with older mothers (that is forty-plus years old)

Dyslexia   A learning disability common in males that affects the ability to read; words become difficult to see, which affects the ability to comprehend meaning as well as verbal capabilities

Eczema   A chronic skin condition characterized by rashes, itching, and scaly patches on the skin; many factors can cause the condition (genetics, chemicals, and other); it is generally accepted as an immune reaction in the body

Elective surgery   A surgical procedure usually not deemed necessary for survival or health but often performed to enhance one's sense of physical or emotional health and wellness; for example, a face lift or liposuction

Emotional intelligence   The ability, capacity, and skills needed to appropriately process one's own emotions and perceptions of other people's emotions

Emotions   Psychophysiological reactions to various life experiences; help to process experiences as good, bad, healthy, unhealthy, or dangerous, examples include anger, fear, happiness, and sadness

Empathy   The ability to share in other people's feelings and experiences

Empirical   A basic concept in science that uses observation, evidence, and other scientific means to advance the study of a topic and answer research questions and/or hypotheses

Enamel   The hard outer covering of teeth that serves to protect the sensitive underlying structures (dentin, nerve roots, and blood vessels); breach in the integrity of this substance is usually a result from dental caries (cavities)

Enculturation A process where a person becomes familiar with the roles and common practices of a given social group or organization

Encopresis The voluntary or involuntary passage of stool in children who are potty trained (usually over age four) causing a soiling of clothes and bedding; there may be several causes, such as physical illness or emotional distress

Endocrinologist A physician who specializes in disorders of the endocrine system; mainly focuses on issues with hormonal dysfunction and metabolic disorders such as diabetes

Enuresis Involuntary urination usually at night while asleep in the bed; also known as *bedwetting*

Epidemic When number of cases of disease increase beyond that which was expected; deviates beyond the norm for a given condition or circumstance

Epidemiology The systematic study of rates and other statistics as they pertain to tracking indicators of health in populations

Epistemological A branch of philosophy concerned with the nature and scope of knowledge, such as questioning what people know, how they come to know something, and what it actually means to know something

Erection A physiological reaction in males whereby the penis engorges with blood causing it to elongate, increase in girth, and overall become stiffer; prepares the penis for sexual activity; often caused by manual or psychological stimulation as well as the hormone testosterone

Etiology The cause of something; the source

Excise Removal of something; usually surgically such as skin or tissue

Extrapolate Taking data or findings from a smaller sample of research and applying them to the greater population

Fiber The indigestible portion of plant foods included in many products; there are two forms, soluble and insoluble; soluble helps regulate cholesterol and blood profiles, whereas insoluble provides roughage that aids in digestion and movement of solid waste products out of the body

Fibroblasts   Cells that form the structure of biological tissues

Flaccid   Referring to a non-erect penis; limp

Fratricide   Murder of one's own brother

Fluoride   A chemical derivative of fluorine that helps to enhance the strength of teeth by bonding to the outer surfaces of the enamel; commonly added to drinking water supplies and offered as a dental treatment in young children in order to prevent cavities

Gender   Sociocultural determinants of how a person expresses his or her sex, such as through masculine or feminine traits

Gender studies   A sector of academic studies that focuses on sociobiological influences one how people come to define their experiences based on their sex

Genetic counseling   A process of advising expectant parents or those planning on conceiving on their reproductive options; often used in couples who have a higher risk for abnormal pregnancies

Geriatric   A descriptive term used to characterize older people; the elderly

Glaucoma   A disease of the eye resulting in damage to the optic nerve affecting vision; usually associated with factors that increase pressure in the eye, such as hypertension

Gout   An inflammatory medical condition characterized by red, swollen, and inflamed joints; caused by a buildup of uric acid that crystallizes in joints, tendons, and tissues; gout can be exacerbated by food choices and alcohol consumption

Grass-roots   Referring to a nontraditional movement or effort addressing a particular topic that often arises less out of standard thought and more original thinking and initiatives

Grieve   The process of coming to terms with a loss such as death

Gross domestic product (GDP)   The measure of an economy in a particular locality, such as a country; the total market value of all goods and services provided by a nation in one year

Harm reduction   Public health policies aimed at reducing the harmful effects of a product (such as illegal drugs) by influencing the availability and penalties of the product; for example, therefore, use of a certain drug is decriminalized or safer alternatives of use are promoted, such as free needle exchange for IV drug users so as to decrease hepatitis, HIV, and other blood-borne pathogens and diseases

Hate crimes   Crimes motivated by the extreme dislike or hatred of a person or group of people based on culture, religious beliefs, sexual orientation, race, or any other classification

Health   The general condition of a person based on a balance of many areas, such as physical, emotional, spiritual, intellectual, environmental, financial, and others; not simply the absent of disease or illness

Health disparity   Any factor, variable, or condition that causes some people to experience good health status when others do not; for example, socioeconomic status often underpins health disparities

Health literacy   The ability of individuals to be able to locate, understand, and act on basic health and health-related information so as to better individual or community health

Health promotion   Helping people take charge of their health by enabling knowledge, attitudes, and skills to improve determinants of health

Health-related quality of life (HRQoL)   A person's or group's perceived mental, physical, and social health status over a period of time; one of the primary goals of public health is to enhance HRQoL

Health risk assessment (HRA)   Forms such as questionnaires or surveys used as tools to formulate a profile concerning a person's relative health status; results of the assessment can be used to make positive health changes

Hernia   Protrusion of an organ or connective tissue (fascia) of an organ through a wall in the body; generally occurs in the abdominal and groin region; the weakened area usually needs to be surgically repaired to avoid further tissue disruption; examples include inguinal (groin) and umbilical (belly button) hernias

Heteronormative   A social perspective that assumes heterosexual orientation is the norm and is to be expected by assuming people will fall into traditional classifications of gender and sex roles

Hippocratic Oath   An oath taken by doctors and those who practice medicine; the premise of the oath is to practice in an ethically responsible manner while proclaiming to "do no harm"

Homeostasis   A state of the body being in balance

Homicide   Murder of another person

Hormones   Chemicals release by some cells in the body to affect other target cells; hormones such as testosterone and estrogen help certain body functions to occur

Human chorionic gonadotropin (HCG)   A hormone produced during pregnancy by the developing embryo that helps protect the developing baby; affects the influence of hormonal tolerance during pregnancy; also can be used as a marker to identify developing tumors

Human rights   Basic freedoms and rights as afforded to all human beings regardless of any other criteria; for example, the right to pursue happiness and to be free of harm

Hygiene   A set of practices aimed at enhancing one's health, such as bathing, oral health, and any other activities geared at maintaining good overall health

Hypermasculine   Over-representing one's masculinity; often viewed as a compensatory mechanism to hide a defect or flaw

Hypovolemic shock   The body's response to a severe reduction in overall fluid content such as blood volume; a person with this condition is in danger of multiple organ failure and possibly death if not treated immediately

Iatrogenic   Of or related to, disease, illness, or dysfunction caused by medicine versus another pathology

Ideology   A set of ideas; a way of thinking

Illicit drugs   Also referred to as *hard drugs* or *street drugs* that are considered illegal in most municipalities and carry with them fines and possible imprisonment; examples include heroin, cocaine, methamphetamine, marijuana

Immunizations   The process of helping to fortify one's own immune system from various biological agents and processes; various chemicals and proteins from known illnesses and diseases can be introduced into the system so as to cause the body's natural immune response to identify and develop immunity from the agent but not enough to make a person sick; usually given during younger childhood

Impotence   Also referred to as *erectile dysfunction;* lacking the ability to maintain a consistent erection due to physical factors, psychological factors, or both

Incarceration   The process of serving time in prison, usually as a form of punishment for a crime

Incidence   An epidemiologic term used to describe the risk of developing or experiencing a condition (illness, injury, disease) over a period of time

Industrialized nations   Countries that have advanced or well-developed socioeconomic infrastructures; often viewed as having more materialistic power and capital; usually countries of the Western world

Infant mortality   The death of a baby within the first year of life

Insulin   A hormone produced and secreted by the pancreas that helps to regulate energy and glucose metabolism; failure to produce this hormone is referred to as type I diabetes mellitus

Intact   Of or referring to an uncircumcised penis

Intentional and unintentional injuries   Causes of injury (bodily harm) from accidents (unintentional) or violence or aggression (intentional);

for example, drowning would be considered an unintentional accident whereas shooting someone would be an intentional injury

Interdependence   Being mutually and physically responsible to others; sharing a common set of values and principles

In utero   A Latin term used to describe the condition of being in the uterus as an embryo or fetus

Ischemic   Pertaining to tissues lacking oxygen; often provoking pain

Lactose   A natural sugar found in milk and milk products, such as cheese; many people lack the enzyme to break down this sugar, which is referred to as *lactose intolerance*

Laparoscopic   A form of minimally invasive surgery that uses a laparoscope to enter tissues, visualize the site, and perform surgery to correct a problem

Learning style   The way a person best intakes, interprets, and utilizes information; for example, some people learn best by listening (auditory), whereas others depend more on experiencing something (experiential or kinesthetic)

Lethargy   Feelings of tiredness or fatigue

Life span   The entirety of a person's existence from birth until death

Life expectancy   The number of years a person can expect to live based on average ages within various strata of the population

Longitudinal research   Methods of research that are carried out over a defined period of time to note trends and developing patterns; this type of research can span from the present into the future (prospective) or examine data from the present into the past (retrospective); one of the main strengths of this method is that it identifies variables that occur as a result of time rather than during a single instance

Lumpectomy   A surgical term that generally refers to surgery pertaining to breast cancer in which a portion of tissue, tumor, or general mass is remove while sparing the breast

Macronutrients   Referring to the primary constituents for good nutritional health and components the body uses to build and restore itself; including carbohydrates, proteins, and fats along with supportive elements, such as vitamins, minerals, and water

Morbid obesity   A term used to describe people who are 100 pounds (or more) heavier than their ideal body weight; also, a body mass index level of >35 is considered morbidly obese, placing a person at great risk for premature death because of physical complications

Maladies   Factors that cause illness, disease, or otherwise negative effects on a person's health status

Male   A descriptive term used to imply a person is biologically a male (he has an XY chromosome pattern); the term is descriptive of all males rather than specific age categories

Male health   Health viewed from a gender-specific, male perspective, such as how various diseases and patterns, for example, prostate cancer, affect males

Malignant   The tendency of tissues, such as tumors, to become out of control and eventually cancerous

Masculinity   Qualities associated with being male; a gender term usually used to describe being a man

Masculine   Of or pertaining to anything related to male; qualities typically associated with being male that are culture bound; for example, strength is a common masculine quality

Mastectomy   Surgery pertaining to breast cancer where part or all of the breast is removed

Masturbation   The process of sexually pleasing oneself, usually by stimulating one's genitals

Melatonin   A hormone secreted by the pineal gland in humans that helps to regulate sleep patterns

Men   A more specific term used to describe biological males; however, the term is more appropriately used to describe biologically mature males (that is, post adolescents)

Metastatis   The process of cancer cells actively spreading to other parts of the body

Miscarriage   The process of a woman losing an embryo or fetus during the development process in the womb

Morbidity   Factors associated with the cause of illness, injury, and disease

Mortality   Factors associated with a cause of death

Myelin   A material that insulates and lines the outside of neurons of the central nervous system; primarily composed of outgrowths of glial cells and material derived from fats

Nebulous   Referring to something being unclear; not well understood

Neonatal   Of or referring to a newborn baby, usually in the first month of life

Nicotine   An alkaloid substance found in plants such as tobacco; the substance is a psychoactive drug that stimulates the brain; it is highly addictive

Normotensive   Referring to normal ranges in terms of blood pressure

Obesity   Body weight (mass) that is in the excess range of that considered healthy for an individual

Observational studies   Research studies that attempt to draws conclusions based on how subjects react or respond to interventions and treatments that are outside the direct control of the researcher; "seeing what happens"

Occlusion   Referring to a blockage, as with an artery

Osteoarthritis   A form of chronic inflammation of bone and related tissues that mainly affects joints in the body; often related to past injury, trauma, and the effects of aging; also very common in people who are overweight and obese due to the added stress on the joints; characterized by pain and swelling

Outing   Revealing that another person or oneself is homosexual or part of the LGBTQI (lesbian, gay, bisexual, transsexual, queer/questioning, and intersex) community

Palliative Medical care or treatment that aims to reduce disease and illness in severity

Pandemic An epidemic disease infection of large populations that spreads across the world; for example, some forms of the influenza virus (H1N1) have become pandemic infections

Pap test Short for the *Papanicolau test,* which attempts to establish the presence of abnormal cells such as cancers by scraping cells from a suspected site and analyzing them under a microscope; in women, this is routinely performed as part of a gynecological visit and examines cervical cells; however, pap tests also can be done using anal or rectal tissues in both sexes to assess forms of anal or rectal cancer

Paradigm A way of thinking

Paradox A true statement or group of statements that leads to the contradiction of a situation; defies intuition

Paternalism An attitude or ideology that refers to a hierarchy governed by male dominance

Patriarchy A sociocultural system of beliefs that culture or society is headed by males; the concept is very popular in traditional cultures and societies

Pediatrician A physician who specializes in care and treatment of infants, babies, young children, and in some cases, younger adults

Pigment Substances in humans that give color (or lack of) to various biological tissues such as the eyes and skin; pigment functions to absorb and reflect light

Plaques A buildup of products such as proteins, fats such as cholesterol in the body; can lead to blockages or impair physical and psychological functioning

Populace A group of people that comprise a population of a specific place, location, or locality

Postindustrial Referring to a nation's process and progress away from a manufacturing-based economy and more toward one based on information, innovation, commerce, and other high technology

Postmortem   After death

Potty training   A training process usually initiated during early childhood or toddler years that assists a child in gaining control over his or her bowel and bladder functions

Precocious   Occurring earlier or sooner than expected

Prepuce (foreskin)   Tissue that covers or surrounds the glans of the penis; helps to lubricate and protect the sensitive glans; comprised of various layers, including a mucosa; sometimes surgically removed during circumcision

Prevalence   The quantity or amount of a disease, illness, or injury in a population over a period of time

Preventative health care   Measures taken to decrease instances of disease or illness; for example, proper nutrition or routinely going to the dentist

Primary prevention   The highest level of preventing disease and illness; focuses on avoiding disease and illness from developing; for example, using good nutrition to prevent heart disease and some cancers

Proliferate   To become more; increase the presence of something

Psychosomatic   Referring to how the mind affects the body

Public health   A combination of art and science in fostering the health and well-being of a community of people through various initiatives and levels of prevention

Resiliency   An attribute of character whereby a person is able to offset negativity, insults, and otherwise overcome challenges; the process of being resilient

Resilient   The characteristic or property of being able to resist or restore oneself from physical or emotional insult

Retardation   A process of being slowed down, often used to describe people who have psychological or emotion developmental issues; condition of being mentally challenged

Retrospective   The process of looking back at something; something that happened in the past

Satiety   A feeling of completeness or fullness; refers to the consumption of a meal

Schemas   A psychological term used to describe mental structures that give meaning to some worldly experience; schemas help people make sense of what they experience based on prior experiences, context, and values

Self-confidence   Assuredness in one's abilities, judgments, and power in accomplishing various tasks or experiences

Self-efficacy   The belief in one's own abilities to accomplish something

Self-esteem   A person's overall self-appraisal of his or her value or worth; can be positive or negative

Self-perception   How a person processes his or her own abilities in life

Self-reliance   A feeling of confidence in a person's own abilities to take action; ability to rely on him- or herself

Semen   Fluids produced by males in the reproductive system that contribute to the ejaculate carrying a man's gametes (sperm); a number of glands secrete fluids to this mixture, including the Cowper's glands and prostate gland

Senility   Mental and physical deterioration associated with aging

Social action   The decisions and choices, such as policies, made by individuals and the groups aimed at influencing a cause

Septicemia   A pathological condition whereby the body becomes inundated with bacteria or other pathogens; if left untreated, the condition can prove fatal

Sex linked   Usually used to describe genetic processes, when a trait or variable is passed on via the male or female (or both) genetic material (chromosomes)

Sex-role strain   Feeling stress because of one's sex due to social and personal expectations related to being a male or female

Sexual abuse   Also referred to as *molestation;* forcing sexual behaviors on another person without that person's approval or consent

Sexuality   The ways people experience sex and erotic stimuli as well as how they express themselves as sexual creatures

Sociobiological   Referring to factors that influence or contribute to a person's health from the person's biology (physical health) as well as external (social) influences, such as the environment

Somatic   Of or referring to the human body

Somatoform   A disease or condition of the body often characterized by pain and dysfunction that has its true origins in the mind and psychological processes of the individual

Spectrum disorders   A variety of diseases and illnesses (usually psychological) that range from mild to severe; examples include autism and Asperger's syndrome; some people are profoundly affected by the disorder, whereas others are high functioning and barely diagnosable

Standard of care   The defined or expected level of health care and measures that are generally accepted by the majority of medical and health professionals in a society; this is usually guided by evidence-based research and methods

Stenosis   A condition pertaining to the narrowing of something, such as an artery or vertebral canal

Stereotypes   Commonly held opinions or beliefs about a person, group of people, or organization based on assumptions rather than facts; often used to demean the person, group, or organization

Stillborn   A full-term baby that is born dead

Stoicism   Approach or philosophy of a person who is removed from his or her emotions or expressions

Stress   A psychobiological consequence of interactions with oneself and the environment; stress does not have to be bad, but it provokes mental and physical changes such as increased heart rate, blood pressure, and sweating

Sudden infant death syndrome (SIDS)   A condition whereby infants suddenly die (usually in a crib or while sleeping); cause was unknown for many years, but recent research suggests a genetic component as well as baby positioning while sleeping

Supplements   Products used to aid in the normal dietary regimen of people; various vitamins, minerals, and substances can be used to augment a person's health profile; example is vitamin C and immunological system functioning

Sutures   "Stitches"; material (often thread) used to close a wound or surgical site

Tantrums   Emotional outbursts often characterized by intense emotions and actions such as yelling, screaming, physical violence, crying, defiance, and otherwise unacceptable types of behaviors; commonly in younger children

Toddler   A young child between the stages of infancy and childhood; usually ages one to four years old; hallmarks include potty training, walking, and speaking and language use

Tolerance   An attitude of allowing something to be or occur; for example, tolerating a person's beliefs does not necessarily mean accept them; physically, when the body builds up familiarity to a substance to achieve an effect or response

Traumatic brain injury (TBI)   Damage to the brain and its related structures when an external force causes jarring to these tissues; also known as an *intracranial injury;* generally results from accidents or injuries such as concussions

Truancy   The intentional unauthorized absence from school

Tunica albuginea   The fibrous, white covering of the testes and corpora cavernosa of the penis in males

Urinalysis   A diagnostic procedure that uses urine to determine the presence of drugs, bacteria, blood, and other substances and diseases

Uropathic   A disease or something of harm to the urogenital system

Ultrasonography   A medical imaging technique that uses sound waves to create an image of internal structures of the body; commonly used to view a baby in the womb

Upper respiratory tract   Part of the respiratory system consisting of the nasal passages, sinuses, oral cavity, trachea, and right and left bronchi that lead to the lungs; often implicated in infections such as bronchitis

Urethra   An anatomical tubelike structure that helps guide urine from the bladder (and semen in males) to the outside of the body; in males, the urethra terminates on the distal end of the penis

Vaccinations   Immunizations used to prevent certain diseases and illness

Vector   A living organism that carries and transmits disease; for example, humans can be a vector for tuberculosis, and mosquitoes are a vector for malaria

Vernacular   The common language and terminology of a defined group or culture

Victorian Era   A period of time commemorating the rule of Queen Victoria of England from 1837 until 1901; several architectural styles, fashions, and social movements are described by this term; the period is strongly characterized by modesty, temperance, and culture

Visceral   Referring to the internal organs of the body such as the heart, lungs, digestive organs, and others

Wellness   A unified process of balanced health that can lead to feelings of comfort and ease of the mind and body

Wisdom   A deeper understand of people, relationships, and life events based on cumulative life experiences; allows people to make better decisions and choices; often associated with advanced age

REFERENCES

Acierno, R., Hernandez, M. A., Amstadter, A. B., Resnick, H. S., Steve, K., Muzzy, W., et al. (2010). Prevalence and correlates of emotional, physical, sexual, and financial abuse and potential neglect in the United States: the National Elder Mistreatment Study. *American Journal of Public Health*, *100*(2), 292–297.

Adams, N., Cox, T., & Dunstan, L. (2004). I am the hate that dare not speak its name: Dealing with homophobia in secondary schools. *Educational Psychology in Practice*, *20*, 259–269.

Addis, M. E., & Mahalik, J. R. (2003). Men, masculinity, and the contexts of help seeking. *American Psychology*, *58*, 5–14.

Adolescent Substance Abuse Knowledge Base. (2010). *Factors of teen drug use*. http://www.adolescent-substance-abuse.com/. Accessed 3/03/2010.

Agatston, A. (2003). *The South Beach diet*. New York: St. Martin's Griffin.

Agency for Health Care Research Quality. (2010). *Real men wear gowns*. http://www.ahrq.gov/healthymen/. Accessed 6/11/2010.

Allwood, P. B. (2004). "Hand washing among public restroom users at the Minnesota State Fair." Available at: http://www.health.state.mn.us/handhygiene/stats/fairstudy.pdf. Accessed 11/15/09.

American Academy of Family Physicians. (2008). Men tend to delay medical care and overestimate their health. *Vitality*, 3.

American Academy of Pediatrics. (1999). Circumcision policy statement. *Pediatrics*, *103*, 686–693.

American Academy of Pediatrics. (2009). *News highlights: Evidence of food allergies growing among children*. http://www.aap.org/advocacy/. Accessed 1/03/10.

American Academy of Pediatrics. (2009a). *Oral health*. http://www.aap.org/. Accessed 11/14/09.

American Academy of Pediatrics. (2009b). *Toddler health*. http://www.aap.org/. Accessed on 11/11/09.

American Academy of Pediatrics and American Academy of Family Physicians (2004). Clinical practice guidelines: Diagnosis and management of acute otitis media. *Pediatrics*, *113*, 1451–1465.

American Alliance for Health, Physical Education, Recreation and Dance. (2010, May/June). Summer port and health observances. *Update Plus*, 6.

American Cancer Society. (2010). *Breast cancer in men*. http://www.cancer.org/. Accessed 1/23/2010.

American Heart Association. (2010a). *Cigarette smoking statistics*. http://www.adolescent-substance-abuse.com/. Accessed 3/03/2010.

American Heart Association. (2010b). *Heart disease and stroke statistics*. http://americanheart.org/. Accessed 1/24/2010.

American Psychiatric Association. (2000). *Diagnostic and statistical manual of mental disorders* (4th ed., text rev.). Washington, DC: American Psychiatric Association, 898–901.

American Public Health Association. (2010). *Healthiest nation in one generation*. http://generationpublichealth.org/. Accessed 6/11/2010.

American Society for Aesthetic Plastic Surgery. (2010). *Rates of men having plastic surgery.* http://www.surgery.org/. Accessed 4/06/2010.

American Society of Andrology. (2010). http://www.andrologysociety.com/. Accessed 6/10/2010.

Anderson, A. E., Cohn, L., & Holbrook, T. (2000). *Making weight: Men's concerns with food, weight, shape and appearance.* Carlsbad, CA: Gurze Books.

Anderson, R. N., & DeTurk, P. B. (2002). United States life tables, 1999. *National Vital Statistics Report, 50,* 33.

Anikeeva, O., Braunack-Mayer, A., & Rogers, W. (2009). Requiring influenza vaccination for health care workers. *American Journal of Public Health, 99*(1), 24–29.

Araujo, A. B., Esche, G. R., Kupelian, V., O'Donnell, A. B., Travison, T. G., Williams, R. E., et al. (2007). Prevalence of symptomatic androgen deficiency in men. *Journal of Clinical Endocrinology Metabolism, 92,* 4241–4247.

Aveline, D. (2006). Did I have blinders on or what?": Retrospective sense making by parents of gay sons recalling their son's earlier years. *Journal of Family Issues, 27,* 777–802.

Bacon, C. G., Mittleman, M. A., Kawachi, I., Giovannucci, E., Glasser, D. B., & Rimm, E. B. (2003). Sexual function in men older than 50 years of age: Results from the Health Professionals Follow-up Study. *Annals of Internal Medicine, 139*(3), 161–168.

Badger Herald Staff. (2007). Masturbation key to health, functional sexual relationships. *The Badger Herald* (Madison, WI). http://badgerherald.com/. Accessed 2/24/2010.

Badinter, E. (1995). *XY: On masculine identity.* New York: Columbia University Press, 130.

Bailey, R. C., Moses, S., et al. (2007). Male circumcision for HIV prevention in young men in Kisumu, Kenya: A randomized controlled trial. *The Lancet, (369)*9562, 643–656.

Baker, R. L. (1979). Newborn male circumcision: Needless and dangerous. *Sexual Medicine Today, 3*(11), 35–36.

Banaszak-Holl, J., & Copen, C. (2002). Gender differences in social support in the nursing home setting. *Abstracts of the Academy of Health Services Research Health Policy Meeting, 19,* 4.

Bandura, A. (1977). *Social learning theory.* New York: General Learning Press.

Baraff, A. (1991). *Men Talk: How men really feel about women, sex, relationships, and themselves.* New York: Plume.

Barkley, R. A. (1997). Behavioral inhibition, sustained attention, and executive functions: Constructing a unifying theory of ADHD. *Psychological Bulletin, 121,* 65–94.

Barsky, A. J., Peekna, H. M., & Borus, J. F. (2001). Somatic symptom reporting in women and men. *Journal of General Internal Medicine, 16,* 266–275.

Baskin, M. L., Ard, J., Franklin, F., & Allison, D. B. (2005). Prevalence of obesity in the United States. *Obesity Reviews, 6*(1), 5–7.

Bayram, C., Fahridin, S., & Britt, H. (2009). Men and mental health. *Australian Family Physician, 38,* 91.

Bazelon, E. (2009, October 11). The tiny differences in the littlest brains. *The Washington Post.*

Beaver, K. M., DeLisi, M., Vaughn, M. G., & Barnes, J. C. (2010). Monoamine oxidase A genotype is associated with gang membership and weapon use. *Comprehensive Psychiatry, 51,* 130–134.

Becker, V. D., Kendrick, D. T., Neuberg, S. L., Blackwell, K. C., & Smith, D. M. (2007). The confounded nature of angry men and happy women. *Journal of Personality and Social Psychology, 92,* 179–190.

Bembo, S. A. (2004). Gynecomastia: Its features, and when and how to treat it. *Cleveland Clinic Journal of Medicine, 71,* 511–517.

Bertoia, C., & Drakich, J. (1993). The fathers' rights movement: contradictions in rhetoric and practice. *Journal of Family Issues, 14,* 592–615.

Bhasin, S. Cunningham, G. R., Hayes, F. J., Matsumoto, A. M., Snyder, P. J., Swerdloff, R. S., & Montori, V. M. (2006). Testosterone therapy in adult men with androgen deficiency syndromes: An endocrine society clinical practice guideline. *Journal of Clinical Endocrinology Metabolism, 91,* 1995–2010.

Bhasin, S., Storer, T. W., Berman, N., Callegari, C., Clevenger, B., Phillips, J., et al. (1996). The effects of supraphysiologic doses of testosterone on muscle size and strength in normal men. *New England Journal of Medicine, 335,* 1–7.

Bhasin, S., Woodhouse, L., & Storer, T. W. (2001). Proof of the effect of testosterone on skeletal muscle. *Journal of Endocrinology, 170,* 27–38.

Bicha, P. J., Mamood, E., Sorur, M., Ananthakrishnan, K., & Irwin, P. P. (2008). Public interest warning: Should we ban wooden/ornamental toilet seats for male infants. *British Journal of Urology International, 102,* 1749.

Biddulph, S. (2008). *Raising boys* (2nd ed.). Berkeley, CA: Celestial Arts.

Biggs, W. S., & Dery, W. H. (2006). Evaluation and treatment of constipation in infants and children. *American Family Physician, 73,* 469–477.

Blumenthal, J. A., Sherwood, A., Babyak, M. A., et al. (2005). Effects of exercise and stress management training on markers of cardiovascular risk in patients with ischemic heart disease. *Journal of the American Medical Association, 293,* 1626–1634.

Bojesen, A., Juul, S., & Gravholt, C. H. (2003). Prenatal and postnatal prevalence of Klinefelter syndrome: A national registry study. *Journal of Clinical Endocrinology and Metabolism, 88*(2), 622–626.

Bordo, S. (1999). *The male body: A look at men in public and in private.* New York: Farrar, Straus & Giroux.

Boulding, E. (2000). *Cultures of peace: The hidden side of history.* Syracuse, NY: Syracuse University Press, 124–127.

Bowman, M. C., Archin, N. M., & Margolis, D. M. (2009). Pharmaceutical approaches to eradication of persistent HIV infection. *Expert Reviews in Molecular Medicine, 11,* e6.

Boyle, G. J., Goldman, R., Svoboda, J. S., & Fernandez, E. (2002). Male circumcision: pain, trauma, and psychosexual sequelae. *Journal of Health Psychology, 7,* 329–343.

Brach, C., & Fraser, I. (2000). Can cultural competency reduce racial and ethnic health disparities? A review and conceptual model. *Medical Care Research and Review, 57,* 181–217.

Brakke, D. (1995). The problematization of nocturnal emissions in early Christian Syria, Egypt, and Gaul. *Journal of Early Christian Studies, 3*(4), 419–460.

Branum, A. M., & Lukacs, S. L. (2009). Food allergy among children in the United States. *Pediatrics, 124,* 1549–1555.

Braithwaite, R. L., Taylor, S. E., & Treadwell, H. M. (Eds.) (2009). *Health issues in the Black community* (3rd ed.). San Francisco: Jossey-Bass.

Braunstein, G. D. (1993). Gynecomastia. *New England Journal of Medicine, 328*(7), 490–495.

Brower, K. J. (2009). Anabolic steroid abuse and dependence in clinical practice. *The Physician and Sports Medicine, 37*(4), doi:10.3810/psm.2009.12.1751.

Brownhill, S., Wilhelm, K. A., Barclay, L., & Schmeid, V. (2005). "Big build": Hidden depression in men. *Australian and New Zealand Journal of Psychiatry, 39,* 921–931.

Brownlee, S. (2007). *Overtreated: Why Too Much Medicine is Making Us Sicker and Poorer.* London: Bloomsbury.

Brown-Trask, B., van Sell, S., Carter, S., & Kindred, C. (2009). Circumcision care. *RN, 72*(2), 22–29.

Brun, C. C., Nicolson, R., Lepore, N., Chou, Y., Vidal, C. N., DeVito, T. J., et al. (2009). Mapping brain abnormalities in boys with autism. *Human brain mapping* [Epub].

Bruno, J. J., Senderoff, D. M., Fracchia, J. A., & Armenakas, N. A. (2007). Reconstruction of penile wounds following complications of AlloDerm-based augmentation phalloplasty. *Plastic and Reconstructive Surgery, 119*(1), 1e–4e.

Buckley, W. A., Yesalis, C. E., Friedl, K. E., Anderson, W., Striet, A., & Wright, J. (1988). Estimated prevalence of anabolic steroid use among male high school seniors. *Journal of the American Medical Association, 260*, 3441–3445.

Buie, M. E. (2005). Circumcision: The good, the bad, and American values. *American Journal of Health Education, 36*, 102–108.

Bureau of Justice Statistics. (2010). http://bjs.ojp.usdoj.gov/. Accessed 2/23/2010.

Buss, D. M. (1994). *The evolution of desire: Strategies of human mating.* New York: Basic Books.

Byrd, R. S., Weitzman, M., Lanphear, N. E., & Auinger, P. (1996). Bed-wetting in U.S. children: Epidemiology and related behavior problems. *Pediatrics, 98*(3), 414–419.

Caldwell, C. H., Wright, J. C., Zimmerman, M. A., Walsemann, K. M., Williams, D., & Isichei, P.A.C. (2004). Enhancing adolescent health behaviors through strengthening non-resident father-son relationships: A model for intervention with African American families. *Health Education Research: Theory and Practice, 19*, 644–656.

Carretero, O. A., & Oparil, S. (2000). Essential hypertension. Part I: definition and etiology. *Circulation, 101*(3), 329–335.

Cash, T. F., & Pruzinsky, T. (Eds.) (2004). *Body image: A handbook of theory, research, and clinical practice.* New York: Guilford.

Cash, T. F., Winstead, B. A., & Janda, L. H. (1997, April). The great American shape-up. *Psychology Today*, 30–35.

Cassidy, S. (2004). Learning styles: an overview of theories, models, and measures. *Educational Psychology, 24,* 419–444.

Castle, P. E., & Scarinci, I. (2009). Should HPV vaccine be given to men? *British Medical Journal, 339*(7726), 872–873.

CBS News. (2010). Boy, 9, found hanged in Texas school. http://www.cbsnews.com/. Accessed 1/26/2010.

Centers for Disease Control and Prevention. (2000). *Growth charts for boys, 2 to 20 years.* http://www.chartsgraphsdiagrams.com/. Accessed 12/28/09.

Centers for Disease Control and Prevention. (2002). *National Vital Statistics Report, 50*(12), 11.

Centers for Disease Control and Prevention. (2005). *Web-based Injury Statistics Query and Reporting System* (WISQARS). National Center for Injury Prevention and Control, CDC (Producer). http://www.cdc.gov/ncipc/. Accessed 5/28/2010.

Centers for Disease Control and Prevention. (2006a). *Life expectancy in the United States.* http://www.cdc.gov/. Accessed 5/23/2010.

Centers for Disease Control and Prevention. (2006b). *Ten leading causes of death.* http://www.cdc.gov/. Accessed 1/17/2010.

Centers for Disease Control and Prevention. (2007). *Causes of non-fatal injuries treated in hospital emergency departments.* http://www.cdc.gov/. Accessed 1/17/2010.

Centers for Disease Control and Prevention. (2007, April). Youth Risk Behavior Surveillance System 2007. *Morbidity and Mortality Weekly Review.*

Centers for Disease Control and Prevention. (2008). *Health, United States, 2008.* http://www.cdc.gov/. Accessed 5/31/2010.

Centers for Disease Control and Prevention. (2009). *Recommended immunization schedule for persons aged 0 through 6 years—United States 2009.* http://www.cdc.gov/. Accessed 11/14/09.

Centers for Disease Control and Prevention, NCHHSTP. (2009). *HIV and AIDS among gay and bisexual men*. http://www.cdc.gov/NCHHSTP/. Accessed 2/04/2010.

Centers for Medicare and Medicaid Services (CMS) Office of the Actuary, National Health Statistics Group. (2010). *Projected data from NHE Projections 2008–2018*. http://www.cms.hhs.gov/. Accessed 5/31/2010.

Central Intelligence Agency [CIA]. (2010). *The world factbook*. https://www.cia.gov/. Accessed 1/19/2010.

Chandy, J. M., Blum, R. W., & Resnick, M. D. (1996). Gender-specific outcomes for sexually abused adolescents. *Child Abuse and Neglect, 20*, 1219–1231.

Chen, J., Gefen, A., Greenstein, A., Matzkin, H., & Elad, D. (2000). Predicting penile size during erection. *International Journal of Impotence Research, 12*(6), 328–333.

Chiarella, T. (2006). The problem with boys. *Esquire*. http://www.esquire.com/. Accessed 1/6/2010.

Chobanian, A. V., Bakris, G. L., Black, H. R., *et al.* (2003). Seventh report of the Joint National Committee on Prevention, Detection, Evaluation, and Treatment of High Blood Pressure. *Hypertension 42* (6), 1206–1252.

Chowdhury, A. N. (1998). One hundred years of Koro: The history of a culture-bound syndrome. *International Journal of Social Psychiatry, 44*(3), 181–188.

Chung, B. (2001). Muscle dysmorphia: A critical review of the proposed criteria. *Perspectives in Biology and Medicine, 44*, 565–574.

Cohane, G. H., & Pope, H. G. (2001). Body image in boys: A review of the literature. *International Journal of Eating Disorders, 29*(4), 373–379.

Cooke, D. W., & Plotnick, L. (2008). Type I diabetes mellitus in pediatrics. *Pediatrics Review, 29*(11), 374–384.

Cooper, Z., & Fairburn, C. G. (2003). Refining the definition of binge eating disorder and non-purging bulimia nervosa. *International Journal of Eating Disorders, 34,* S89–S95.

Cornish, K., Turk, J., & Levitas, A. (2007). Fragile X syndrome and autism: Common developmental pathways. *Current Pediatric Reviews, 3,* 3–4.

Cox, A. J. (2006). *Boys of few words: Raising our sons to communicate and connect.* New York: Guilford.

Circumcision Information Resource Pages. (n.d.). http://www.cirp.org/. Accessed 9/29/09.

Clarke, L., Cooksey, E. C., & Verropoulou, G. (1998). Fathers and absent fathers: Sociodemographic similarities in Britain and the United States. *Demography, 35,* 217–228.

Colapinto, J. (2001). *As nature made him: The boy who was raised as a girl.* New York: Harper Perennial.

College Board. (2010). *2009–2010 college prices.* http://www.collegeboard.com/. Accessed 2/21/2010.

Crooks, R., & Baur, K. (2005). *Our sexuality* (9th ed.). Pacific Grove, CA: Thompson Wadsworth.

Crosby, R. A., Benitez, J., & Young, A. (2008). Correlates of intent to be vaccinated against HPV: An exploratory study of rural and urban young males. *Health Educator, 25*(2), 18–20.

Cunningham, R. M., Walton, M. A., Roahen-Harrison, S., Resko, S. M., Stanley, R., Zimmerman, M., et al. (2009). Past-year intentional and unintentional injury among teens treated in an inner-city emergency department. *Journal of Emergency Medicine* [ePub ahead of print].

Daling, J. R., Doody, D. R., Sun, X., Trabert, B. L., Weiss, N. S., Chen, C., et al. (2009). Association of marijuana use and the incidence of testicular germ cell tumors. *Cancer, 115*(6), 1215–1223.

Ensrud, K. E., Lewis, C. E., Lambert, L. C., Taylor, B. C., Fink, H. A., Barrett-Connor, E., et al. (2006). O.F.I.M.M.S. Research Group.

Endogenous sex steroids, weight change and rates of hip bone loss in older men: The MrOS study. *Osteoporosis International, 17,* 1329–1336.

Darby, R. (2005). The riddle of the sands: Circumcision, history, and myth. *New Zealand Medical Journal, 118*(1218), U1564.

Darby, R. (2003). The masturbation taboo and the rise of routine male circumcision: A review of the historiography. *Journal of Social History, 36,* 737–759.

Davis, B., & Carpenter, C. (2009). Proximity of fast-food restaurants to schools and adolescent obesity. *American Journal of Public Health, 99*(3), 505–510.

Davis, L. M., Kilburn, M. R., & Schultz, D. (2009). *Reparable harm: Assessing and addressing disparities faced by boys and men of color in California.* Santa Monica, CA, RAND.

Dawber, T. R., Kannel, W. B., Revotskie, N., Stokes, J. I., Kagan, A., Gordon, T. (1959) Some factors associated with the development of coronary heart disease: Six years' follow-up experience in the Framingham Study. *American Journal of Public Health, 49*(10), 1349–1356.

Dawes, J., & Mankin, T. (2004). Muscle dysmorphia. *Strength and Conditioning Journal, 26,* 24–25.

DeMartino, M. F. (1979). *Human autoerotic practices.* New York: Human Sciences.

Denton, R. E., & Kampfe, C. M. (1994). The relationship between family variables and adolescent substance abuse: A literature review. *Adolescence 114,* 475–495.

De Paepe, A., Devereux, R. B., Dietz, H. C., Hennekam, R. C., & Pyeritz, R. E. (1996). Revised diagnostic criteria for the Marfan syndrome. *American Journal of Medical Genetics, 62*(4), 417–426.

Diamond, J. (1998). *Male menopause.* Naperville, IL: Sourcebooks.

Diamond, T., Sambrook, P., Williamson, M., Flicker, L., Nowson, C., Fiatarone-Singh, et al. (2001). Men and osteoporosis. *Australian Family Physician, 30,* 781–785.

Dillon, B. E., Chama, N. B., & Honig, S. C. (2008). Penile size and penile enlargement surgery: A review. *International Journal of Impotence Research, 20,* 519–529.

Dishion, T. J., Capaldi, D., Spracklen, K. M., & Li, F. (1995). Peer ecology of male adolescent drug use. *Development and Psychopathology, 7,* 803–824.

Doak, C., Heitmann, B. L., Summerbell, C., & Lissner, L. (2009). Prevention of childhood obesity: What type of evidence should we consider relevant? *Obesity Reviews, 10,* 350–356.

Doheny, K. (2009). *Phthalates affect the way young boys play.* http:// children.webmd.com/. Accessed 1/18/2010.

Donnan, G. A., Fisher, M., Macleod, M., & Davis, S. M. (2008). Stroke. *Lancet, 371*(9624), 1612–1623.

Drum, C., Horner-Johnson, W., & Krahn, G. L. (2008). Self-rated health and healthy days: Examining the disability paradox. *Disability and Health Journal, 1*(2), 71–78.

Drummond, J. (Ed.). (2008). For men: Doctors are good for your health. *Vitality, 3,* 30.

Dubensky, T. W., & Reed, S. G. (2010). Adjuvants for cancer vaccines. *Seminars in Immunology, 22*(3), 155–161.

Duke, S. (2007). Banning boyhood. *American Thinker.* http:// www.americanthinker.com/. Accessed 1/6/2010.

Duncan, G. E. (2006). Prevalence of diabetes and impaired fasting glucose level among U.S. adolescents. *Archives of Pediatric and Adolescent Medicine, 160,* 523–528.

Dunne, E. F., Unger, E. R., & Sternburg, M. (2007). Prevalence of HPV infection among females in the United States. *Journal of the American Medical Association, 297*(8), 813–819.

Dutton, K. R. (1995). *The perfectible body: The Western ideal of male physical development.* New York: Continuum.

Eastwood, J., & Doering, L. V. (2005). Gender differences in coronary artery disease. *Journal of Cardiovascular Nursing, 20*(5), 340–345.

Eberst, R. M. (1984). Defining health: A multidimensional model. *Journal of School Health, 54*(3), 99–104.

Eliot, L. (2009). *Pink brain blue brain.* Boston: Houghton Mifflin Harcourt.

Erikson, E. H. (1959). *Identity and the life cycle.* New York: International Universities Press.

Erwin, C. L. (2006). *The everything parent's guide to raising boys.* Avon, MA: Adams Media.

Etcoff, N. (1999). *Survival of the prettiest: The science of beauty.* New York: Doubleday.

Euringer, A. (2007). *Foreskin face cream and other beauty products of the future.* http://www.alternet.org/. Accessed 9/29/09.

Faludi, S. (1999). *Stiffed.* New York: Morrow.

Family Doctor. (2009). *Enuresis (bed-wetting).* http://familydoctor.org/. Accessed 1/6/2010.

Farzin, F., Perry, H., Hessl, D., et al. (2006). Autism spectrum disorders and attention deficit hyperactivity disorder in boys with the fragile X permutation. *Journal of Developmental and Behavioral Pediatrics, 27,* 137S–144S.

Fathers.com. (n.d.). The consequences of fatherlessness. http://www.fathers.com/. Accessed 10/6/09.

Fay, R. E., Turner, C. F., Klassen, A. D., & Gagnon, J. H. (1989). Prevalence and patterns of same-gender sexual contact among men. *Science, 243*(4889), 338–348.

Feldman, H. A., Longcope, C., Derby, C. A., Johannes, C. B., Araujo, A. B., Coviello, A. D., et al. (2002). Age trends in the level of serum testosterone and other hormones in middle-aged men: Longitudinal results from the Massachusetts Male Aging Study. *Journal of Clinical Endocrinology and Metabolism, 87,* 589–598.

Ferguson, F., & Bloch, H. R. (1989). *Misogyny, misandry, and misanthropy.* Berkeley: University of California Press.

Fillion, K. (2008). *How to fix boys.* http://www.macleans.ca/. Accessed 1/6/2010.

Fineran, S. (2001). Peer sexual harassment in high school. *Journal of School Social Work, 11*(2), 50–69.

Fink, K. S., Carson, C. C., & DeVellis, R. F. (2002). Adult circumcision outcomes study: Effect on erectile function, penile sensitivity, sexual activity and satisfaction. *Journal of Urology, 167,* 2113–2116.

Fisher, T. L., Burnet, D. L., Huang, E. S., Chin, M. H., & Cagney, K. A. (2007). Cultural leverage: Interventions using culture to narrow racial disparities in health care. *Medical Care Research and Review, 64*(5), Supp., 243S–282S.

Flaherty, J. A. (1980). Circumcision and schizophrenia. *Journal of Clinical Psychiatry, 41,* 96–98.

Franzoi, S., & Chang, Z. (2002). The body esteem of Hmong and Caucasian young adults. *Psychology of Women Quarterly, 26,* 89–91.

Frisbie, W. P., Cho, Y., & Hummer, R. A. (2001). Immigration and the health of Asian and Pacific Islander adults in the United States. *American Journal of Epidemiology, 153*(4), 372–380.

Fuller, S. J., Tan, R. S., & Martins, R. N. (2007). Androgens in the etiology of Alzheimer's disease in aging men and possible therapeutic interventions. *Journal of Alzheimer's Disease, 12*(2), 129–142.

Garibaldi, G. (2006). *The feminized American classroom—and how it hurts boys.* http://www.manhattan-institute.org/. Accessed 2/28/2010.

Garrett, B. E., Dube, S. R., Trosclair, A., Caraballo, R. S., & Pechacek, T. F. (2011). Cigarette smoking: United States, 1965–2008. *Morbidity and Mortality Weekly Reports, 60,* Supp. 109–113.

Gazi, M. A., Ankem, A. K., Pantuck, A. J., Han, K. R., Firoozi, F., & Barone, J. G. (2001). Management of penile toilet seat injury: Report of two cases. *Canadian Journal of Urology, 8,* 1293–1294.

Gearhart J. P., & Rock, J. A. (1989). Total ablation of the penis after circumcision with electrocautery: A method of management and long-term follow-up. *Journal of Urology, 142,* 799–801.

Gee, G. C., Spencer, M. S., Chen, J., & Takeuchi, D. (2007). A nationwide study of discrimination and chronic health conditions among Asian Americans. *American Journal of Public Health, 97*(7), 1275–1282.

Gerharz, E. W., & Haarmann, C. (2000). The first cut is the deepest? Medicolegal aspects of male circumcision. *British Journal of Urology International, 86,* 332–338.

Gerressu, M., Mercer, C. H., Graham, C. A., Wellings, K., & Johnson, A. M. (2007). Prevalence of masturbation and associated factors in a British national probability survey. *Archives of Sexual Behavior, 37*(2), 266–278.

Geyer, J., Ellsbury, D., et al. (2002). An evidence-based multidisciplinary protocol for neonatal circumcision pain management. *Obstetrics and Gynecological Neonatal Nursing, 31*(4), 403–410.

Gibbons, A. (2004). American Association of Physical Anthropologists meeting. Tracking the evolutionary history of warrior gene. *Science, 304*(5672), 818.

Gilgal Society. (2004). *Preparation and after-care for your child's circumcision.* http://www.circinfo.com/. Accessed 9/29/09.

Gilmore, D. D. (1990). *Manhood in the making: Cultural concepts of masculinity.* New Haven: Yale University Press.

Ginsburg, K. R. (2007). The importance of play in promoting healthy child development and maintaining strong parent–child bonds. *Pediatrics, 119,* 182–191.

Glanz, K., Rimer, B. K., & Marcus-Lewis, F. (eds.) (2002). *Health behavior and health education: Theory, research, and practice* (3rd ed.). San Francisco: Jossey-Bass, pgs. 165–184.

Glasgow, R. E., Litchenstein, E., & Marcus, A. C. (2003). Why don't we see more translation of health promotion research to practice? Rethinking the efficacy-to-effectiveness transition. *American Journal of Public Health, 93,* 1261–1267.

Gleitman, H., Fridlund, A. J., & Reisberg, D. (2004). *Psychology* (6th ed.). New York: Norton.

Goldman, R. (1999). The psychological impact of circumcision. *BJU International, 83*(1), 93–102.

Goldstein, L. B., & Simel, D. L. (2005). Is this patient having a stroke? *Journal of the American Medical Association, 293*(19), 2391–2402.

Gollust, S. E., Thompson, R. E., Gooding, H. C., & Biesecker, B. B. (2003). Living with achondroplasia in an average-sized world: An assessment of quality of life. *American Journal of Medical Genetics. Part A 120A*(4), 447–458.

Goodman, A. (2008). The long wait for male birth control. *Time.* http://www.time.com/. Accessed 3/27/2010.

Gordon, S. (2009). Circumcision guards against STDs. *U.S. News and World Report.* http://health.usnews.com/. Accessed 9/22/2009.

Graber, J. A., Peterson, A. C., & Brooks-Gunn, J. (1996). Pubertal processes: Methods, measures, and models. In J. A. Graber, A. C. Peterson, & J. Brooks-Gunn (Eds.), *Transitions through adolescence: Interpersonal domains and context* (pp. 23–53). Mahwah, NJ: Erlbaum.

Gray, J. (1992). *Men are from Mars, women are from Venus.* New York: HarperCollins.

Gray, R. H., Wawer, M. J., Kigozi, G., & Serwadda, D. (2008). Commentary: Disease modeling to inform policy on male circumcision for HIV prevention. *International Journal of Epidemiology, 37,* 1253–1254.

Gremillion, D. (2004). Personal communication [lecture] by the Men's Health Network.

Grigsby-Bates, K. (2007). Student with Asperger syndrome charged in murder. http://www.npr.org/. Accessed 1/7/2010.

Gremillion, D. (2004). Personal communication [lecture] by the Men's Health Network.

Grubin, D., & Beech, A. (2010). Chemical castration for sex offenders. *British Medical Journal, 340,* c74.

Gutmann, M. C. (2009). The missing gamete? Ten common mistakes or lies about men's sexual destiny. In M. C. Inhorn, T. Tjornhoj-Thomsen, H. Goldberg, & M. la Cour Mosegaard. *Reconceiving the second sex: Men, masculinity, and reproduction* (pp. 21–44). London: Berghahn.

Hackshaw, A. K., Law, M. R., & Wald, N. J. (1997). The accumulated evidence on lung cancer and environmental tobacco smoke. *British Medical Journal, 315,* 980–988.

Hagerman, R. J., Berry-Kravis, E., Kaufmann, W. E., et al. (2009). Advances in the treatment of fragile X syndrome. *Pediatrics, 123*(1), 378–390.

Haldeman, D. (1994). The practice and ethics of sexual orientation conversion therapy. *Journal of Consulting and Clinical Psychology, 62,* 221–227.

Hamilton, C. J., & Mahalik, J. R. (2009). Minority stress, masculinity, and social norms predicting gay men's health risk behaviors. *Journal of Counseling Psychology, 56,* 132–141.

Hankey, G. J. (1999). Smoking and risk of stroke. *Journal of Cardiovascular Risk, 6*(4), 207–211.

Harman, S. M., Metter, E. J., Tobin, J. D., Pearson, J., & Blackman, M. R. (2001). Longitudinal effects of aging on serum total and free testosterone levels in healthy men. Baltimore Longitudinal Study of Aging. *Journal of Clinical Endocrinology and Metabolism, 86,* 724–731.

Hardy, L. (2009). Encopresis: A guide for psychiatric nurses. *Archives of Psychiatric Nursing, 23,* 351–358.

Harris, R. H. (1994). *It's perfectly normal: Changing bodies, growing up, sex, and sexual health.* Miami, FL: PapaMedia.com.

Haskell, W. L., Lee, I. M., Pate, R. R., Powell, K. E., Blair, S. N., Franklin, B. A., et al. (2007). Physical activity and public health: Updated recommendation for adults for the American College of Sports Medicine and the American Heart Association. *Medicine and Science in Sports and Exercise, 39*(8), 1423–1434.

Hawks, S. R., Smith, T., Thomas, H. G., Christley, H. S., Meinzer, N., & Pyne, A. (2008). The forgotten dimensions in health education research. *Health Education Research, 23,* 319–324.

Hadziselimovic, F. (2002). Cryptorchidism: Its impact on male fertility. *European Urology, 411,* 21–23.

Heavey, S. (2010). *Radiation for prostate cancer lacks data: U.S. panel.* Reuters. http://www.reuters.com/. Accessed 4/22/2010.

Helgoe, L. A., & Helgoe, B. M. (2008). *The complete idiot's guide to raising boys.* Indianapolis, IN: Alpha Books.

Heller, C. G., & Myers, G. B. (1944). The male climacteric: Its symptomatology, diagnosis and treatment. *Journal of the American Medical Association, 126,* 472–477.

Heron, M. (2007). Deaths: Leading causes for 2004. *National Vital Statistics Reports, 56*(5), 7–8.

Hettler, (1976). http://www.hettler.com/.

Heru, A. M., Stuart, G. L., Rainey, S., Eyre, J., & Recupero, P. R. (2006). Prevalence and severity of intimate partner violence and associations with family functioning and alcohol abuse in psychiatric inpatients with suicidal intent. *Journal of Clinical Psychiatry, 67,* 23–29.

Hiatt, K., Riebel, L., & Friedman, H. (2007). The gap between what we know and what we do about childhood obesity: A multi-factor model for assessment, intervention, and prevention. *Journal of Social, Behavioral, and Health Sciences, 1,* 1–23.

Hijazi, R. A., & Cunningham, G. R. (2005). Andropause: Is androgen replacement therapy indicated for the aging male? *Annual Reviews of Medicine, 56,* 117–137.

Hill, K. G., Howell, J. C., Hawkins, J. D., & Battin-Pearson, S. R. (1999). Childhood risk factors for adolescent gang membership: Results from the Seattle social development project. *Journal of Research in Crime and Delinquency, 36,* 300–322.

Hill, S. E., & Flom, R. (2007). 18- and 24-month-olds' discrimination of gender-consistent and inconsistent activities. *Infant Behavior and Development, 30,* 168–173.

Hinton, A. E., & Buckley, G. (1988). Parental smoking and middle ear effusions in children. *Journal of Laryngology and Otology, 102,* 992–996.

Hiss, J., Horowitz, A., & Kahana, T. (2000). Fatal hemorrhage following male ritual circumcision. *Journal of Clinical Forensic Medicine, 7,* 32–34.

Hodges, F. M. (2001). The ideal prepuce in ancient Greece and Rome: Male genital aesthetics and their relation to *Lipodermos,* circumcision, foreskin restoration, and the *Kynodesme. Bulletin of the History of Medicine, 75,* 375–405.

Hoffman, J. (2008). Vaccinating boys for girls' sake? *New York Times.* http://www.nytimes.com/. Accessed 2/4/2010.

Hoffman, J. R., Kraemer, W. J., Bhasin, S., Storer, T., Ratamess, N. A., Haff, G. G., et al. (2009). Position stand on androgen and human growth hormone use. *Journal of Strength and Conditioning Research, 23*(5), S1–S59.

Hogervorst, E., Williams, J., Budge, M., Barnetson, L., Combrinck, M., & Smith, A. D. (2001). Serum total testosterone is lower in men with Alzheimer's disease. *Neuroendocrinology Letters, 22,* 163–168.

Holmes, R. M., & Holmes, S. T. (2002). Pedophilia and psychological profiling. In R. M. Holmes & S. T. Holmes (Eds.), *Profiling violent crimes: An investigative tool* (3rd ed., pp. 158–171). Thousand Oaks, CA: Sage.

Holmes, W. C. & Slap, G. B. (1998). Sexual abuse of boys: Definition, prevalence, sequelae, and management. *Journal of the American Medical Association, 280,* 1855–1872.

Holtgrave, D. R., Hall, I. H., Rhodes, P. H., & Wolitski, R. J. (2009). Updated annual HIV transmission rates in the United States, 1977–2006. *Journal of Acquired Immune Deficiency Syndromes, 50,* 236–238.

Hong, G. S., & White-Means, S. L. (1993). Do working mothers have healthy children? *Journal of Family and Economic Issues, 14,* 163–186.

Hormone Foundation. (n.d.). *Pituitary disorders overview.* http://www.hormone.org/. Accessed 1/16/2010.

Horner, M. J., Ries, L.A.G., Krapcho, M., Neyman, N., Aminou, R., Howlader, N., Altekruse, S. F., Feuer, E. J., Huang, L., Mariotto, A., Miller, B. A., Lewis, D. R., Eisner, M. P., Stinchcomb, D. G., & Edwards, B. K. (Eds). (2008). *SEER Cancer Statistics Review, 1975–2006.* Bethesda, MD: National Cancer Institute.

Hu, J. C., Gu, X., Lipsitz, S. R., Barry, M. J., D'Amico, A. V., Weinberg, A. C., & Keating, N. L. (2009). Comparative effectiveness of minimally invasive vs. open radical prostatectomy. *Journal of the American Medical Association, 302*(14), 1557–1564.

Huang, W., Qiu, C., Winblad, B., & Fratiglioni, L. (2002). Alcohol consumption and incidence of dementia in a community sample aged 75 years and older. *Journal of Clinical Epidemiology, 55,* 959–964.

Hudson, J. I., Hiripi, E., Pope, H. G., & Kessler, R. C. (2007). The prevalence and correlates of eating disorders in the National Comorbidity Survey Replication. *Biological Psychiatry, 61*(3), 348–358.

Iggulden, C., & Iggulden, H. (2007). *The dangerous book for boys.* New York: Harper Collins.

Insurance Institute for Highway Safety. (2008). *Fatality facts, older people.* Arlington, VA: IIHS. http://www.iihs.org/. Accessed 6/01/2010.

International Data Base, U.S. Census Bureau. (2008). http://www.census.gov/. Accessed 12/20/2008.

International Men's Health Week. (2009). http://www.menshealthmonth.org/. Accessed 8/24/2009.

Jack, L. (2005). Toward a men's health research agenda in health education: Examining gender, sex roles, and health-seeking behaviors in context. *American Journal of Health Education, 36,* 309–312.

Jacques, E. (1965). Death and the midlife crisis. *International Journal of Psychoanalysis, 46,* 502–514.

Jadad, A. R., & O'Grady, L. (2008). How should health be defined? *British Medical Journal, 337,* a2900.

Jayson, S. (2010, January 26). Truth about sex: 60 percent of young men, teen boys lie about it. *USA Today.*

Jemal, A., Siegel, R., Ward, E., Hao, Y., Xu, J., Murray, T., et al. (2008). Cancer statistics, 2008. *Cancer Journal of Clinicians, 58,* 71–96.

Jernigan, D. H., & Wright, P. A. (1996). Media advocacy: Lessons from community experiences. *Journal of Public Health Policy, 17*(3), 306–330.

Johnson, A. M., Wadsworth, J., Wellings, K., Bradshaw, S., & Fields, J. (1992). Sexual lifestyles and HIV risk. *Nature, 360*(6403), 410–412.

Johnson, C. K. (2009). Autism rates: Government studies find 1 in 100 children has autism disorders. *The Huffington Post.* http://www.huffingtonpost.com/. Accessed 1/7/2010.

Jones, M. (2003, March 16). The weaker sex. *The New York Times.*

Jones, D. C., Vigfusdottir, T. H., & Lee, Y. (2004). Body image and the appearance culture among adolescent girls and boys. *Journal of Adolescent Research, 19*(3), 323–339.

Jordan, G. H. (2006). Peyronie's disease. In J. J. Mulcahy (Ed.), *Male sexual functioning: A guide to clinical management* (2nd ed., pp. 401–417). New York: Humana.

Judge, T. A., & Cable, D. M. (2004). The effect of physical height on workplace success and income: Preliminary test of a theoretical model. *Journal of Applied Psychology, 89,* 428–441.

Juhn, M. S. (2003). Popular sports supplements and ergogenic aids. *Sports Medicine, 33*, 921–939.

Juul, A., & Skakkebaek, N. E. (2002). Testosterone treatment of elderly men. The so called andropause doesn't exist. (in Danish). *Ugeskrift for Laeger, 164*(42): 4941–4942.

Kaiser Family Foundation. (2009). *Trends in health care costs and spending.* www.kff.org. Accessed 5/12/2010.

Kampmeier, R. H. (1972). The Tuskegee study of untreated syphilis. *Southern Medical Journal, 65*, 1247–1251.

Kanayama, G., Cohane, G. H., Weiss, R. D., & Pope, H. G. (2003). Past anabolic-androgenic steroid use among men admitted for substance abuse treatment: An underrecognized problem? *Journal of Clinical Psychiatry, 64*, 156–160.

Kanayama, G., Gruber, A. J., Pope, H. G., Borowiecki, J. J., & Hudson, J. I. (2001). Over-the-counter drug use in gymnasiums: An underrecognized substance abuse problem? *Psychotherapy and Psychosomatics, 70*, 137–40.

Kanayama, G., Hudson, J. I., & Pope, H. G. (2008). Long-term psychiatric and medical consequences of anabolic-androgenic steroid abuse: A looming public health concern? *Drug and Alcohol Dependence, 98*(1–2), 1–12.

Kanayama, G., Pope, H. G., & Hudson, J. I. (2001). "Body image" drugs: A growing psychosomatic problem. *Psychotherapy and Psychosomatics, 70*, 61–65.

Karch, D., Crosby, A., Simon, T. (2006). Toxicology testing and results for suicide victims: Thirteen states, 2004. *Morbidity and Mortality Weekly Reports, 55*, 1245–1248.

Katz, R. V., Kegeles, S. S., Kressin, N. R., et al. (2006). The Tuskegee Legacy Project: Willingness of minorities to participate in biomedical research. *Journal of Health Care of the Poor and Underserved, 17*(4), 698–715.

Kazem, M., Hosseini, R., & Alizadeh, F. (2005). A vacuum device for penile elongation: Fact or fiction? *British Journal of Urology International, 97*(4), 777–778.

Kelishadi, R. (2007). Childhood overweight, obesity, and the metabolic syndrome in developing countries. *Epidemiologic Reviews, 29*, 62–76.

Kemp, G., Segal, J., & Cutter, D. (2009). *Learning disabilities in children.* http://helpguide.org/ Accessed 10/20/09.

Kendirci, M., Nowfar, S., & Hellstrom, W. J. (2005). The impact of vascular risk factors on erectile function. *Drugs Today, 41*(1), 65–74.

Kenedy, R. (2004). *Fathers for justice: The rise of a new social movement in Canada as a case study of collective identity formation.* Los Angeles: Caravan.

Kennedy, H. (1986). Trauma in childhood: Signs and sequelae as seen in the analysis of an adolescent. *Psychoanalytic Study of the Child, 41*, 209–219.

Kindlon, D., & Thompson, M. (2000). *Raising Cain: Protecting the emotional life of boys.* New York: Random House.

Kirkwood, M. W., Yeates, K. O., & Wilson, P. E. (2006). Pediatric sport-related concussion: A review of the clinical management of an oft-neglected population. *Pediatrics, 117*(4), 1359–1371.

Kim, Y. S., & Leventhal, B. (2008). Bullying and suicide: A review. *International Journal of Adolescent Medicine and Health, 20*(2), 133–154.

Kimbro, R. T., Bzostek, S., Goldman, N., & Rodriguez, G. (2008). Race, ethnicity, and the education gradient in health. *Health Affairs, 27*(2), 361–372.

Kinsey, A. C., Pomeroy, W. B., & Martin, C. E. (1948). *Sexual behavior in the human male.* Indiana University: Saunders, p. 519.

Klein, A. M. (1993). *Little big men.* Albany: State University of New York Press.

Klinefelter, H. F. (1986). Klinefelter's syndrome: Historical background and development. *Southern Medical Journal, 79*, 1089–1093.

Klinefelter, H. F., Reifenstein, E. C., & Albright, J. R. (1942). Syndrome characterized by gynecomastia, aspermatogenesis without a-Leydigism and increased excretion of follicle-stimulating hormone. *Journal of Clinical Endocrinology and Metabolism, 2*, 615–624.

Knoesen, N. (2009). To be superman: The male looks obsession. *Australian Family Physician, 38*(3), 131–133.

Knowler, W. C., Barrett-Conner, E., Fowler, S. E., Hamman, R. F., Lachin, J. M., Walker, E. A., et al. (2002). Reduction in the incidence of type 2 diabetes with lifestyle intervention or metformin. *New England Journal of Medicine, 346*(6), 393–403.

Kohlstädt, S. (2010). *Prostate cancer: Risk increases with the number of affected family members.* http://www.eurekalert.org/. Accessed 4/26/2010.

Kokkinos, P., Myers, J., Kokkinos, J. P., Pittaras, A., Narayan, P., Manolis, A., et al. (2008). Exercise capacity and mortality in Black and White men. *Circulation, 117*, 614–622.

Korenman, S. G. (2004). Epidemiology of erectile dysfunction. *Endocrine, 23*, 87–91.

Kotz, D. (2009, August 31). Should circumcision become public health policy? *U.S. News & World Report.* http://health.usnews.com/. Accessed 9/29/09.

Koutsky, L. A., & Kiviat, N. B. (1999). Genital human papillomavirus. In K. Holmes, P. Sparling, P. Mardh et al. (Eds), *Sexually transmitted diseases* (3rd ed., pp. 347–359). New York: McGraw-Hill.

Kozol, J. (1991). *Savage inequalities: Children in America's schools.* New York: Harper Perennial.

Kraemer, S. (2000). The fragile male. *British Medical Journal, 321*(7276), 1609–1612.

Kronenke, K., & Spitzer, R. L. (1998). Gender differences in the reporting of physical and somatoform symptoms. *Psychosomatic Medicine, 60*(2), 150–155.

Kruger, A. (1994). The mid-life transition: crisis or chimera? *Psychological Reports, 75,* 1299–1305.

Kung, H. C., Hoyert, D. L., Xu, J., & Murphy, S. L. (2008). Deaths: Final data for 2005. *National Vital Statistics Reports, 56*(10), 2, 25–26.

Kurlan, R., Como, G., Miller, B., et al. (2002). The behavioral spectrum of tic disorders. *Neurology, 59,* 414–420.

Lachman, M. (2004). Development in midlife. *Annual Review of Psychology, 55,* 305–331.

Lane, T. (2002). Male circumcision reduces risk of both acquiring and transmitting human papillomavirus infection. *International Family Planning Perspectives, 28,* 179–180.

Laumann, E. O., Masi, C. M., & Zuckerman, E. W. (1997). Circumcision in the United States. *Journal of the American Medical Association, 277,* 1052–1057.

Laurentani, F., Bandinelli, S., Russo, C. R., Maggio, D., Di Iorio, A., Cherubini, A., et al. (2006). Correlates of bone quality in older persons. *Bone, 39,* 915–921.

Law, J., Garrett, Z., & Nye, C. (2003). Speech and language therapy interventions for children with primary speech and language delay or disorder. *Cochrane Database Systematic Reviews, 3,* CD004110.

Laws, D. R., & O'Donohue, W. T. (2008). *Sexual deviance: Theory, assessment, and treatment.* New York: Guilford.

Lean, G. (2008). It's official: Men really are the weaker sex. *The Independent.* http://www.independent.co.uk/. Accessed 10/6/2009.

Lefebvre, R. C., & Flora, J. A. (1988). Social marketing and public health intervention. *Health Education Quarterly, 15*(3), 300–301.

Legato, M. J. (2006, June 17). The weaker sex. *The New York Times.* http://www.nytimes.com/. Accessed 10/6/09.

Leit, R. A., Gray, J. J., & Pope, H. G. (2001). Cultural expectations of muscularity in men: The evolution of the *Playgirl* centerfolds. *International Journal of Eating Disorders, 22*, 90–93.

Lenehan, P. (2003). *Anabolic steroids and other performance-enhancing drugs.* London: Taylor & Francis, 50–51.

Leone, J. E. (2003). Be forthright with athletes about supplements. *NATA News*, 26–28.

Leone, J. E., & Fetro, J. V. (2007). Perceptions and attitudes toward androgenic-anabolic steroid usage among two age categories: A qualitative inquiry. *Journal of Strength and Conditioning Research, 21*, 532–537.

Leone, J. E., Fetro, J. V., Kittleson, M. J., Welshimer, K. J., Partridge, J. A., & Robertson, S. L. (2011). Predictors of adolescent male body image dissatisfaction: Implications for negative health practices and consequences for school health from a regionally representative sample. *Journal of School Health, 81*(4), 174–184.

Leone, J. E., Gray, K. A., & Sedory, E. J. (2005). Helping athletes: Recognition and treatment of muscle dysmorphia and related body image disorders. *Journal of Athletic Training, 40*, 352–359.

Lever, J., Frederick, J. A., & Peplau, L. A. (2006). Does size matter? Men's and women's views on penis size across the lifespan. *Psychology of Men and Masculinity, 7*, 129.

Levin, B., Lieberman, D. A., McFarland, B., Smith, R. A., Durado, B., Andrews, K. S., et al. (2008). Screening and surveillance for the early detection of colorectal cancer and adenomatous polyps. A joint guideline from the American Cancer Society, the US Multi-Society Task Force on Colorectal Cancer, and the American College of Radiology. *Cancer Journal for Clinicians, 58*, 130–160.

Levine, L. A., Estrada, C. R., Storm, D. W., & Matkov, T. G. (2003). Peyronie's disease in younger men: Characteristics and treatment results. *Journal of Andrology, 24*(1), 27–32.

Levy, B., et al. (2007). Older persons' exclusion from sexually transmitted disease risk-reduction clinical trials. *Sexually Transmitted Diseases*, *34*(8), 541–544.

Lindau, S. T., Schumm, P., Laumann, E. O., Levinson, W., O'Muircheartaigh, C. A., & Waite, L. J. (2007). A study of sexuality and health among older adults in the United States. *New England Journal of Medicine*, *357*(8), 762–774.

Lipinski, J. P., & Pope, H. G. (2002). Body ideals in young Samoan men: A comparison with men in North America and *Europe. International Journal of Men's Health*, *1*, 163–171.

Lloyd-Jones, D., Adams, R. J., Brown, T. M., et al. (2010). Heart disease and stroke statistics—2010 update: A report from the American Heart Association Statistics Committee and Stroke Statistics Subcommittee. *Circulation*, *121*, e1–e170.

Lochary, M. E., Lockhart, P. B., & Williams, W. T. (1998). Doxycycline and staining of permanent teeth. *Pediatric Infectious Disease Journal*, *17*, 429–431.

Lorson, B., Melgar-Quinonez, H., & Taylor, C. (2009). Correlates of fruit and vegetable intakes in U.S. children. *Journal of the American Dietetic Association*, *109*, 474–478.

Lottrup, G., Andersson, A. M., Leffers, H., Mortensen, G. K., Toppari, J., Skakkebaek, N. E., et al. (2006). Possible impact of phthalates on infant reproductive health. *International Journal of Andrology*, *29*(1), 172–180.

Luciano, L. (2001). *Looking good: Male body image in modern America*. New York: Hill & Wang.

Luquis, R., & Perez, M. (2006). Cultural competency among school health educators. *Journal of Cultural Diversity*, *13*(4), 218–222.

MacGillivray, I. K. (2000). Educational equity for gay, lesbian, bisexual, transgendered, and queer/questioning students: The demands of democracy and social justice for America's schools. *Education of Urban Society*, *32*(3), 303–323.

Mahmoud, A., & Comhaire, F. H. (2006). Mechanisms of disease: Late-onset hypogonadism. *Nature Clinical Practice Urology*, *3*(8), 430–438.

Maida, D. M., & Armstrong, S. L. (2005). The classification of muscle dysmorphia. *International Journal of Men's Health*, *4*, 73–91.

Mainous, A. G., Everett, C. J., Liszka, H., King, D. E., & Egan, B. M. (2004). Prehypertension and mortality in a nationally representative cohort. *American Journal of Cardiology*, *94*(12), 1496–1500.

Mallants, C., & Casteels, K. (2008). Practical approach to childhood masturbation: A review. *European Journal of Pediatrics*, *167*(10), 1111–1117.

Malcher, G. (2009). Engaging men in health care. *Australian Family Physician*, *38*, 92–95.

Mandoki, M. W., & Sumner, G. S. (1991). Klinefelter syndrome: The need for early identification and treatment. *Clinical Pediatrics*, *30*(3), 161–164.

Marcell, A. V. (2007). Adolescence. In R. M. Kliegman, R. E. Behrman, H. B. Jenson, & B. F. Stanton (Eds.), *Nelson textbook of pediatrics* (18th ed., chap 12). Philadelphia: Saunders Elsevier.

Marshall, W. A., & Tanner, J. M. (1970). Variations in the pattern of pubertal changes in boys. *Archives of Disorders in Children*, *45*, 13–23.

Martin, J. P., & Bell, J. (1943). A pedigree of mental defect showing sex-linkage. *Journal of Neurology, Neurosurgery, and Psychiatry*, *6*, 154–157.

Martin, S. A., Haren, M. T., Taylor, A. W., Middleton, S. M., & Wittert, G. A. (2008). Chronic disease prevalence and associations in a cohort of Australian men: The Florey Adelaide Male Aging Study (FAMAS). *BMC Public Health*, *8*, 261.

Maruschak, L. M., & Beavers, R. (2009, December). HIV in prisons 2007–2008. *Bureau of Justice Statistics Bulletin* [U.S. Department of Justice], NCJ 228307.

Master, V. A., & Turek, P. J. (2001). Ejaculatory physiology and dysfunction. *Urology Clinics of North America, 28*(2), 363–375.

Mathers, M. J., Sperling, H., Rübben, H., & Roth, S. (2009). The undescended testis: Treatment and long term consequences. *Deutches Ärtzeblatt International, 106*(33), 527–532.

Maurer-Starks, S. S., Clemons, H. L., & Whalen, S. L. (2008). Managing heteronormativity and homonegativity in athletic training: In the classroom and beyond. *Journal of Athletic Training, 43*(3), 326–336.

Mayo Clinic. (n.d.a). *Living wills and advance directives for medical decisions.* http://www.mayoclinic.com/. Accessed 4/14/2011.

Mayo Clinic. (n.d.b). *Nutrition for kids: Guidelines for a healthy diet.* http://www.mayoclinic.com/. Accessed on 10/16/09.

Mayo Clinic Staff. (n.d.c). *Undescended testicle (cryptorchidism).* http://www.mayoclinic.com/. Accessed 11/14/09.

McCreary, D. R., & Sasse, D. K. (2000). An exploration of the drive for muscularity in adolescent boys and girls. *Journal of American College Health, 48*, 297–304.

McDermott, R. J., Wilson, D. D., & Marty, P. J. (1982). Neonatal circumcision. *Patient Counseling and Health Education, 3*, 132–136.

McGrath, E. (2002). Teen depression: Boys. *Psychology Today.* http://www.psychologytoday.com/. Accessed 1/18/2010.

McKee, A. C., Cantu, R. C., Nowinski, C. J., et al. (2009). Chronic traumatic encephalopathy in athletes: Progressive tauopathy after repetitive head injury. *Journal of Neuropathology and Experimental Neurology, 68*, 709–735.

MedicineNet. (n.d.). *Male breast cancer.* http://www.medicinenet.com/. Accessed 1/25/2010.

Mehrotra, R. (2005). *The essential Dalai Lama: His important teachings.* New York: Viking, 8.

Mellström, D., Johnell, O., Ljunggren, O., Eriksson, A. L., Lorentzon, M., Mallmin, H., et al. (2006). Free testosterone is an independent predictor of BMD and prevalent fractures in elderly men: MROS Sweden. *Journal of Bone Mineral Research, 21,* 529–535.

Menczer, J. (2003). The low incidence of cervical cancer in Jewish women: Has the puzzle finally been solved? *Israel Medical Association Journal, 5,* 120–123.

Men's Health Network. (2009). http://www.menshealthnetwork.org/. Accessed 10/18/2009.

Meryn, S., & Jadad, A. R. (2001). The future of men and their health. *British Medical Journal, 323,* 1013–1014.

Mikkonen, P., Leino-Arjas, P., Remes, J., Zitting, P., Taimela, S., & Karppinen, J. (2008). Is smoking a risk factor for low back pain in adolescents?: A prospective cohort study. *Spine, 33*(5), 527–532.

Miller, M., Barber, C., Azrael, D., Calle, E. E., Lawler, E., Mukamal, K. J. (2009). Suicide among U.S. veterans: A prospective study of 500,000 middle-age and elderly men. *American Journal of Epidemiology, 170*(4), 494–500.

Mills, M. V., Henley, C. E., Barnes, L. L., Carreiro, J. E., & Degenhardt, B. F. (2003). The use of osteopathic manipulative treatment as adjuvant therapy in children with recurrent acute otitis media. *Archives of Pediatric Adolescent Medicine, 157,* 861–866.

Mishkind, M. E., Rodin, J., Silberstein, L. R., & Streigel-Moore, R. H. (1986). The embodiment of masculinity: Cultural, psychological, and behavioral mechanisms. *American Behavioral Scientist, 29*(5), 545–562.

Mohr, B. A., O'Donnell, A. B., & McKinlay, J. B. (2004). Do changes in obesity affect total testosterone levels? Longitudinal results from the Massachusetts male aging study. *Annals of Epidemiology, 14*(8), 598.

Mohr, J. P., Choi, D., Grotta, J., & Wolf, P. (2004). *Stroke: Pathophysiology, diagnosis, and management.* New York: Churchill & Livingstone.

Molland, J. (n.d.). *Curbing toddler biting.* http://pediatrics.about.com/. Accessed 12/27/09.

Mooradian, A. D., & Korenman, S. G. (2006). Management of the cardinal features of andropause. *American Journal of Therapeutics, 13*(2), 145–160.

Moore, K. L., Dalley, A. F., & Agur, A. M. (2009). *Clinically oriented anatomy* (6th ed.). Philadelphia: Lippincott, Williams, & Wilkins.

Morbidity and Mortality Weekly Review. (2007). Reproductive health data and statistics. *Morbidity and Mortality Weekly Review, 56*(33), 852.

Morris, M. C., Evans, D. A., Bienias, J. L., et al. (2003). Consumption of fish and n-3 fatty acids and risk of incident Alzheimer's disease. *Archives of Neurology, 60*, 940–946.

Moscucci, O. (1996). *Clitordectomy, circumcision, and the politics of sexual pleasure in mid-Victorian Britain.* Sexualities in Victorian Britain. Bloomington: Indiana University Press.

Moses, S., Bailey, R. C., & Ronald, A. R. (1998). Male circumcision: Assessment of health benefits and risks. *Sexually Transmitted Infections, 74*, 368–373.

Moses, S., Plummer, F. A., Bradley, J. E., et al. (1994). The association between lack of male circumcision and risk for HIV infection: A review of the epidemiological data. *Sexually Transmitted Diseases, 21*, 201–210.

Myers, D. G. (1998). Adulthood's ages and stages. *Psychology, 5*, 196–197.

Myers, E. R., McCrory, D. C., Nanda, K., Bastian, L., & Matchar, D. B. (2000). Mathematical model for the natural history of human papillomavirus infection and cervical carcinogenesis. *American Journal of Epidemiology, 151*(12), 1158–1171.

Nabarro, J.D.N. (2008). Acromegaly. *Clinical Endocrinology, 26*(4), 481–512.

National Cancer Institute. (2009a). http://www.nci.nih.gov/ cancertopics/ types/prostate. Accessed 9/6/2009.

National Cancer Institute. (2009b). *Testicular cancer treatment.* http://www.cancer.gov/. Accessed 2/17/2010.

National Center for Health Statistics. (2005). http://marchofdimes.com. Accessed 11/17/2008.

National Center for Health Statistics. (2006, 2008). http://www.cdc.gov/nchs/. Accessed 8/22/2009.

National Center for Injury Prevention and Control. (2006). *CDC injury fact book.* Atlanta: Centers for Disease Control and Prevention.

National Survey of Children's Health. (2007). *Data analysis provided by the Child and Adolescent Health Measurement Initiative, Data Resource Center.* http://www.childhealthdata.org/. Accessed 1/18/2010.

Niedziela, M. (2007). Endocrine disorders of puberty. *Endocrine Abstracts, 14,* S18.1.

Nelson, H. D., Nygren, P., Walker, M., & Panoscha, R. (2006). Screening for speech and language delay in preschool children: Systematic evidence review for the U.S. Preventive Services Task Force. *Pediatrics, 117,* e298–e319.

Nilsson, P. M., Moller, L., & Solstad, K. (2009). Adverse effects of psychosocial stress on gonadal function and insulin levels in middle-aged males. *Journal of Internal Medicine, 237*(5), 479–486.

Nussbaum, D. (2003, December 21). Kindergarten can wait. *The New York Times.* http://www.nytimes.com/. Accessed 1/4/10.

Oberne, A., & McDermott, R. J. (2010). How many steps does it take to put on a condom? A commentary. *Journal of School Health, 80*(5), 211–213.

O'Brien, M. A., Prosser, L. A., Paradise, J. L., et al. (2009). New vaccines against otitis media: Projected benefits and cost-effectiveness. *Pediatrics, 123,* 1452–1463.

Odhiambo, J., Williams, H., Clayton, T., Robertson, C., & Asher, M. (2009). Global variations in prevalence of eczema symptoms in children from ISAAC Phase Three. *Journal of Allergy and Clinical Immunology, 124,* 1251–1258.e23.

Olivardia, R. (2001). Mirror, mirror on the wall, who's the largest of them all? *Harvard Review of Psychiatry, 9,* 254–259.

Oppenheimer, M. (2005). *Thirteen and a day: The bar and bat mitzvah across America.* New York: Farrar, Straus, & Giroux.

Opie, I., & Opie, P. (1997). *The Oxford dictionary of nursery rhymes* (2nd ed., pp. 100–101). Oxford, UK: Oxford University Press.

Orom, H., Kiviniemi, M. T., Underwood, W., Ross, L., & Shavers, V. L. (2010). Perceived cancer risk: Why is it lower among non-Whites than Whites? *Cancer Epidemiology Biomarkers and Prevention, 19*(3), 746.

Osler, M., McGue, M., Lund, R., & Christensen, K. (2008). Marital status and twins' health and behavior: An analysis of middle-aged Danish twins. *Psychosomatic Medicine, 70,* 482–487.

Palmore, E., & Luikart, C. (1972). Health and social factors related to life satisfaction. *Journal of Health and Social Behavior, 13*(1), 68–80.

Panek, P. E., & Hayslip, B. (1989). *Adult development and aging.* San Francisco: Harper & Row.

Parker-Pope, T. (2008, April 23). Boy or girl? The answer may depend on mom's eating habits. *The New York Times.* http://well.blogs.nytimes.com/. Accessed 10/18/2009.

Parkin, J. (2007). Stop feminizing our schools, our boys are suffering. *Mail Online.* http://www.dailymail.co.uk/. Accessed 1/6/2010.

Parsons, J. (2009). Not mission impossible. *Australian Family Physician, 38,* 3.

Pascoe, C. J. (2007). *Dude, you're a fag: Masculinity and sexuality in high school.* Berkeley: University of California Press.

Pawlowski, B., Dunbar, R.I.M., & Lipowicz, A. (2000). Tall men have more reproductive success. *Nature, 403*(13), 156.

Peate, I. (2005). The effects of smoking on the reproductive health of men. *British Journal of Nursing, 14*(7), 362–366.

Perry, A., & Schacht, M. (2001). *American Medical Association Complete Guide to Men's Health*. New York: John Wiley & Sons, Inc., pgs. 430–431.

Phillips, K. A. (1998). *The broken mirror: Understanding and treating body dysmorphic disorder*. New York: Oxford University Press, 199–208.

Phillips, K. A., & Castle, D. J. (2001). Body dysmorphic disorder in men. *British Medical Journal, 323,* 1015–1016.

Pinthus, J. H., Pacik, D., & Ramon, J. (2007). Diagnosis of prostate cancer. In J. Ramon & L. J. Denis (Eds.), *Prostate cancer* (pp. 83–99). New York: Springer.

Pirke, K. M., & Doerr, P. (1973). Age related changes and interrelationships between plasma testosterone, oestradiol, and testosterone-binding globulin in normal adult males. *Acta Endocrinology (Copenhagen), 74,* 792–800.

Planned Parenthood. (n.d.). *Safer sex [Safe sex]*. http://www.plannedparenthood.org/. Accessed 1/19/2010.

Pope, H. G., & Brower, K. J. (1999). Anabolic-androgenic steroid abuse. In B. J. Sadock & V.A. Sadock (Eds.), *Comprehensive textbook of psychiatry* (7th ed., pp. 1085–1096). Baltimore: Lippincott, Williams & Wilkins.

Pope, H. G., Cohane, G. H., Kanayama, G., Siegel, A. J., & Hudson, J. I. (2003). Testosterone gel supplementation for men with refractory depression: a randomized, placebo-controlled trial. *American Journal of Psychiatry, 160,* 105–111.

Pope, H. G., Gruber, A. J., Mangweth, B., Bureau, B., deCol, C., Jouvent, R., et al. (2000). Body image perception among men in three countries. *American Journal of Psychiatry, 157,* 1297–1301.

Pope, H. G., & Katz, D. L. (1994). Psychiatric and medical effects of anabolic-androgenic steroid use: A controlled study of 160 athletes. *Archives of General Psychiatry, 51,* 375–382.

Pope, H. G., Katz, D. L., & Hudson, J. I. (1993). Anorexia nervosa and "reverse anorexia nervosa" among 108 male bodybuilders. *Comprehensive Psychiatry, 34*, 406–409.

Pope, H. G., Olivardia, R., Borowiecki, J. J., & Cohane, G. H. (2001). The growing commercial value of the male body: A longitudinal survey of advertising in women's magazines. *Psychotherapy and Psychosomatics, 70*, 189–192.

Pope, H. G., Olivardia, R., Gruber, A. J., & Borowiecki, J. (1999). Evolving ideals of male body image as seen through action toys. *International Journal of Eating Disorders, 26*, 65–72.

Pope, H. G., Phillips, K. A., & Olivardia, R. (2000). *The Adonis complex: The secret crisis of male body obsession.* New York: Free Press.

Porche, D. (2009). Men's health: Integration into the national health care policy agenda. *American Journal of Men's Health, 3*, 5.

Powers, M. (2005). Performance-enhancing drugs. In J. Houglum, G. Harrelson, & D. Leaver-Dunn (Eds.), *Principles of pharmacology for athletic trainers* (pp. 327–332). Thorofare, NJ: Slack.

Queer Foundation. (2006). *Being gay is not a choice: Is homosexuality innate or a learned behavior?* http://queerfoundation.org/. Accessed 2/16/2010.

Rabenberg, V. S., Ingersoll, C. D., Sandrey, M. A., & Johnson, M. T. (2002). The bactericidal and cytotoxic effects of antimicrobial wound cleansers. *Journal of Athletic Training, 37*, 51–54.

Rando, R. A., Rogers, J. R., & Brittan-Powell, C. (1998). Gender role conflict in college men's sexually aggressive attitudes and behavior. *Journal of Mental Health Counseling, 20*, 359–369.

Raynor, M. C., Carson, C. C., Pearson, M. D., & Nix, J. W. (2007). Androgen deficiency in the aging male: a guide to diagnosis and testosterone replacement therapy. *Canadian Journal of Urology, 14*, Supp. 1, 63–68.

Rebora, A. (2004). Pathogenesis of androgenetic alopecia. *Journal of the American Academy of Dermatology, 50*(5), 777–779.

Redelmeier, D. A., & Singh, S. M. (2001). Survival in Academy Award-winning actors and actresses. *Annals of Internal Medicine, 134,* 955–962.

Remafedi, G., Farrow, J. A., & Deisher, R. W. (1991). Risk factors for attempted suicide in gay and bisexual youth. *Pediatrics, 87*(6), 869–875.

Reynolds, K., Lewis, B., Nolen, J. D., et al. (2003). Alcohol consumption and risk of stroke: A meta-analysis. *Journal of the American Medical Association, 289*(5), 579–588.

Reynolds, M. D., Tarter, R., Kirisci, L., Kirillova, G., Brown, S., Clark, D. B., et al. (2007). Testosterone levels and sexual maturation predict substance use disorders in adolescent boys: A prospective study. *Biological Psychiatry, 61*(11), 1223–1227.

Richardson, L. C., Wingo, P. A., Zack, M. M., Zahran, H. S., & King, J. B. (2008). Health-related quality of life (HRQoL) in cancer survivors between 20 and 64: Population-based estimates from the Behavioral Risk Factor Surveillance System (BRFSS). *Cancer, 112,* 1380–1389.

Ridings, H., & Amaya, M. (2007). Male neonatal circumcision: An evidence-based review. *Journal of the American Academy of Physician Assistants, 20,* 32–34, 36.

Rietschel, P., Corcoran, C., Stanley, T., Basgoz, N., Klibanski, A., & Grinspoon, S. (2000). Prevalence of hypogonadism among men with weight loss related to human immunodeficiency virus infections who were receiving highly active antiretroviral therapy. *Clinical Infectious Disease, 31,* 1240–1244.

Robson, W.L.M. (2009). Evaluation and management of enuresis. *New England Journal of Medicine, 360,* 1429–1436.

Robertson, K., & Murachver, T. (2009). Attitudes and attributions associated with female and male partner violence. *Journal of Applied Social Psychology, 39,* 1481.

Robertson, M. M. (2000). Tourette syndrome, associated conditions and the complexities of treatment. *Brain*, *123*, 425–462.

Rodin, J., Silberstein, L., & Striegel-Moore, R. (1984). Women and weight: a normative discontent. *Nebraska Symposium on Motivation*, *32*, 267–307.

Rolland, K., Farnill, D., & Griffiths, R. A. (1997). Body figure perception and eating attitudes among Australian school children age 8 to 12 years. *International Journal of Eating Disorders*, *21*, 273–278.

Ropelato, J. (n.d.). *Internet pornography statistics.* http://internet-filter-review.toptenreviews.com/. Accessed 2/25/2010.

Rosenstock, I. M., Strecher, V. J., & Becker, M. H. (1988). Social learning theory and the Health Belief Model. *Health Education Quarterly*, *15*(2), 175–183.

Rother, K. I. (2007). Diabetes treatment: Bridging the divide. *New England Journal of Medicine*, *356*(15), 1499–1501.

Rovet, J., Netley, C., Keenan, M., Bailey, J., & Stewart, D. (1996). The psychoeducational profile of boys with Klinefelter syndrome. *Journal of Learning Disabilities*, *29*(2), 180–196.

Rowe, J. W., & Kahn, R. L. (1997). Successful ageing. *Gerontologist*, *37*(4), 433–440.

Rowe, J. W., & Kahn, R. L. (1987). Human ageing: Usual and successful. *Science*, *237*(4811), 143–149.

Ruohola, A., Meurman, O., Nikkari, S., et al. (2006). Microbiology of acute otitis media in children with tympanostomy tubes: Prevalence of bacteria and viruses. *Clinical Infectious Diseases*, *43*, 1417–1422.

Russell, D. B. (2009). The newly single man. *Australian Family Physician*, *38*(3), 98–100.

Russell, W. D. (2002). Comparison of self-esteem, body satisfaction, and social physique anxiety across males of different exercise frequency and racial background. *Journal of Sport Behavior*, *25*, 74–90.

Ruxton, S. (2009). *Man made: Men, masculinities, and equality in public Policy*. London: Coalition on Men and Boys.

Sanchez, G. R., Sanchez-Youngman, S., Murphy, A.A.R., Goodin, A. S., Santos, R., & Valdez, R. B. (2011). Explaining public support (or lack thereof) for extending health coverage to undocumented immigrants. *Journal of Health Care to the Poor and Underserved, 22*(2), 683–699.

Sanderson, S. K. (2001). *The evolution of human sociality*. Lanham, MD: Rowman & Littlefield, p. 198.

Savitz, D. A., Schwingl, P. J., & Keels, M. A. (1991). Influence of paternal age, smoking, and alcohol consumption on congenital anomalies. *Teratology, 44*, 429–440.

Scarborough, H. S., & Dobrich, W. (1990). Development of children with early language delay. *Journal of Speech and Hearing Research, 33*, 70–83.

Schilder, P. (1935). *The image and appearance of the human body*. New York: International Universities Press.

Schmid, T. E., Eskenazi, B., Baumgartner, A., Marchetti, F., Young, S., Weldon, R., et al. (2007). The effects of male age on sperm DNA damage in healthy non-smokers. *Human Reproduction, 22*(1), 180–187.

Schmithorst, V. J., Holland, S. K., & Dardzinski, B. J. (2008). Developmental differences in white matter architecture between boys and girls. *Human Brain Mapping, 29*, 696–710.

Schonfeld, W. A. (1943). Primary and secondary sexual characteristics: study of their development in males from birth through maturity, with biometric study of penis and testes. *Archives of Pediatrics & Adolescent Medicine, 65*(4), 535–549.

Schum, T. R., Kolb, T. M., McAuliffe, T. L., Simms, M. D., Underhill, R. L., & Lewis, M. (2002). Sequential acquisition of toilet-training skills: A descriptive study of gender and age differences in normal children. *Pediatrics, 109*, e48.

Schwartz, J. P., & Tylka, T. L. (2008). Exploring entitlement as a moderator and mediator of the relationship between masculine gender role conflict and men's body esteem. *Psychology of Men and Masculinity*, *9*(2), 67–81.

Schwingl, P. J., & Guess, H. A. (2000). Safety and effectiveness of vasectomy. *Fertility and Sterility*, *73*(5), 923–936.

Schworm, P. (2009, June 8). Pressure mounts to test elder drivers. *Boston Globe*. http://www.boston.com/. Accessed 3/3/2010.

Serrant-Green, L., & McLuskey, J. (2008). *The sexual health of men*. Oxom, UK: Radcliffe Publishing.

Shain, B. N. (2007). Suicide and suicide attempts in adolescents. *Pediatrics*, *120*(3), 669–676.

Shang, C., Shur-Fen Gau, S., & Soong, W. (2006). Association between childhood sleep problems and perinatal factors, parental mental distress and behavioral problems. *Journal of Sleep Research*, *15*, 63–73.

Shavers, V. L., & Brown, M. L. (2002). Racial and ethnic disparities in the receipt of cancer treatment. *Journal of the National Cancer Institute*, *94*, 334–357.

Sherwood, L. (1997). *Human physiology: From cells to systems*. Belmont, CA: Wadsworth.

Shonkoff, J. P., Boyce, W. T., & McEwen, B. S. (2009). Neuroscience, molecular biology, and the childhood roots of health disparities: Building a new framework for health promotion and disease prevention. *Journal of the American Medical Association*, *301*(21), 2252–2259.

Silva, P. A., Williams, S. M., & McGee, R. (1987). A longitudinal study of children with developmental language delay at age three: later intelligence, reading and behavior problems. *Developmental Medical Child Neurology*, *29*, 630–640.

Silva, R. O., Brandão, S.A.B., Izar, M.C.O., Helfenstein, T., Santos, A. O., Monteira, C.M.C., et al. (2007). Hypertension and erectile dysfunction. *International Journal of Arthrosclerosis*, *2*(2), 156–161.

Simmons, C. A., Lehmann, P., & Cobb, N. (2008). A comparison of women versus men charged with intimate partner violence: General risk factors, attitudes regarding using violence, and readiness to change. *Violence and Victims*, *23*(5), 571–585.

Singh-Manoux, A., Guéguen, A., Ferrie, J., Shipley, M., Martikainen, P., Bonenfant, S., et al. (2008). Gender differences in the association between morbidity and mortality among middle-aged men and women. *American Journal of Public Health*, *98*(12), 2251–2257.

Skakkebaek, N. E., et al. (2001). Testicular dysgenesis syndrome: An increasingly common developmental disorder with environmental aspects. *Human Reproduction*, *5*, 972–978.

Slatcher, R. B., Mehta, P. H., Josephs, R. A. (2011). Testosterone and self-reported dominance interact to influence human mating behavior. *Social Psychological and Personality Science*, doi: 10.1177/1948550611400099.

Slowik, G. (2009). *Middle ear infection.* http://www.ehealthmd.com/. Accessed 11/14/09.

Small, E. J., Schellhammer, P. F., Higano, C. S., Redfern, C. H., Nemunaitis, J. J., Valone, F. H., et al. (2006). Placebo-controlled phase III trial of immunologic therapy with sipuleucel-T (APC8015) in patients with metastatic, asymptomatic hormone refractory prostate cancer. *Journal of Clinical Oncology*, *24*(19), 3089–3094.

Smedley, A., & Smedley, B. D. (2005). Race as biology is fiction, racism as a social problem is real. *American Psychologist*, *60*(1), 16–26.

Smith, J. A., Braunack, M., Wittert, G. A., & Warin, M. J. (2008). Qualities men value when communicating with general practitioners: Implications for primary care settings. *Medical Journal of Australia*, *189*, 618–621.

Solanas, V. (1967). *The S.C.U.M. Manifesto.* http://gos.sbc.edu. Accessed 6/11/2010.

Sorrells, M. L., Snyder, J. L., Reiss, M. D., Eden, C., Milos, M. F., Wilcox, N., & Van Howe, R. S. (2007). Fine-touch pressure thresholds in the adult penis. *BJU International*, *99*, 864–869.

Stanton, W. R., Oci, T.P.S., & Silva, P. A. (1994). Sociodemographic characteristics of adolescent smokers. *International Journal of the Addictions, 7*, 913–925.

Stengers, J., & van Neck, A. (2001). *Masturbation: The history of the great terror.* New York: Palgrave.

Stibbe, A. (2004). Health and the social construction of masculinity in men's health magazines. *Men and Masculinities, 7*(1), 31–51.

Stinchecum, A. M. (1993). *Everyone poops: My body science.* Brooklyn, NY: Kane/Miller.

Striegel-Moore, R. H., & Franko, D. L. (2004). Body image issues among girls and women. In T. F. Cash & T. Pruzinsky (Eds.), *Body image: A Handbook of theory, research, and clinical practice* (pp. 183–191). New York: Guilford.

Stromps, J. P., Kolios, G., & Cedidi, C. C. (2009). Hypertrophic scar and keloid formation after male circumcision: A case report. *European Journal of Plastic Surgery, 32*, 213–215.

Subotnik, R. B., & Harris, G. G. (2005). *Surviving infidelity: Making decisions, recovering from the pain.* Avon, MA: Adams Media.

Szabo, R. K., & Short, J. S. (2000). How does male circumcision protect against HIV infection? *BMJ, 320*, 1592–1594.

Taichman, R. S., Loberg, R. D., Mehra, R., & Pienta, K. J. (2007). The evolving biology and treatment of prostate cancer. *Journal of Clinical Investigation, 117*(9), 2351–2361.

Tan, Z. S. (2005). *Age-proof your mind.* New York: Warner Books.

Tel Aviv University. (2009, April 1). Are men the "weaker" sex? Pregnancy with male fetus riskier, study claims. *Science Daily.* http://www.sciencedaily.com/. Accessed 10/6/09.

Testicular Cancer Resource Center. (n.d.). *How to do a testicular sel- exam.* http://tcrc.acor.org/tcexam.html. Accessed 2/16/2010.

Thacker, P. D. (2004). Biological clock ticks for men, too. *Journal of the American Medical Association, 291*, 1683–1685.

Thompson, D. (2008, June 14). HPV vaccine for boys? It just might happen. *The Washington Post.* http://www.washingtonpost.com/. Accessed 2/12/2010.

Tiggemann, M. (2005). Television and adolescent body image: The role of program content and viewing motivation. *Journal of Social Clinical Psychology, 24,* 361–381.

Tiggemann, M., & Lynch, J. E. (2001). Body image across the lifespan in adult women: The role of self-objectification. *Developmental Psychology, 37,* 243–253.

Tjaden, P. (2003). Symposium on integrating responses to domestic violence: Extent and nature of intimate partner violence as measured by the National Violence Against Women Survey, 47 *Loy. L. Rev.* 41–54.

Treadwell, H. M., & Ro, M. (2003). Poverty, race, and the invisible men. *American Journal of Public Health, 93,* 705–707.

Treptow, C. (2009). U.K. government encourages teen masturbation? http://abcnews.go.com/. Accessed 2/2/2010.

Trope, M. (2002). Clinical management of the avulsed tooth: Present strategies and future directions. *Dental Traumatology, 18,* 1–11.

Tsigos, C., & Chrousos, G. P. (2002). Hypothalamic-pituitary-adrenal axis, neuroendocrine factors, and stress. *Journal of Psychosomatic Research, 53,* 865–871.

Tudiver, F., & Talbot, Y. (1999). Why don't men seek help? Family physicians perspective on help-seeking behavior in men. *Journal of Family Practice, 48,* 47–52.

Twenge, J. M., & Nolen-Hoeksema, S. (2002). Age, gender, race, socioeconomic status, and birth cohort differences on the children's depression inventory: A meta-analysis. *Journal of Abnormal Psychology, 111,* 578–588.

U.S. Agency for Healthcare Research. (2008). http://www.ahrq.gov/. Accessed 8/25/2009.

U.S. Bureau of Labor Statistics. (n.d.). http://www.bls.gov/. Accessed 7/02/2009.

U.S. Census Bureau. (2003). *Children's living arrangements and characteristics: March 2002*, P20–547, Table C8. Washington, DC: Government Printing Office.

U.S. Department of Health and Human Services. (2004). *Bone health and osteoporosis: A report of the surgeon general.* http://www.surgeongeneral.gov/. Accessed 2/2/2010.

U.S. Department of Health and Human Services. (2009). *Sexually transmitted disease surveillance 2008.* http://www.cdc.gov/. Accessed 2/5/2010.

U.S. Department of Health and Human Services, Office of Disease Prevention and Health Promotion. (2010). *Healthy People 2020: The road ahead.*

van de Mortel, T., Bourke, R., McLoughlin, J., Nonu, M., & Reis, M. (2001). Gender influences hand washing rates in the critical care unit. *American Journal of Infection Control, 29,* 395–399.

Van Howe, R. S., & Robson, W.L.M. (2007). The possible role of circumcision in newborn outbreaks of community-associated methicillin-resistant *Staphylococcal aureus. Clinical Pediatrics, 46,* 356–358.

Van Ryzin, L. (2000). The circumcision debate. *American Journal of Nursing, 100,* 24A–24B.

Van Wijk, C. M., & Kolk, A. M. (1997). Sex differences in physical symptoms: The contribution of symptom perception theory. *Social Science and Medicine, 45,* 231–246.

Vastag, B. (2009). Tenacious STD: Drug-resistant gonorrhea is spreading. *Science News, 171*(16), 245–246.

Vernon, P. A., Petrides, K. V., Bratko, D., & Schermer, J. A. (2008). A behavioral genetic study of trait emotional intelligence. *Emotion, 8,* 635–642.

Virtanen, M., Ferrie, J. E., Singh-Manoux, A., Shipley, M. J., Vahtera, J., Marmot, M.G., & Kivimäki, M. (2010). Overtime work and incident coronary heart disease: The Whitehall II prospective cohort study. *European Heart Journal, 31*(14), 1737–1744.

Wallner, L. P., Sarma, A. V., Lieber, M. M., St. Sauver, J. L., Jacobson, D. J., McGree, M. E., et al. (2008). Psychosocial factors associated with an increased frequency of prostate cancer screening in men ages 40 to 79 years: The Olmstead County study. *Cancer Epidemiology Biomarkers & Prevention, 17*, 3588–3592.

Waldinger, M. D., Quinn, P., Dilleen, M., Mundayat, R., Schweitzer, D. H., & Boolell, M. (2005). A multinational population survey of intravaginal ejaculation latency time. *Journal of Sexual Medicine, 2*, 492–497.

Walsh, B. (2009). He's a connector. *Bostonia.* http://www.bu.edu/bostonia/. Accessed 1/7/2010.

Wang, Y., & Lobstein, T. (2006). Worldwide trends in childhood overweight and obesity. *International Journal of Pediatric Obesity, 1*(1), 11–25.

Wannamethee, S. G., Shaper, A. G., Whincup, P. H., & Walker, M. (1995). Smoking cessation and the risk of stroke in middle-aged men. *Journal of the American Medical Association, 274*(2), 155–160.

Wan-Qing, W., Xiao-Ou, S., Steinbuch, M., Severson, R. K., Reaman, G. H., Buckley, J. D., & Robison, L. L. (2000). Paternal military service and risk for childhood leukemia in offspring. *American Journal of Epidemiology, 151*, 231–240.

Wardle, J., Haase, A. M., Steptoe, A., Nillapun, M., Jonwutiwes, K., & Bellisle, F. (2004). Gender differences in food choice: the contribution of health beliefs in dieting. *Annals of Behavioral Medicine, 27*, 107–116.

Watkins, B., & Bentovim, A. (1992). The sexual abuse of male children and adolescents: A review of current research. *Journal of Clinical Psychology and Psychiatry, 33*, 197–248.

WebMD. (n.d.a). http://my.webmd.com/. Accessed 10/20/2009.

WebMD. (n.d.b). *Sleep disorders health center.* http://www.webmd.com/. Accessed 6/30/2009.

WebMD. (n.d.c). *Understanding thyroid problem: The basics.* http:// women.webmd.com/. Accessed 1/21/2010.

Weinstock, H., Berman, S., & Cates, W. (2004). Sexually transmitted disease among American youth: Incidence and prevalence estimates, 2000. *Perspectives on Sexual and Reproductive Health, 36,* 6–10.

Weiss, R. A. (1993). How does HIV cause AIDS? *Science, 260*(5112), 1273–1279.

Wessells, H., Lue, T., & McAninch, J. (1996). Penile length in the flaccid and erect states: guidelines for penile augmentation. *Journal of Urology, 156,* 995–997.

Westmoreland-Corson, P., & Anderson, A. E. (2004). Body image issues among boys and men. In T. F. Cash & T. Pruzinsky (Eds.), *Body image: A handbook of theory, research, and clinical practice* (pp. 192–199). New York: Guilford.

Wetzstein, C. (2010, March 2). Psychiatrists mull new sex disorders. *The Washington Times.* http://washingtontimes.com/. Accessed 3/2/2010.

Wild, S., Roglic, G., Green, A., Sicree, R., & King, H. (2004). Global prevalence of diabetes: Estimates for 2000 and projections for 2030. *Diabetes Care, 27*(5), 1047–1053.

Wilhelm, K. A. (2009). Men and depression. *Australian Family Physician, 38*(3), 102–105.

Williams, G. I. (2002). *"Fathers' Rights Movement." Historical and Multicultural Encyclopedia of Women's Reproductive Rights in the United States.* Westport, Connecticut: Greenwood Press, pgs. 81–83.

Williams, D. R. (2003). The health of men: Structured inequalities and opportunities. *American Journal of Public Health, 93,* 724–731.

Williams, N., & Kapila, L. (1993). Complications of circumcision. *British Journal of Surgery, 80,* 1231–1236.

Winkleby, M. A., Jatulis, D. E., Frank, E., & Fortmann, S. P. (1992). Socioeconomic status and health: How education, income, and occupation contribute to risk factors for cardiovascular disease. *American Journal of Public Health, 82*(6), 816–820.

Wodka, E. L., Loftis, C., Mostofsky, S. H., Prahme, C., Gidley-Larson, J. C., Denckla, M. B., & Mahone, E. M. (2008). Prediction of ADHD in boys and girls using the D-KEFS. *Archives of Clinical Neuropsychology, 23*, 283–293.

Woodside, D. B., Garfinkel, P. E., Goering, P., Kaplan, A., Goldblum, D. S., & Kennedy, S. H. (2001). Comparisons of men with full or partial eating disorders, men without eating disorders and women with eating disorders in the community. *American Journal of Psychiatry, 158*, 570–574.

World Health Organization. (2002). *Sexual and reproductive health*. http://www.who.int/. Accessed 2/2/2010.

Worobey, M., Gemmel, M., Teuwen, D. E., et al. (2008). Direct evidence of extensive diversity of HIV-1 in Kinshasa by 1960. *Nature, 455*(7213), 661–664.

Wroblewska, A. M. (1997). Androgenic-anabolic steroids and body dysmorphia in young men. *Journal of Psychosomatic Research, 42,* 225–234.

Yano, H., Okitsu, N., Hori, T., et al. (2009). Detection of respiratory viruses in nasopharyngeal secretions and middle ear fluid from children with acute otitis media. *Acta Oto-laryngologica, 129,* 19–24.

Xanthos, C. (2008). The secret epidemic: Exploring the mental health crisis affecting adolescent African-American males. *Community Voices: Healthcare for the Underserved,* 1–16.

Xu, F., Sternberg, M., Kottiri, B., McQuillan, G., Lee, F., Nahmias, A., et al. (2006). National trends in herpes simplex virus type 1 and type 2 in the United States: Data from the National Health and Nutrition Examination Survey (NHANES). *Journal of the American Medical Association, 296,* 964–973.

Youth Risk Behavior Surveillance System. (2008). http://www.cdc.gov/HealthyYouth/yrbs/index.htm. Accessed 3/2/2010.

INDEX

Page references followed by *fig* indicate an illustrated figure; followed by *t* indicate a table.

Height norms, 145

Heightism, 146

Hematuria, 286

Hemorrhagic stroke, 297

Hernias, 72

Heteronormative concept, 245

Heterosexist health care, 370–371

Hippocratic Oath, 51

Hispanic males: diabetes risk of, 299, 300; HIV/AIDS
rates in, 20; juvenile offenders and incarceration
among, 211; *machismo* attitude of the, 21; obesity
among, 128; routine infant circumcision not
practiced by, 424. *See also* Racial/ethnic
differences

HIV/AIDS: circumcision impact on development of,
46–47, 57; education efforts for prevention of,
176–177, 220; homosexuality and rates of, 196;
incarcerated populations and rates of, 214; increasing
problem during adolescence, 170; male health
disparities related to, 20; overview of, 174–177;
racial/ethnic disparities in, 175–176*t*, 369;
recommendations related to, 177; rising rates among
people over fifty, 321. *See also* AIDS-related complex
(ARC); Sexually transmitted infections (STIs)

Homeostatic relationships, 144

Homicide: age-adjusted rates of, 2; black young adults
and risk for, 221; gender differences in rates of, 15;
young adult males and, 220–221. *See also* Violence

Homophobia, 197

Homophobic bullying, 191, 197

Homosexuality: acceptance of, 194; adolescence and,
192–193; adolescent suicide related to, 197–198;
bisexual men, 20, 175; bullying issue of, 191, 197;
conversion therapy to "cure," 193–194; domestic
violence related to, 196; eating disorders and, 226;
health issues related to, 196; HIV/AIDS rates and,
196; incarcerated populations and, 194; nature vs.
nurture debate over, 195; STIs rates related to, 57,
171–173, 178, 196. *See also* Men who have sex with
men (MSM); Sexual orientation

Hormone replacement therapy (HRT), 144,
317–319

Hormones: ADS and diminishing levels of, 314–316;
cortisol, 49, 225, 265; influence on behavior, 100;
regulating homeostatic relationships, 144; sex,
144–145. *See also* Testosterone

Huffing, 210

Human chorionic gonadotropin (HCG), 87

Human growth hormone (hGH), 272

Human papilloma virus (HPV), 46, 57, 177–179

Human papilloma virus (HPV) vaccinations, 179–181

Human rights, 368

Hygiene: as circumcision benefit, 44–45; hand-washing
practice for, 91–92; phimosis due to inadequate, 46;
teaching toddlers and young children, 90

Hypercholesterolemia, 282

Hypergonadism, 139

Hypermasculine male models, 12

Hypertension (HTN): description and treatment of,
294–297; as stroke risk, 297–298

Hyperthyroidism, 147–148

Hypogonadal, 143, 318

Hypogonadism, 139, 316

Hypothyroidism, 147–148

Hypovolemic shock, 50

I

"I" statements, 115

Iatrogenic disease, 51

Ideology (gang), 213–214

Ileostomy, 293

Illicit drugs: adolescent use of, 210–211; emotional
issues leading to, 167. *See also* Drug and alcohol
abuse

Immunizations: description of, 84; human papilloma
virus (HPV), 179–181; recommendations for
toddlers/young child, 85*t*–86; school-aged boys and,
107

Impotence, 316. *See also* Erectile dysfunction (ED)

In utero ultrasonagraphy, 70

Inadequacy feelings, 150–151

Incarcerated populations: HIV/AIDS and other diseases
among, 214; homosexuality in, 194; juvenile
offenders, 211–215; state rates of, 214. *See also* U.S.
penal system

Incidence, 20

Industrialized nations: men as at-risk group in,
371–372; risk of male fetuses and infants in, 32.
See also United States

Infant mortality rates: health risk and male, 30–33;
higher rates of male, 55; racial/ethnic differences in,
18. *See also* Mortality rates

Infections: from circumcisions, 50–51; middle ear,
87–90. *See also* Sexually transmitted infections (STIs)

Infertility, 230–233

Infidelity, 304–305

Influenza virus, 91

Inguinal canal (or ligament), 86

Social stigma challenges: gender role conflict model on, 10*fig*; male heights outside of the norm, 145–147

Social support, 325, 326, 327

Sociobiological perspective: examining life stage using, 3; on gender differences, 64

Sociocultural development: costs of not preventing gender disparities in early childhood, 78–79; gender emotional disparities and, 76–77; gender physical disparities and, 72–76; nutrition and diet role in, 68–70; parental role in, 65–67; sexual health and, 70–71; social paradigm shift in how we approach, 75–76

Sociocultural perspectives: ageism bias, 332; erectile dysfunction (ED) and, 235–238; implications of being born male, 33–35; normative discontent concept, 237–238; single-parent and nontraditional families, 35–39; young adult social health, 247–249. *See also* Cultural perspectives; Culture; Masculine values

Socioeconomic status (SES): health-related disparities and, 2; as predictor of health-related outcomes, 85; single-parent/nontraditional families and lower, 35

Somatoform disorders, 254

South Beach Diet, 223, 224

Spectrum disorders, 122. *See also* Autism spectrum disorders (ASDs)

Spermatorrhoea, 187

Spiritual health, definition of, 5*fig*, 6

Sports: cost barriers to participation in certain, 129–130; school-age social development through, 125–127. *See also* Physical activity

"Stage fright," 92–93

Stand by Me (film), 154

Standard of care, 22–23

Status issue, 75

Stenosis (plumonic), 72

Stereotypes: gender behavior, 100–101; of men and emotions, 97

Stillborn risk, 31

Stoicism, 9

Stress: bedwetting caused by, 108; cortisol levels due to, 49, 225, 265; divorce and infidelity, 305; erectile dysfunction (ED) and, 235; eustress and distress forms of, 265; examining impacts of job, 3; low testosterone levels correlated to, 316; sleep disorders due to job, 267; type A personality, heart disease, and, 282; weight management by controlling, 225; young adult emotional health and, 265–266

Stroke (cerebrovascular accident), 297–299

Substance abuse. *See* Drug and alcohol abuse

Sudden infant death syndrome (SIDS), 15

Suicide rates: elderly adult males, 336; of gay adolescent males, 197–198; gender differences in preadolescent, 152–153; older adult males, 325; rising black male, 19

"Supermale" media image, 253

Surgeries: circumcision, 39–58, 156; cosmetic, 259–262*t*, 302, 304; erectile dysfunction (ED) treatments using, 240–242; hair transplants, 262–265

Survival of the Prettiest: The Science of Beauty (Etcoff), 259

Sutures (circumcision), 43

Syphilis (*Treponema pallidum*), 172–173

Systolic pressure, 295*t*

T

T-cell levels, 175

T-cells, 16

Tallness, 145

Tanner stages of physical development, 139–141, 144, 162–163

Tantrums, 84

Tara Klamp method, 43–44

Tel Aviv University, 30, 32

Tertiary prevention: resources and cost of, 222*fig*; testicular cancer and, 164

Testicular cancer, 163–164, 231

Testicular self-exams (TSEs), 163–164, 324

Testis, 231–232

Testosterone: adolescent levels of, 200; ADS and diminishing levels of, 314–316; benign prostatic hyperplasia (BPH) development role of, 286; breast tissue growth suppressed by, 166; to combat effects of depression, 318; genetically defined males and, 11; hearing loss due to high levels of, 16; hormonal fluctuations during the day, 100; hormone replacement therapy (HRT) of, 144, 317–319; masturbation and levels of, 189, 190; middle adulthood, midlife crisis, and loss of, 303; stress levels correlated to lower levels of, 316. *See also* Hormones

Testosterone replacement therapy, 144, 317–319

Therapies: cognitive behavioral therapy (CBT), 202; conversion, 193–194; hormone replacement therapy (HRT), 144, 317–319

"Threatened masculinity" theory, 11–12

Thyroid disorders, 147–148